Stroke Prevention in Atrial Fibrillation

Stroke Prevention in Atrial Fibrillation

GREG FLAKER, MD
Professor of Medicine
Medicine
University of Missouri
Columbia, MO, United States

ELSEVIER

ELSEVIER

3251 Riverport Lane
St. Louis, Missouri 63043

STROKE PREVENTION IN ATRIAL FIBRILLATION   ISBN: 978-0-323-55429-9

Content Strategist: Kayla Wolfe
Content Development Manager: Kathy Padilla
Content Development Specialist: Jennifer Horigan
Publishing Services Manager: Deepthi Unni
Project Manager: Nadhiya Sekar
Designer: Gopalakrishnan Venkatraman

Working together
to grow libraries in
developing countries

Printed in United States of America

Last digit is the print number: 9   8   7   6   5   4   3   2   1

www.elsevier.com • www.bookaid.org

List of Contributors

Arnold J. Greenspon, MD
Professor of Medicine
Director
Cardiac Electrophysiology Laboratory
Cardiology
Sidney Kimmel Medical College at Thomas
    Jefferson University
Philadelphia, PA, United States

Paul P. Dobesh, PharmD
Professor of Pharmacy Practice
College of Pharmacy
University of Nebraska Medical Center
Omaha, NE, United States

Zachary A. Stacy, PharmD
Associate Professor of Pharmacy Practice
St. Louis College of Pharmacy
St. Louis, Missouri, United States

Christopher B. Granger, MD
Director, Coronary Care Unit
Duke University Medical Center
Durham, NC, United States

David A. Manly, MD
Cardiovascular Medicine Fellow
Duke University Medical Center
Durham, NC, United States

Farhan Shahid, MBBS, BSc
Research Fellow
Institute of Cardiovascular Sciences
University of Birmingham
Birmingham, United Kingdom

Eduard Shantsila, PhD
Postdoctoral Research Fellow
Institute of Cardiovascular Sciences
University of Birmingham
Birmingham, United Kingdom

Mikhail S. Dzeshka, MD
Research Fellow
Department of Internal Medicine I
Grodno State Medical University
Grodno, Belarus

Gregory Y.H. Lip, MD, FRCP, FACC, FESC
Professor
Cardiovascular Medicine Adjunct Professor of
    Cardiovascular Sciences Thrombosis Research Unit
Aalborg University
Denmark;
University of Birmingham
Birmingham, United Kingdom

Renato D. Lopes, MD, MHS, PhD
Professor of Medicine
Medicine/Cardiology
Duke University Medical Center
Durham, NC, United States

Anne Rose, PharmD
Manager of Patient Care Services: Cardiology,
Internal Medicine and Anticoagulation
University of Wisconsin Health
Madison, WI, United States

Geno J. Merli, MD, MACP, FSVM, FHM
Professor of Medicine & Surgery
Sydney Kimmel Medical College
Thomas Jefferson University
Philadelphia, PA, United States

Michael C. Giudici, MD, FACC, FACP, FHRS
Professor of Medicine
Director of Arrhythmia Services
Department of Internal Medicine
University of Iowa Hospitals and Clinics
Iowa City, IA, United States

Sandeep Gautam, MD, MPH
Assistant Professor of Medicine
Director, Cardiac Electrophysiology
University of Missouri
Columbia, MO, United States

Joshua Payne, MD, MPH
Cardiovascular Medicine Fellow
University of Missouri,
Columbia, MO, United States

Robert G. Hart, MD
Professor of Medicine (Neurology)
McMaster University
Hamilton, ON, Canada

Luciana Catanese, MD
Assistant Professor
Vascular Neurology
McMaster University
Hamilton, ON, Canada

Chad Ward, MD
Cardiovascular Medicine Fellow
University of Iowa Hospital & Clinics
Iowa City, IA, United States

Bria Giacomino, DO
Cardiovascular Medicine Fellow
University of Iowa Hospital & Clinics
Iowa City, IA, United States

Michael Walsh, MD, PhD
Associate Professor
Medicine and Health Research Methods,
    Evaluation & Impact
McMaster University
Hamilton, ON, Canada

David Collister, MD
Clinical Scholar
Medicine and Health Research Methods,
    Evaluation & Impact
McMaster University
Hamilton, ON, Canada

Lynda Thomson, PharmD
Advanced Practice Pharmacist
Jefferson Vascular Center
Thomas Jefferson University Hospital
Philadelphia, PA, United States

John U. Doherty, MD, FACC
Professor of Medicine (Cardiology)
Director, Clinical Services
Division of Cardiology
Jefferson Heart Institute
Sidney Kimmel School of Medicine
Philadelphia, PA, United States

William J. Hucker, MD, PhD
Research Fellow in Electrophysiology
Massachusetts General Hospital
Harvard Medical School
Boston, MA, United States

Mitul Kanzaria, MD
Fellow in Interventional Cardiology
Jefferson Heart Institute
Sidney Kimmel School of Medicine
Philadelphia, PA, United States

Richard Weachter, MD
Associate Professor of Clinical Medicine
University of Missouri
Columbia, MO, United States

Abhinav Sharma, MD, FRCPC
Duke Clinical Research Institute and Mazankowski
    Alberta Heart Institute
University of Alberta
Edmonton, Alberta, Canada

Foreword

Atrial fibrillation (AF) is the most frequently encountered cardiac arrhythmia beyond isolated extrasystoles and a powerful risk factor for ischemic stroke. More than 2.5 million Americans are known to have AF, rising to at least 12 million people worldwide, and likely millions more in whom it has not been diagnostically identified, such that the true prevalence of AF is underestimated. According to the Global Burden of Disease survey, the burden of morbidity associated with AF, as measured in terms of disability, adds to the costs borne by individuals, health systems, and national economies. The toll is inherently linked to hospitalizations, reduced tolerance for physical effort, impaired quality of life, exacerbation of heart failure, and most pertinently to stroke and mortality. Strokes associated with AF are typically severely disabling, making primary prevention the paramount goal. This goal was first realized about three decades ago in clinical trials of anticoagulation, and the uniformity and strength of evidence made antithrombotic therapy the standard of care for stroke prevention in patients with AF.

Early studies in Denmark, Canada, and the United States confirmed that the vitamin K antagonist warfarin, when administered and regulated within a limited therapeutic range, reduces stroke by about 68% in patients with AF. The efficacy of aspirin, at best about 20% by prevention of mainly smaller, atherothrombotic strokes, is no more than half that of warfarin, and both the relative and absolute benefits of warfarin are greater for high-risk patients than for those at lower risk. Until the introduction of target-specific nonwarfarin oral anticoagulants (NOACs), the crux of the clinical matter was that warfarin reduced ischemic stroke far more than aspirin among patients with AF, yet the net benefit was limited to selected high-risk patients, who can be identified using risk stratification schemes based on readily available demographic variables such as age, prior stroke, hypertension, and heart failure. For those at lower risk of thromboembolism, the risk of bleeding during treatment with vitamin K antagonists, and especially the risk of intracerebral hemorrhage, becomes prohibitive, considering that such events in an anticoagulated patient are usually permanently disabling or fatal.

Without a doubt, effective antithrombotic prophylaxis has been established for most patients with AF, tailored to their inherent risks for stroke and bleeding.

Perhaps a third of patients with AF are not at sufficient stroke risk to benefit from long-term anticoagulation, and reliable estimates of treatment efficacy combined with characterization of stroke risk enable clinicians to estimate the magnitude of benefit conferred by anticoagulation. This net benefit is generally amplified when a NOAC is prescribed in preference over a vitamin K antagonist. The equation becomes more nuanced in special situations, as for patients undergoing cardioversion or catheter-based ablation procedures intended to restore or maintain sinus rhythm, for patients with clinically silent AF in whom the very presence of the arrhythmia is detected by one or another type of electrocardiographic rhythm monitoring apparatus, or for patients with specific comorbidities, such as coronary artery disease, prior hemorrhagic stroke, or intolerance of anticoagulation.

Dr. Gregory Flaker has been involved in the evolution of this field almost since its inception. As a participant in each of the federally funded Stroke Prevention in Atrial Fibrillation trials, in studies of the first NOAC as an alternative to warfarin, and in numerous other broad-based clinical investigations, he has amassed a fulsome experience and unique perspective that guided the development of this book. The result is a clinically relevant, evidence-based approach to optimizing the care of patients with AF as harbors of the cause of the most preventable type of stroke. In this effort, he blends vast experience as a cardiac electrophysiologist, trialist, and pragmatic physician, from whom much can be learned that translates directly and forcefully to clinical practice. As patients live longer with more advanced forms of cardiovascular disease, the prevalence of AF will continue to increase. At the least, readers of this book will be comprehensively well informed. At best, clinical application during this epidemic AF, the most serious of which is severely disabling stroke, will facilitate delivery of optimum preventive therapy to a large proportion of the population a risk and prevent countless strokes.

Jonathan L. Halperin, MD
Robert and Harriet Heilbrunn Professor
of Medicine (Cardiology)
Icahn School of Medicine at Mount Sinai
New York, NY, United States

Contents

CHAPTER 1

An Economic Analysis of Stroke and Atrial Fibrillation

ARNOLD J. GREENSPON, MD

A 67-year-old accountant is sitting at his desk, idly staring at his computer screen. He should be focusing on the balance sheet and the delay in accounts receivable. Instead, he suddenly can't remember what day it is, what time it is. Is it morning, is it evening? In fact, he can't remember where he is. He looks to his left and tries to speak but only garbled words come out. His coworker looks at him with alarm as he becomes more confused and disoriented. Soon, he is on the floor, as coworkers feverishly scramble and call 911 for help. He is having an acute stroke.

We often measure the outcome of an acute event by analyzing the patient's response and initial reaction to therapy, such as days in the intensive care unit or hospital. These treatment costs can be easily measured. We can also easily measure in-hospital or 30-day mortality as a measurement of outcome. With stroke, outcome measures are more difficult to define. This is partly because patients might survive their initial stroke but then go on to have significant residual disability that affects both their clinical and economic capacity. Disability incurs significant rehabilitation costs and affects the future ability of the patient to function and earn income. These effects are more difficult to measure.

Atrial fibrillation (AF) is a major risk factor for ischemic stroke.[1-3] Strategies to reduce the risk for stroke in AF patients involve chronic oral anticoagulation.[4-6] Warfarin is the traditional oral anticoagulant given for stroke protection. It is a drug that is difficult to use because of its complex pharmacokinetics and drug interactions. Warfarin has a narrow therapeutic index that also makes it difficult to use. A target INR (international normalized ratio) of 2–3 must be achieved to protect a high-risk AF patient from stroke.[7,8] An INR that is very low indicates the patient is at risk for stroke; an INR that is very high indicates the patient is at risk for bleeding. The direct oral anticoagulants (DOACs) were developed to improve outcomes in at-risk AF patients because they do not possess the disadvantages of warfarin.[9,10] However, the advantages of DOACs come at higher price. The question is whether these advantages are worth the additional cost.

This chapter will review the economic costs of acute stroke and analyze the impact of AF. The economic savings of stroke prevention will be presented along with an analysis of the potential impact of the new DOAC drugs.

INTRODUCTION

Stroke is one of the most significant medical problems encountered in the United States. Despite significant progress in the treatment of stroke, it remains the fifth leading cause of death in the United States and the leading cause of major disability.[11,12] This is down from the third leading cause of death, likely because of advances in acute stroke care.[13] Each year, approximately 795,000 people experience a stroke, 610,000 of whom have their first attack. The National Center for Health Statistics estimates that strokes are responsible for about 1 of every 20 deaths in the United States.[11]

The age-adjusted stroke death rate has actually fallen. Between 2003 and 2013 the stroke-related death rate declined by 33.7% while the actual number of stroke-related deaths declined by 18.2% during this period.[11] This suggests that more patients are surviving their stroke. Despite improved survival, approximately 50% of these patients are left with some degree of cognitive or functional impairment.

It is estimated that there are 6.6 million Americans older than 20 years of age who have survived a stroke. Using NHANES 2008–12 data, the overall stroke prevalence is estimated at 2.6%.[14] Because the majority of strokes occur in the elderly population, it is assumed that the prevalence of stroke will increase dramatically over the coming years with the aging of the US population. It is projected that by 2030, an additional 3.4 million people in the United States will have had a stroke, which represents an increase of 20% from 2012.[15] Some of this increase will be due to the projected improved survival from the initial stroke. Patients who survive their stroke will continue to incur medical costs associated with their rehabilitation and continuing care.

Stroke is a devastating disease. It is associated with not only significant mortality but also potentially life-altering cognitive and motor disability. The American Heart Association estimates that the lifetime cost of ischemic stroke is $140,048.[11] Any economic assessment of stroke has to take into account not only the effects of mortality but also the major impact on both cognitive and functional ability. The costs associated with the loss of productivity may be close to the cost of treating the acute stroke.[16] Between 2011 and 2012, the direct cost of treating stroke was estimated at $17.2 billion while the indirect costs including lost productivity were estimated at $15.8 billion.[11] Studies comparing the cost of stroke show that approximately 0.27% of gross domestic product or 3% of total national health-care expenditures is spent on the treatment of stroke.[17] Although the total annual costs associated with stroke are now estimated at between $36.5 and $65 billion, the costs associated with stroke treatment are only expected to grow so that by 2030 these costs may exceed $240 billion.[15]

Based on these estimates, it is clear that the treatment of stroke is costly. However, some of these costs are difficult to measure. To better understand the economics of stroke, it is useful to divide these costs into three separate categories: direct costs, indirect costs, and the intangibles (Fig. 1.1).

DIRECT COST OF STROKE

The direct cost of stroke measures the direct amount of care required to treat a patient who has suffered a stroke.[18] The majority of this cost relates to in-patient hospital care, including intensive care and interventional procedures. Direct cost of stroke also includes rehabilitation, nursing home care, and prescription drugs. Analyses of the direct costs associated with acute stroke include retrospective studies of in-patient databases from academic centers and larger studies of administrative databases such as the Nationwide In-patient Sample, which sample more than one million patients. In these studies, hospitalization costs range

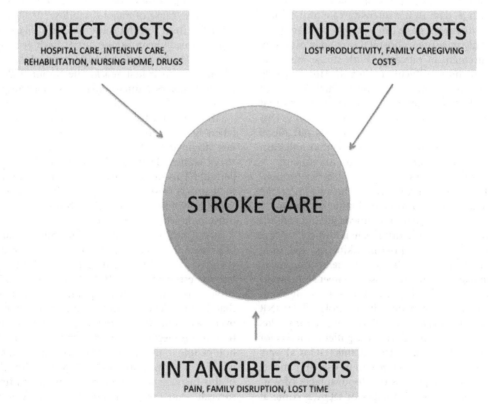

FIG. 1.1 The total cost of stroke care may be divided into the direct costs, the indirect costs, and the intangible costs.

from $8000 to $23,000 (converted to 2008 dollars) with an average hospital stay of 4.6–12.4 days.[19]

Studies on the cost of acute stroke care identify early critical care as a major component of hospital cost.[20] In a study by Demaerschalk and Durocher, one-third of the total in-hospital costs of treating acute ischemic stroke with tissue plasminogen activator (rt-PA) were due to acute critical care.[21] Other in-patient costs involve diagnostic radiology, drugs, laboratory tests, and general in-patient care. The cost of interventional vascular procedures now utilized to treat acute stroke must also be factored into the final analysis of acute cost.

The majority of the direct costs associated with acute stroke treatment are attributable to the initial hospitalization.[22] However, it appears that the costs associated with initial hospitalization for stroke are actually decreasing over time. In 1990 Taylor found that 70% of direct costs in the first year following an acute stroke were from the initial hospitalization.[23] These costs decreased to 62% in a review of administrative claims data from 2002 to 2003[24] and subsequently to approximately 50% in a review of MarketScan Commercial and Medicare Database from 2009 to 2012.[25] There are two explanations for this trend. Improved survival could be due to advances in interventional therapy for acute stroke and neurologic intensive care. An alternative explanation for the shifting of costs is the escalating costs and complexity of poststroke discharge care and rehabilitation.

Significant costs are encountered in the year following acute stroke. Johnson and coworkers studied retrospective claims from 20,314 commercially insured and 31,037 Medicare beneficiaries in the year postadmission for acute ischemic stroke between January 2009 and December 2012.[25] Total average costs were $61,354 and $44,929, respectively. Most studies have shown that the highest costs occur in the 1–3 months following an acute stroke.[26-28] This may relate to the high rate of hospital readmission postdischarge from acute stroke.[25,29-31] Previous studies have shown that the 30-day readmission rate ranges from 14% to 28%. This climbs to as high as 35% at 90 days postdischarge.[31] Most readmissions appear to be related to the sequelae of the acute stroke. In a study of healthcare utilization poststroke, 71.7% of 12,042 Medicare readmissions within 30 days of discharge were due to stroke-related sequelae.[25] This resulted in an average inpatient cost of $12,000 per patient or $104 million for the group. These data suggest that improvements in the management of patients during their initial hospitalization for stroke may reduce the economic burden in the year post–acute stroke if hospital readmissions are targeted.

INDIRECT COST OF STROKE

Indirect cost of stroke measures the value of loss of productivity due to disability, as well as the costs of caregiving by unpaid family members. Indirect costs may sometimes exceed the direct costs of treating the acute stroke. In the study by Taylor in 1996, indirect costs accounted for $23.6 billion or 58% of the total lifetime stroke-related costs.[23] Subsequently, Joo and coworkers summarized the results of 31 studies between 1990 and 2012 evaluating the indirect cost of stroke.[32] They highlighted the difficulty in precisely establishing the true indirect cost of stroke. This difficulty is due to the range of study methods, types of data, and the definitions of indirect costs. In their review, indirect costs, depending on the definition, represented a median of 32% of the total cost of treating stroke.

Two examples highlight the difficulty in precisely measuring the indirect cost of stroke. First, the cost of informal caregiving by family members following acute stroke is difficult to quantify. Although many studies mention the importance of informal caregiving in the rehabilitation of a stroke patient, there is no accepted method to measure the cost of lost wages or productivity by involved family members. A second area where measurement may be inexact is estimating the true cost of lost productivity due to illness and disability. This is a particularly difficult area to analyze since many stroke patients are older than 65 years and, while not in full-time positions, are still contributing to the workforce on a part-time or volunteer basis. Therefore, because there is no consensus on how to measure indirect cost, further study is necessary to better understand and assess the impact of indirect costs. But, there can be no doubt that indirect costs represent a substantial proportion of the total economic burden of stroke.

INTANGIBLE COSTS

These costs might include items that are generally not considered in the evaluation of disease states such as the cost of pain and suffering of the victim or his/her family members. Intangible costs might also include disruption in a family member's ability to be fully employed or fully productive. Lost time and lost wages are difficult to track. Intangible costs are difficult, if not impossible, to accurately measure. Nonetheless, they have an important impact on the true cost of stroke.

IMPACT OF ATRIAL FIBRILLATION ON STROKE-RELATED COSTS

AF is associated with strokes that are larger and more severe, resulting in more prolonged hospital stays and higher mortality.[33] Stroke severity is measured using various clinical tools such as the Scandinavian Stroke Scale and the National Institute of Health Stroke Scale. Multiple studies show that patients with AF are three to four times more likely to have severe strokes and higher degrees of functional impairment.[34-37] These strokes are associated with higher in-hospital, 30-day, and 1-year mortality. In a study of 1185 acute stroke patients, Jørgensen and coworkers found that AF patients had a higher in-hospital mortality (odds ratio = 1.84) and more prolonged hospital stays (50.4 vs. 39.8 days, $P < .001$).[38] Twelve studies compared the 30-day mortality in acute stroke patients with and without AF[34-36,38-46] (Table 1.1). These studies show that, on average, mortality in AF patients was approximately two times higher than their counterparts without AF (30-day AF mortality 11.3%–27% vs. no AF mortality 3.4%–12.2%). The higher mortality rate in AF patients extended 1 year post–hospital discharge (AF mortality 31.7%–63% vs. no AF mortality 13.7%–34%).

The costs associated with the care of AF stroke patients are also higher. Ali and coworkers evaluated the direct medical costs associated with acute stroke care in consecutive patients.[47] Direct medical costs were 50% greater for those patients with AF compared with those in sinus rhythm (£9083 vs. £5729, $P < .001$). Multivariate analysis in this study confirmed that AF is an independent predictor of acute care costs. Other studies have confirmed these findings including a MarketScan analysis of the medical treatment of 160,456 stroke patients for 1 year. In their analysis, Sussman et al. found that adjusted mean incremental costs (index plus 12-month postindex) for AF patients were $4726 higher than those for non-AF, a difference of approximately 20%.[48] These data provide further evidence of the impact of AF on stroke-related healthcare costs. Targeting AF patients could, therefore, have a major economic impact on the costs associated with overall stroke care.

COST-EFFECTIVENESS OF TREATMENTS FOR STROKE PREVENTION IN ATRIAL FIBRILLATION

AF is the most common arrhythmia encountered in clinical practice. Its prevalence ranges from 0.4% to 1.1% of the United States population.[49] The presence of AF increases with age, affecting approximately 10% of patients over the age of 80 years.[50] The risk for

TABLE 1.1
Influence of Atrial Fibrillation (AF) on Stroke Survival

Study		SAMPLE SIZE		30-DAY MORTALITY (%)			1-YEAR MORTALITY (%)		
		AF	No AF	AF	No AF	Sig.	AF	No AF	Sig.
Candelise[40]	1991	221	837	27	14	<0.05			
Britton[39]	1985	92	196	26	5	<0.05			
Broderick[41]	1992	318	1064	23	8	<0.001	44	18	<0.001
Sandercock[42]	1992	115	560	23	8	<0.05			
Lin[34]	1996	103	398	25	14	<0.05	63	34	<0.05
Jørgensen[38]	1996	968	217	33	17	<0.001			
Lamassa[35]	2001	803	3659	19	12	<0.001			
Kimura[43]	2005	3335	12,496	11	3	<0.001			
Ghatnekar[44]	2008	1619	4992	13	7	<0.01			
Thygesen[45]	2009	741	3108	15	6	<0.05	32	14	<0.05
Hannon[36]	2010	177	391	15	12	NS			
Saposnik[46]	2013	2185	10,501	22	10	<0.001	37	20	<0.01

embolic stroke is estimated to be at least five times higher in those patients with AF compared with the general population.[1] In addition to age, clinical risk factors, such as diabetes, hypertension, congestive heart failure, vascular disease, and history of prior stroke or transient ischemic attack (TIA), identify those patients with AF who are at higher risk for stroke. The CHADS$_2$-Vasc score was validated as a useful clinical tool to identify those patients most likely to benefit from anticoagulation.[51]

Randomized clinical trials have shown that the vitamin K antagonist warfarin significantly reduces strokes in high-risk AF patients. Hart and coworkers performed a metaanalysis on data from 16 randomized trials testing warfarin to prevent stroke in AF.[4] Warfarin was associated with a 62% relative risk reduction (95% CI 48%–72%) when compared with placebo. The major limitation of warfarin is bleeding, with intracranial bleeding being the most serious potential complication.[52] When compared with aspirin, warfarin almost doubles the risk of major bleeding (2.2 vs. 1.3 events per 100 patient-years).[53] Any economic evaluation of anticoagulant therapy in stroke prevention must consider the benefit of anticoagulation therapy against the risk of bleeding.

ECONOMIC ANALYSIS OF ANTICOAGULATION FOR STROKE PREVENTION

Economic analyses have validated the cost-effectiveness of warfarin in preventing stroke. Any economic analysis has to take into account the potential health gain of a therapy and balance it against the cost and potential adverse events associated with that therapy. Health gain may be measured by determining the response to treatment and subtracting the adverse events. There are several ways in which these effects can be evaluated: cost reduction studies, cost-effectiveness studies, and finally, cost utility studies.

Cost reduction studies compare the direct costs of treatment. As previously described, direct costs include hospitalizations, medications, and overall medical resources. In a study of the economic impact of warfarin on stroke prevention, Caro and coworkers found that warfarin was associated with lower direct medical costs as compared with no therapy ($2599 per patient-year vs. $4113 per patient-year).[54] These findings were based on the assumption that warfarin reduced the rate of thromboembolic stroke by 69%, an estimated stroke rate of 14.3/1000 warfarin patients versus 46.7/1000 patients not anticoagulated.

Cost-effectiveness studies are another method to evaluate the economic impact of an intervention. These studies are often reported as the cost per unit of outcome such as dollars per year of life saved or cost of preventing one stroke. The cost-effectiveness of anticoagulation in nonrheumatic AF was modeled utilizing the costs from a UK anticoagulation clinic, meta-analyses from clinical trial data of anticoagulation such as the Boston Area Anticoagulation Trial for Atrial Fibrillation, and UK National Health data.[55] The discounted cost of anticoagulation for one subject over 10 years was £4760 compared with £17,820 for the treatment of stroke for one subject over 10 years. This translated into a cost per year of life gained of £1751–£13,221, depending on the case scenario.

Cost utility studies measure the effectiveness of a therapy over a time horizon in the target population. This is usually expressed by using the term quality-adjusted life year (QALY). The health gain obtained by anticoagulation is, therefore, the benefit of stroke prevention minus the costs associated with bleeding. Economists have used various methods to determine whether a therapy is cost-effective. The incremental cost-effectiveness ratio (ICER) is expressed as the difference in cost between two therapies divided by the difference in health gain or QALY. An ICER less than $50,000/QALY is felt to be cost-effective.

Gage and coworkers used decision analysis to model the effects of anticoagulation on patient outcomes in nonvalvular AF.[56] Stroke prevention was considered in the context of clinical variables along with adverse outcomes such as major hemorrhage. In patients over 65 years of age with one additional risk factor for stroke (hypertension, diabetes mellitus, heart disease, or prior stroke/TIA) who are considered at medium risk for stroke, warfarin costs $8000 per QALY saved. However, if one considered anticoagulation in a 65-year-old with nonvalvular atrial fibrillation (NVAF) and no risk factors, the QALY saved rose to $370,000. Other investigators have modeled the cost-effectiveness of warfarin depending on the clinical scenario of warfarin monitoring.[57] They found that the economic benefit of warfarin declined as INR control became less optimal as compared with clinical trials. This type of analysis allows one to conclude that warfarin therapy is most cost-effective when it is dosed appropriately in those at high risk for stroke.

LIMITATIONS OF COST ANALYSIS STUDIES

It is always problematic to extrapolate the results of carefully conducted clinical trials to real-world experience. The efficacy of warfarin in reducing stroke in nonvalvular AF is well established. However, economic analysis relies on a number of assumptions that may not apply in clinical practice. First, the number of AF patients at risk for stroke who are actually treated with anticoagulation is low. In a 2011 study of Medicare patients, only 41.5% of nonvalvular AF patients were on warfarin.[58] Second, patient adherence is low. Fang and colleagues found that 26.3% of Medicare patients discontinued warfarin treatment despite a low risk for hemorrhage.[59] Third, warfarin is a difficult drug because of differences in bioavailability, drug and food interactions, and a narrow therapeutic index. Patients must achieve an INR of 2–3 to achieve therapeutic efficacy.[60] Patients are often unable to maintain a therapeutic INR. In a study of 138,319 AF patients undergoing INR monitoring, the time in therapeutic range (TTR) averaged 53.7%.[61] Similarly, in ORBIT, a registry of AF patients, only 59% of the INR measurements were between 2 and 3, with a median TTR of 68%.[62] Previous studies have shown that a high TTR correlates with improved outcomes.[63] Therefore, some of these limitations will influence the assumptions used in the economic models and affect the precision of any cost analysis.

COST-EFFECTIVENESS OF THE NEW ANTICOAGULANTS

Cost analysis has been applied to the newer DOACs, dabigatran, rivaroxaban, apixaban, and edoxaban. Clinical trials have shown that these agents are at least as effective as warfarin in reducing stroke in NVAF.[9] These new drugs, however, come at a higher cost than warfarin, which is relatively inexpensive. On the other hand, the DOACs do not incur the expense of routine laboratory monitoring. The question is whether these newer agents are worth the cost.

The cost-effectiveness of these agents compared with the standard therapy of warfarin anticoagulation has been evaluated in numerous studies[64-66] (Table 1.2). These economic evaluations utilize Markov modeling to simulate clinical outcomes based on the input of a number of variables. These variables include the expected efficacy of a DOAC, based on the results of clinical trials, the expected TTR for the warfarin group, and baseline stroke risk factors, generally derived from the CHADS$_2$-Vasc score. Other factors, such as patient age, the expected time horizon for therapy, and drug cost may be entered into these models. In addition, the negative impact of significant hemorrhage is factored into the results. Although warfarin

is consistently found to be the least costly drug, all of the newer agents are more cost-effective than dose-adjusted warfarin.

Healthcare professionals and payers need to evaluate any new therapy when it becomes available. Is the new therapy, which often comes at a higher acquisition cost, associated with better outcomes? In simple terms, is the new therapy worthwhile? When reviewing the results of the economic analyses of the DOACs, it is apparent that there are variable outcome measurements. In addition, the outcome of these models must be kept in perspective because the QALY difference between apixaban, the best performer, and rivaroxaban, the weakest performer, is only 50 days. The QALY, overall cost, and ICER vary from study to study. This is because each model is based on different assumptions. The model tested assumes different patient characteristics, drug compliance or TTR if the patient is on warfarin, and the rate of bleeding or significant hemorrhage. The outcome of the model will be significantly affected if the assumptions are changed. It is clear from previous studies on the cost-effectiveness of warfarin that the target population must have a significant risk for stroke in order for the treatment to be cost-effective.[56] Therefore, any model can only approximate what will happen in the "real world" when patients are not selected for a clinical trial or their risk factors are not carefully screened and drug pricing is not rigidly controlled. The cost-effectiveness of the DOACs will also depend on the effectiveness of warfarin control in a given population. However, it must be emphasized that the consistent message of these economic analyses is the superiority of the DOACs for stroke prevention. Improved pricing will only improve the economic advantage.

The question then becomes, which of the DOACs is the most cost-effective? In the most recent analysis, Shah and coworkers developed a Markov model for the five available oral anticoagulants—warfarin, dabigatran, rivaroxaban, apixaban, and edoxaban.[66] The model utilized a US commercial population and modeled the cost-effectiveness of treatment over a lifetime horizon. Similar to previous studies, they found that warfarin costs were the lowest ($46,241, 95% CI $44,499–47,874) and rivaroxaban costs were the highest ($58,889, 95% CI $57,467–60,444). Of the agents studied, apixaban had the highest QALY (9.38, 95% CI 9.24–9.48), which corresponds to an ICER of $25,816/QALY when compared with warfarin. This study demonstrates that apixaban is cost-effective given an ICER of less than $50,000, which is generally the accepted value for a favorable effect.

TABLE 1.2
Cost-effectiveness of Direct Oral Anticoagulants Compared With Warfarin

Study	Year	Drug	Dose	QALY	Cost	ICER/QALY
Freeman[67] $US 2008	2011	WAR		10.28	143,193	_____
		DAB	110 mg bid	10.70	164,576	51,229
			150 mg bid	10.84	168,398	45,372
Shah[68] $US 2010	2011	WAR		8.40	44,300	_____
		DAB	110 mg bid	8.54	43,700	150,000
			150 mg bid	6.68	40,169	86,000
Sorenson[69] $CAN 2010	2011	WAR		6.82	44,379	_____
		DAB	110 mg bid	6.86	41,324	29,994
			150 mg bid	7.08	42,946	9041
Gonzalez-Juanatey[70] € 2012	2012	WAR		8.45	10,343	_____
		DAB	150 mg bid	8.73	15,195	17,581
Kamel[71] $US 2011	2012	WAR		3.91		_____
		DAB		4.19		25,000
Lee[72] $US 2011	2012	WAR		9.81	88,544	_____
		RIVA	20 mg daily	10.03	94,456	27,498
Kamel[73] $US 2011	2012	WAR		3.91	378,000	_____
		APIX	5 mg bid	4.19	381,700	11,4000
Harrington[64] $US 2013	2013	WAR		7.97	77,813	_____
		DAB	150 mg bid	8.41	82,719	11,150
		RIVA	20 mg daily	8.26	78,738	3190
		APIX	5 mg bid	8.47	85,326	15,026
Shah[66] $US 2015	2016	WAR			46,241	_____
		DAB	150 mg bid	9.35	56,425	31,435
		RIVA	20 mg daily	9.24	58,879	57,434
		APIX	5 mg bid	9.38	55,455	25,816
		EDOX	60 mg daily	9.31	54,159	27,643

APIX, apixaban; *DAB*, dabigatran; *EDOX*, edoxaban; *ICER*, incremental cost-effectiveness ratio; *QALY*, quality-adjusted life year; *RIVA*, rivaroxaban; *WAR*, warfarin.

CONCLUSION

Stroke remains a devastating disease with high morbidity and mortality. This chapter has pointed out that the economic impact of stroke is profound, but difficult to quantitate. Anticoagulation can significantly reduce the risk for stroke. Economic analysis has shown that warfarin is highly cost-effective despite problems with compliance and achieving an adequate TTR. The newer agents offer the promise of reducing stroke and being cost-effective.

REFERENCES

1. Wolf PA, Abbott RD, Kannel WB, et al. Atrial fibrillation as an independent risk factor for stroke: the Framingham study. *Stroke*. 1991;22:983–988.
2. Wolf PA, Dawber TR, Thomas Jr HE, et al. Epidemiologic assessment of chronic atrial fibrillation and risk of stroke: the Framingham study. *Neurology*. 1978;28:973–977.
3. Wolf PA, Abbott RD, Kannel WB, et al. Atrial fibrillation: a major contributor to stroke in the elderly: the Framingham study. *Arch Intern Med*. 1987;147:1561–1564.

4. Hart RG, Benavente O, McBride R, et al. Antithrombotic therapy to prevent stroke in patients with atrial fibrillation. *Ann Intern Med.* 2003;131:492–501.

5. January CT, Wann LS, Alpert JS, et al. 2014 AHA/ACC/HRS guidelines for the management of patients with atrial fibrillation. *Circulation.* 2014;10:e199–e267.

6. You JJ, Singer DE, Howard PA, et al. Antithrombotic therapy and prevention of thrombosis, 9th edition: American College of Chest Physicians evidence-based clinical practice guidelines. *Chest.* 2012;141(suppl 2):e531S–e575S.

7. Hylek EM, Skates SJ, Sheehan MA, et al. An analysis of the lowest effective intensity of prophylactic anticoagulation for patients with nonrheumatic atrial fibrillation. *N Engl J Med.* 1996;335:540–546.

8. Hylek EM, Go AS, Chang Y, et al. Effect of intensity of oral anticoagulation on stroke severity and mortality in atrial fibrillation. *N Engl J Med.* 2003;349:1019–1026.

9. Dentali F, Rivera N, Crowther M, et al. Efficacy and safety of the novel oral anticoagulants in atrial fibrillation: a systematic review and meta-analysis of the literature. *Circulation.* 2012;126:2381–2391.

10. Halperin JL, Dorian P. Trials of novel oral anticoagulants for stroke prevention in patients with non-valvular atrial fibrillation. *Curr Cardiol Rev.* 2014;10:297–302.

11. Mozzaffarian D, Benjamin EJ, Go AS, et al. Executive summary: heart disease and stroke statistics-2016 update. *Circulation.* 2016;133:447–454.

12. National Vital Statistics Report. https://www.cdc.gov/nchs/data/nvsr/nvsr65/nvsr65_05.pdf.

13. Towfighi A, Saver JL. Stroke declines from third to fourth leading cause of death in the United States: historical perspective and challenges ahead. *Stroke.* 2011;42:2351–2355.

14. Centers for Disease Control and Prevention (CDC). Prevalence of stroke- United States, 2006–2010. MMWR *Morb Mortal Wky Rep.* 2012;61:379–382.

15. Ovbiagele B, Goldsten LB, Higashida RT, et al. Forecasting the future of stroke in the United States: a policy statement from the American Heart Association and American Stroke Association. *Stroke.* 2013;44:2361–2375.

16. Demaerschalk BM, Hwang HM, Leung G. US cost burden of ischemic stroke: a systematic literature review. *Am J Manag Care.* 2010;16:525–533.

17. Evers SM, Struijs JN, Ament AJ, et al. International comparison of stroke cost studies. *Stroke.* 2004;35:1209–1215.

18. Taylor TN. The medical economics of stroke. *Drugs.* 1997;54(suppl 3):51–58.

19. Qureshi AI, Suri MF, Nasar A, et al. Changes in cost and outcome among US patients with stroke hospitalized in 1990 to 1991 and those hospitalized in 2000 to 2001. *Stroke.* 2007;38:2180–2184.

20. Diringer MN, Edwards DF, Mattson DT, et al. Predictors of acute hospital costs for treatment of ischemic stroke in an academic center. *Stroke.* 1999;30:724–728.

21. Demaerschalk BM, Durocher DL. How diagnosis-related group 559 will change the US Medicare cost reimbursement ratio for stroke centers. *Stroke.* 2007;38:1309–1312.

22. Wang G, Joo H, Tong X, et al. Hospital costs associated with atrial fibrillation for patients with ischemic stroke aged 18-64 years in the United States. *Stroke.* 2015;46:1314–1320.

23. Taylor TN, Davis PH, Torner JC, et al. Lifetime cost of stroke in the United States. *Stroke.* 1996;27:1459–1466.

24. Engel-Nitz NM, Sander SD, Harley C, Rey GG, Shah H. Costs and outcomes of noncardioembolic ischemic stroke in a managed care population. *Vasc Health Risk Manag.* 2010;6:905–913.

25. Johnson BH, Bonafede MM, Watson C. Short- and longer-term healthcare resource utilization and costs associated with acute stroke. *Clinicoecon Outcomes Res.* 2016;8:53–61.

26. Samsa GP, Bian J, Lipscomb J, Matchar DB. Epidemiology of recurrent cerebral infarction: a Medicare claims–based comparison of first and recurrent strokes on 2-year survival and cost. *Stroke.* 1999;30:338–349.

27. Sloss EM, Wickstrom SL, McCaffrey DF, et al. Direct medical costs attributable to acute myocardial infarction and ischemic stroke in cohorts with atherosclerotic conditions. *Cerebrovasc Dis.* 2004;18:8–15.

28. Lipscomb J, Ancukiewicz M, Parmigiani G, et al. Predicting the cost of illness: a comparison of alternative models applied to stroke. *Med Decis Making.* 1998;18(suppl 2):S39–S56.

29. Fonarow GC, Smith EE, reeves MJ, et al. Get with the Guidelines Steering Committee and Hospitals. Hospital level variation in mortality and rehospitalization for Medicare beneficiaries with acute ischemic stroke. *Stroke.* 2011;42:159–166.

30. Lichtman JH, Leifheit-Limson EC, Jones SB, et al. Preventable readmissions within 30 days of ischemic stroke among Medicare beneficiaries. *Stroke.* 2013;44:3429–3435.

31. Fehnel CR, Lee Y, Wendell LC, et al. Post-acute care for predicting readmission data after ischemic stroke: a nationwide cohort analysis using the minimum data set. *J Am Heart Assoc.* 2015;4:e002145.

32. Joo H, George MG, Fang J, et al. A literature review of indirect costs associated with stroke. *J Stroke Cerebrovasc Dis.* 2014;23:1753–1763.

33. Censori B, Camerlingo M, Casto L, et al. Prognostic factors in first-ever stroke in the carotid artery territory seen within 6 hours after onset. *Stroke.* 1993;24:532–535.

34. Lin HJ, Wolf PA, Kelly-Hayes M, et al. Stroke severity in atrial fibrillation: the Framingham study. *Stroke.* 1996;27:1760–1764.

35. Lamassa M, Di Carlo A, Pracucci G, et al. Characteristics, outcome, and care of stroke associated with atrial fibrillation in Europe: data from a multicenter multinational hospital-based registry (The European Community Stroke Project). *Stroke.* 2001;32:392–398.

36. Hannon N, Sheehan O, Kelly L, et al. Stroke associated with atrial fibrillation – incidence and early outcomes in the North Dublin population stroke study. *Cerebrovasc Dis.* 2010;29:43–49.

37. Hannon N, Daly L, Murphy S, et al. Acute hospital, community, and indirect costs of stroke associated with atrial fibrillation- population-based study. *Stroke*. 2014;45:3670–3674.

38. Jørgensen HS, Nakayama H, Reith J, et al. Acute stroke with atrial fibrillation: the Copenhagen stroke study. *Stroke*. 1996;27:1765–1769.

39. Britton M, Gustafsson C. Non-rheumatic atrial fibrillation as a risk factor for stroke. *Stroke*. 1985;16:182–188.

40. Candelise L, Pinardi G, Morabito A. Mortality in acute stroke with atrial fibrillation. The Italian acute stroke study group. *Stroke*. 1991;22:169–174.

41. Broderick J, Phillips S, Ofallen W, et al. Relationship of cardiac disease to stroke occurrence, recurrence, and mortality. *Stroke*. 1992;23:1250–1256.

42. Sandercock P, Bamford J, Dennis M, et al. Atrial fibrillation and stroke: prevalence in different types of stroke and influence on early and long-term prognosis. *BMJ*. 1992;305:1460–1465.

43. Kimura K, Minematsu K, Yamaguchi T. Atrial fibrillation as a predictive factor for severe stroke in early death in 15,831 patients with acute ischaemic stroke. *J Neurol Neurosurg Psychiatry*. 2005;76:679–683.

44. Ghatnekar O, Glader E. The effect of atrial fibrillation on stroke-related inpatient cost in Sweden: a 3 year analysis of registry data from 2001. *Value Health*. 2008;11:862–868.

45. Thygesen K, Frost L, Eagle K, et al. Atrial fibrillation in patients with ischemic stroke: a population based study. *Clin Epidemiol*. 2009;1:55–65.

46. Saposnik G, Gladstone D, Raptis R, et al. Atrial fibrillation in ischaemic stroke: predicting response to thrombolysis and clinical outcomes. *Stroke*. 2013;44:99–104.

47. Ali AN, Abdel-Hafiz. Cost of acute stroke care for patients with atrial fibrillation compared with those in sinus rhythm. *Pharmacoeconomics*. 2015;33:511–520.

48. Sussman M, Menzin J, Lin I, et al. Impact of atrial fibrillation on stroke-related healthcare costs. *J Am Heart Assoc*. 2013;2:e000479.

49. Go AS, Hylek EM, Phillips KA, et al. Prevalence of diagnosed atrial fibrillation in adults: national implications for rhythm management and stroke prevention: the AnTicoagulation and Risk factors in atrial fibrillation (ATRIA) study. *JAMA*. 2001;285(18):2370–2375.

50. Piccini JP, Hammill BG, Sinner MF, et al. Incidence and prevalence of atrial fibrillation and associated mortality among Medicare beneficiaries, 1993–2007. *Circ Cardiovasc Qual Outcomes*. 2012;5:85–93.

51. Olesen JB, Lip GY, Hansen ML, et al. Validation of risk stratification schemes for predicting stroke and thromboembolism in patients with atrial fibrillation: nationwide cohort study. *BMJ*. 2011;342:d124.

52. Garcia DA, Regan S, Crowther M, et al. The risk of hemorrhage among patients with warfarin-associated coagulopathy. *J Am Coll Cardiol*. 2006;47:804–808.

53. van Walraven C, Hart RG, Singer DE, et al. Oral anticoagulants vs aspirin in nonvalvular atrial fibrillation: an individual patient meta-analysis. *JAMA*. 2002;288:2441–2448.

54. Caro JJ, O'Brien JA, Klittich W, et al. The economic impact of warfarin prophylaxis in non-valvular atrial fibrillation. *Dis Mang Clin Outcomes*. 1997;1:54–60.

55. Lightowlers S, McGuire A. Cost-effectiveness of anticoagulation in nonrheumatic atrial fibrillation in the primary prevention of stroke. *Stroke*. 1998;29:1827–1832.

56. Gage BF, Cardinalli AB, Albers G, et al. Cost-effectiveness of warfarin and aspirin for prophylaxis of stroke in patients with nonvalvular atrial fibrillation. *JAMA*. 1995;274:1839–1845.

57. Soensen SV, Dewilde S, Singer DE, et al. Cost-effectiveness of warfarin: trial versus "real-world" stroke prevention in atrial fibrillation. *Am Heart J*. 2009;157:1064–1073.

58. Mercaldi CJ, Ciarametaro M, Hahn B, et al. Cost efficiency of anticoagulation with warfarin to prevent stroke in Medicare beneficiaries with non valvular atrial fibrillation. *Stroke*. 2011;42:412–418.

59. Fang MC, Go AS, Chang Y, et al. Warfarin discontinuation after starting warfarin for atrial fibrillation. *Circ Cardiovasc Qual Outcomes*. 2010;3:623–631.

60. Hylek EM, Go AS, Chang Y, et al. Effect of intensity of oral anticoagulation on stroke severity and mortality in atrial fibrillation. *N Engl J Med*. 2002;349:1019–1026.

61. Diott JS, George RA, Huang X, et al. National assessment of warfarin anticoagulation treatment for stroke prevention in atrial fibrillation. *Circulation*. 2014;129:1407–1414.

62. Pokorney SD, DaJuanicia NS, Thomas L, et al. Patient time in therapeutic range on warfarin among US patients with atrial fibrillation: results from ORBIT-AF registry. *Am Heart J*. 2015;170:141–148.

63. Connolly SJ, Pogue J, Eikelboom J, et al. Benefit of oral anticoagulation over antiplatelet therapy in atrial fibrillation depends on the quality of international normalized ratio control achieved by centers and countries as measure by time in therapeutic range. *Circulation*. 2008;118:2029–2037.

64. Harrington AR, Armstrong EP, Nolan Jr PE, et al. Cost-effectiveness of apixaban, dabigatran, rivaroxaban, and warfarin for stroke prevention in atrial fibrillation. *Stroke*. 2013;44:1676–1681.

65. von Scheele B, Fernandez M, Hogue SL, et al. Review of economics and cost-effectiveness analyses of anticoagulant therapy for stroke prevention in atrial fibrillation in the US. *Ann Pharmacother*. 2013;47:671–685.

66. Shah A, Shewale A, Hayes CJ, et al. Cost-effectiveness of oral anticoagulants for ischemic stroke prophylaxis among nonvalvular atrial fibrillation patients. *Stroke*. 2016;47:1555–1561.

67. Freeman JV, Zhu RP, Owens DK, et al. Cost effectiveness of dabigatran compared with warfarin for stroke prevention in atrial fibrillation. *Ann Intern Med*. 2011;154:1–11.

68. Shah SV, Gage BF. Cost effectiveness of dabigatran for stroke prophylaxis in atrial fibrillation. *Circulation*. 2011;123:2562–2570.

69. Sorenson SV, Kansal AR, Connolly S, et al. Cost effectiveness of dabigatran etexilate for the prevention of stroke
and systemic embolism in atrial fibrillation: a Canadian
payer perspective. *Thromb Haemost.* 2011;105:908–919.

70. Gonzalez-Juanatey JR, Alvarez-Sabin J, Lobos JM, et al.
Cost effectiveness of dabigatran for stroke prevention in
nonvalvular atrial fibrillation in Spain. *Rev Esp Cardiol.*
2012;65:901–910.

71. Kamel H, Johnston SC, Easton JD, et al. Cost effectiveness
of dabigatran compared with warfarin for stroke prevention in patients with atrial fibrillation and prior stroke or
transient ischemic attack. *Stroke.* 2012;43:881–883.

72. Lee S, Anglade MW, Pham D, et al. Cost-effectiveness of
rivaroxaban compared to warfarin for stroke prevention
and atrial fibrillation. *Am J Cardiol.* 2012;110:845–851.

73. Kamel H, Easton JD, Johnston SC, et al. Cost-effectiveness
of apixaban vs. warfarin for secondary stroke prevention
and atrial fibrillation. *Neurology.* 2012;79:1428–1434.

CHAPTER 2

Pharmacology of Oral Anticoagulants

PAUL P. DOBESH, PHARMD, FCCP, BCPS •
ZACHARY A. STACY, PHARMD, FCCP, BCPS

VITAMIN K ANTAGONISTS

Vitamin K antagonists (VKAs) remain the most commonly used method of oral anticoagulation for a number of clinical settings. Although several VKAs, such as phenprocoumon, acenocoumarol, and flu-indione, are available across the globe, warfarin remains the most commonly used VKA, especially in North America. Despite the differences between VKAs in terms of half-life and metabolism pathways, the mechanism of providing an anticoagulant effect is consistent.

Pharmacology

VKAs provide their anticoagulant effect by interfering with vitamin K recycling and the activation of a number of clotting factors (Fig. 2.1).[1-4] It is necessary to understand the role of vitamin K in the creation of biologically active clotting factors II, VII, IX, and X (vitamin K–dependent factors) to appreciate the inhibitory effects of VKAs.[4] The vitamin K–dependent clotting factors require γ-carboxylation for their procoagulant activity. The reduced form of vitamin K (vitamin KH_2) is necessary for the carboxylation reaction to take place, as well as molecular oxygen, carbon dioxide, and γ-glutamyl carboxylase.[5] After carboxylation, vitamin K is left in an oxidized state as vitamin K epoxide and must undergo two reductase reactions to return to vitamin KH_2 (Fig. 2.1). In the first step, vitamin K epoxide reductase (VCOR) reduces vitamin K epoxide to vitamin K_1. This is the step in which VKAs have their greatest effect because VKOR is significantly inhibited by VKAs.[2,3] Vitamin K_1 is the form of vitamin K found in foods and pharmacologic vitamin K. The second step involves the conversion of vitamin K_1 to vitamin KH_2 by vitamin K reductase. Because vitamin K reductase is less sensitive to inhibition by VKA, the anticoagulant effect of VKAs can be overcome by low-dose phytonadione or dietary vitamin K by bypassing the major inhibitory action of VKAs. Vitamin KH_2 is now again able to take part in γ-carboxylation of the vitamin K–dependent clotting factors. Therefore, by inhibiting the recycling and reduction of vitamin K, the carboxylation of these clotting factors is diminished and the ability for clot formation is reduced.

Carboxylation of these clotting factors is necessary for the binding of these factors to phospholipid membranes.[6-8] In the presence of the divalent cation Ca^{2+}, the two carboxyl groups on these clotting factors provide two negative charges, which promotes binding to the membranes (Fig. 2.2). For clotting factors IX and X, this involves the ability to bind to the surface of the platelet to create the tenase and prothrombinase complexes, respectively. Factor VII binding to the endothelial wall to become activated by tissue factor also requires this process. Finally, thrombin (factor II) must also bind to endothelial cells via this process to interact with thrombomodulin and other phospholipid membranes throughout the clotting cascade. Therefore, the inability of these clotting factors to gain the second carboxyl group through γ-carboxylation due to VKA therapy prevents the binding to these membranes and consequently inhibits coagulation at a number of different locations.[6,8]

Besides inhibiting carboxylation of clotting factors II, VII, IX, and X, VKAs also inhibit carboxylation of proteins C, S, and Z. These proteins assist in the biologic inhibition of thrombosis. Therefore, inhibiting these proteins has the potential to induce thrombosis, especially in the initial days of VKA therapy.[9] This is why patients started on warfarin therapy were initially hospitalized in the past to overlap with intravenous heparin, a practice that is not continued now.

Pharmacokinetics and pharmacodynamics

Warfarin is almost completely and rapidly absorbed from the gastrointestinal (GI) tract and reaches peak blood concentrations within 90 min of oral administration.[10,11] Warfarin is highly water soluble and therefore, does not widely distribute into adipose tissue but is highly protein bound, mainly to albumin.[10] Warfarin exists as a racemic mixture of approximately equal portions of two optically active isomers, or more specifically, enantiomers.[10-12] The S enantiomer (S-warfarin) has approximately four to five times more potent anticoagulant

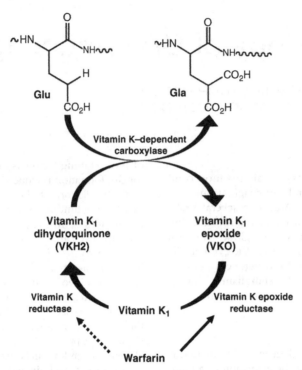

FIG. 2.1 Impact of warfarin on the vitamin K cycle.

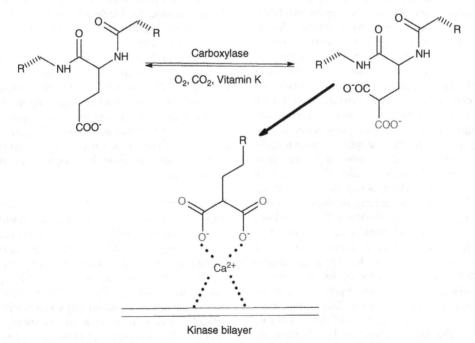

FIG. 2.2 Binding of vitamin K–dependent clotting factors to phospholipid membranes.

activity compared with the R enantiomer (R-warfarin). The half-life of racemic warfarin is 36–42h but is longer for R-warfarin (~45h) compared with S-warfarin (~30h). Racemic warfarin accumulates in the liver where each enantiomer is metabolized by different pathways. S-warfarin undergoes extensive oxidative metabolism (~90%) via the cytochrome P450 (CYP) system, with the CYP2C9 enzyme being the principal metabolism pathway and CYP3A4 contributing to a lesser extent.[13] R-warfarin undergoes approximately 60% oxidative metabolism, with CYP1A2 and CYP3A4 being the major pathways and CYP2C19 contributing to a lesser extent.[13] Metabolism of the remaining amount of both enantiomers is reduction to diastereomeric alcohols. Given these complicated pharmacokinetic properties, it is understandable why direct-acting oral anticoagulants (DOACS) provide a simpler method of anticoagulation.

There are some pharmacokinetic differences with the other less often utilized VKAs. Similar to warfarin, acenocoumarol and phenprocoumon also exist as enantiomers but have distinct stereochemical characteristics. R-acenocoumarol has a shorter elimination half-life of 9h compared with warfarin, with S-acenocoumarol having a half-life of only about 30min.[14] For acenocoumarol, the R enantiomer is more potent than the S enantiomer. R-acenocoumarol is primarily metabolized by CYP2C9 and CYP2C19, whereas S-acenocoumarol is primarily metabolized by CYP2C9.[14] Phenprocoumon has a longer half-life of 5.5 days compared with warfarin, with similar

half-lives for both the R and S enantiomers.[15] This longer half-life makes treatment of bleeding or reversal more challenging. S-phenprocoumon is 1.5–2.5 times more potent than R-phenprocoumon, and both enantiomers are metabolized by CYP2C9.[15] Fluindione is an indandione VKA with a mean half-life of 30–40h.[16] Unlike warfarin, fluindione is not a chiral compound.[16]

The pharmacodynamic response to warfarin is influenced by a number of genetic and environmental factors, making the dose-response relationship difficult to predict. A number of point mutations in the gene coding for the CYP2C9 have been identified.[17] Because CYP2C9 is the primary oxidative metabolism pathway for the more potent S-warfarin, these polymorphisms have a potential significant impact on pharmacodynamic response to warfarin therapy.[18] The most common polymorphisms are CYP2C9*2 and CYP2C9*3, and both are associated with a reduced ability to metabolize S-warfarin, resulting in a decrease in S-warfarin clearance and, as a result, an increased anticoagulant effect of a given dose of warfarin.[17,18] Therefore, patients with either heterozygous or homozygous expression of a variant allele of CYP2C9 require lower doses of warfarin compared with patients who are homozygous for the wild-type allele (CYP2C9*1*1) (Table 2.1).[19,20] These polymorphisms in CYP2C9 have been found to occur in different frequencies in various ethnic groups, which should be considered when selecting an initial warfarin dose.[19,21] The CYP2C9

TABLE 2.1 Warfarin Polymorphisms[19,20]					
CYP2C9 Genetic Alleles	CYP2C9*1	CYP2C9*2	CYP2C9*3	CYP2C9*4	CYP2C9*5
ETHNIC GROUP (%)					
Whites	79–86	8–19.1	6–10	ND	ND
Indigenous Canadians	91	3	6	ND	ND
African-Americans	98.5	1–3.6	0.5–1.5	ND	2.3
Asians	95–98.3	0	1.7–5	0–1.6	0
VCOR genetic haplotype sequence	H CCATCTCTG H2 CCGAGCTCTG			H7 TCGGTCCGCA H8 TAGGTCCGCA H9 TACGTTCGCG	
ETHNIC GROUP (%)					
Europeans	37			58	
Africans	14			49	
Asians	89			10	

VCOR, vitamin K epoxide reductase.

polymorphism affect other VKAs but to a lesser extent compared with warfarin.

Another major genetic influence on the pharmacodynamic effect of warfarin includes mutations in the main target for VKA, VCOR. The gene that encodes for this enzyme encodes for several isoforms of a protein that are collectively termed the vitamin K epoxide complex 1 (VCORC1).[22] Mutations in this gene have been identified leading to VCOR enzymes with varying sensitivities to inhibition by warfarin and subsequently affecting the pharmacodynamics of warfarin.[23-25] Whereas some mutations in VCORC1 produce increased inhibition of the enzyme and an exaggerated anticoagulant effect, resulting in the need for lower doses of warfarin, other mutations lead to reduced ability of warfarin to inhibit the enzyme and a subsequent warfarin resistance, with some patients requiring 5- to 20-fold higher doses compared with typical doses to provide an anticoagulant effect.[26] As with the CYP2C9 polymorphisms, these mutations occur with differing frequencies in various populations (Table 2.1).[19,20]

In addition to genetic factors mentioned above, dietary factors and a number of disease states affect the pharmacodynamic response to the VKA. Fluctuating intake of dietary vitamin K has been demonstrated to have an influence on maintenance of therapeutic international normalized ratio (INR) with long-term warfarin therapy.[27,28] Most dietary vitamin K (vitamin K1) is supplied predominately as phylloquinone in plant material, with a recommended intake of 80 μg/day (based on a 2000-calorie diet).[28] Because dietary vitamin K enters the vitamin K cycle after VCOR and is reduced by vitamin K reductase, which is only weakly inhibited by VKA, the inhibitory impact of VKA can be overcome.[29] The amount of vitamin K from dietary sources can differ significantly based on the type of food and portion size (Table 2.2).[30] Although patients are often counseled to maintain a fairly consistent intake of dietary vitamin K, this may be easier said than done depending on the types and amounts of foods ingested. Dietary vitamin K is also found in multivitamins and other nutritional supplements. Therefore, patients must be educated about checking amounts or informing their clinicians about changes in products or brands of these supplements. During times of illness or poor appetite, there can be a significant reduction in dietary vitamin K intake below average, which may increase the anticoagulant effect of the VKA at that patient's typical dose and increase risk of bleeding.

Disease states such as hepatic dysfunction can affect the pharmacodynamic effect of the VKA. In hepatic dysfunction, there can be an impaired synthesis of clotting factors and impaired metabolism of warfarin, which can potentiate and prolong the anticoagulant effect.[31] Hypermetabolic states such as fever or hyperthyroidism have demonstrated the ability to increase the anticoagulant effect of warfarin by increasing catabolism of vitamin K–dependent clotting factors.[32,33] Patients with heart failure have demonstrated the need for a reduced dose of warfarin, likely due to increased hepatic congestion and increased responsiveness to therapy.[34] Patients with end-stage renal disease have reduced CYP2C9 metabolism activity and therefore, an increased exposure of the more potent S-warfarin, resulting in a higher risk of bleeding.[35]

Drug interactions

There are numerous drug-drug interactions with VKAs with varying degree of clinical significance (Table 2.3).[36-40] Depending on the source, there are over 200 drug-drug interactions listed for warfarin. The challenge to gaining understanding about these drug interactions is that many sources do not contain the same list. One investigation of major drug information sources identified 648 different drug interactions with warfarin, but only 50 interactions were consistent for all of the sources used.[41] This is likely due to different levels of evidence required to document an interaction, with many interactions being registered based on single case reports.

Drug-drug interaction with warfarin can be pharmacokinetic or pharmacodynamic in nature. Most pharmacokinetic interactions involve an impact on absorption or metabolism of warfarin. Cholestyramine is known to inhibit the GI absorption of warfarin, producing a reduced anticoagulant response.[42] Interactions affecting the metabolism of warfarin can be from either inhibition of metabolism, leading to an increased anticoagulant effect with increased risk of bleeding, or an induction of metabolism, leading to a decreased anticoagulant effect with an increased risk of thrombosis. Some agents have the ability to inhibit certain warfarin metabolism enzymes while inducing others, leaving the impact on the anticoagulant effect of warfarin unpredictable. Drug interactions can also be characterized by the enzymes they affect. Inhibition of S-warfarin metabolism (CYP2C9 > CYP3A4) is more important clinically because this isomer is more potent as a VKA than the R-isomer.[43,44] Clearance of S-isomer warfarin is inhibited by a number of agents such as metronidazole and trimethoprim-sulfamethoxazole.[45,46] These agents produce increases in the prothrombin time (PT) and INR, increasing the risk of bleeding without dose adjustment. In contrast, drugs

TABLE 2.2
Vitamin K–Containing Foods

Food	Portion Size	Vitamin K in μg
Artichoke hearts (globe or French), boiled	1 cup	25
Artichokes (globe or French), boiled	1 cup	18
Asparagus spears, frozen, boiled	4	48
Asparagus spears, canned, boiled	4	30
Asparagus spears, boiled	4	30
Avocado, puree, raw	1 cup	48
Beans, snap, green, frozen, microwaved	1 cup	64
Beans, snap, green or yellow, canned or boiled	1 cup	60
Beans, snap, green or yellow, frozen, boiled	1 cup	51
Beans, fava, in pod, raw	1 cup	52
Beans, kidney, red, mature seeds, boiled	1 cup	15
Beet greens, 1″ pieces, boiled	1 cup	697
Blackberries, raw	1 cup	29
Blueberries, frozen sweetened	1 cup	41
Blueberries, raw	1 cup	28
Broccoli, chopped, boiled	1 cup	220
Broccoli, frozen, chopped, boiled	1 cup	162
Broccoli, raw, chopped	1 cup	93
Brussels sprouts, frozen, boiled	1 cup	300
Brussels sprouts, raw	1 cup	156
Cabbage, shredded, boiled	1 cup	163
Cabbage, chopped, raw	1 cup	68
Cabbage, Chinese (pak-choi), boiled	1 cup	58
Cabbage, savoy, raw	1 cup	48
Cabbage, red, chopped, raw	1 cup	34
Carrots, boiled, sliced	1 cup	21
Carrots, frozen, boiled, sliced	1 cup	20
Carrots, raw, grated	1 cup	15
Cauliflower, frozen, boiled	1 cup	21
Cauliflower, boiled	1 cup	17
Cauliflower, raw, chopped	1 cup	17
Celery, boiled, diced	1 cup	57
Celery, raw	1 cup	30
Chard, Swiss, chopped, boiled	1 cup	573
Chard, Swiss, raw	1 cup	299
Collards, frozen, chopped, boiled	1 cup	1059
Collards, chopped, boiled	1 cup	773
Cowpeas (blackeyes), immature seeds, frozen, boiled	1 cup	63

Continued

TABLE 2.2
Vitamin K–Containing Foods—cont'd

Food	Portion Size	Vitamin K in μg
Cowpeas (blackeyes), immature seeds, boiled	1 cup	44
Cress, garden, boiled	1 cup	518
Cress, garden, raw	1 cup	271
Cucumber, with peel, raw	1 large	49
Cucumber, peeled, raw	1 large	20
Dandelion greens, chopped boiled	1 cup	597
Dandelion greens, chopped, raw	1 cup	428
Edamame, frozen, prepared	1 cup	41
Endive, raw	1 cup	116
Escarole, boiled	1 cup	318
Fennel, sliced, raw	1 cup	55
Fish, tuna, light, canned in oil, drained	1 cup	64
Fish, tuna, light, canned in water, drained	1 cup	1
Grapes, red or green, raw	1 cup	22
Kale, frozen, chopped, boiled	1 cup	1147
Kale, chopped, boiled	1 cup	1062
Kale, chopped 1″ pieces, raw	1 cup	113
Kiwifruit, green, sliced, raw	1 cup	73
Kiwifruit, green, raw	1 medium	28
Leeks (bulb and lower leaf portion), boiled	1 cup	26
Lettuce, butterhead, chopped, raw	1 cup	56
Lettuce, cos or romaine, shredded, raw	1 cup	48
Lettuce, green leaf, shredded, raw	1 cup	46
Lettuce, red leaf, shredded, raw	1 cup	39
Lettuce, iceberg, shredded, raw	1 cup	17
Miso	1 cup	81
Mung beans, mature seeds, sprouted, raw	1 cup	34
Mung beans, mature seeds, sprouted, boiled	1 cup	28
Mustard greens, chopped, boiled	1 cup	830
Mustard greens, frozen, chopped, boiled	1 cup	503
Mustard greens, chopped, raw	1 cup	144
Noodles, egg, spinach, cooked, enriched	1 cup	162
Nuts, pine nuts, dried	1 ounce	15
Okra, frozen, sliced, boiled	1 cup	88
Okra, sliced, boiled	1 cup	64
Onions, spring or scallions (tops and bulb), chopped, raw	1 cup	207
Parsley, dried	1 tbsp	22
Parsley sprigs, fresh	10	164

TABLE 2.2
Vitamin K–Containing Foods—cont'd

Food	Portion Size	Vitamin K in µg
Peas, green (baby and LeSueur), canned	1 cup	64
Peas, podded, frozen, boiled	1 cup	48
Peas, green, boiled	1 cup	41
Peas, podded, boiled	1 cup	40
Peas, green, raw	1 cup	36
Peas and carrots, frozen, boiled	10 ounces	52
Pickles, sweet or bread and butter, chopped	1 cup	75
Pickles, sour	1 cup	73
Prunes (dried plums), pitted	1 cup	104
Prunes (dried plums), pitted, stewed	1 cup	65
Prunes (dried plums) raw	5	28
Pumpkin, canned	1 cup	39
Radicchio, shredded, raw	1 cup	102
Raspberries, frozen, red, sweetened	1 cup	16
Rhubarb, frozen, cooked, with sugar	1 cup	51
Sauerkraut, canned, solids and liquid	1 cup	31
Soybeans, mature, sprouted, steamed	1 cup	66
Spinach, frozen chopped or leaf, boiled	1 cup	1027
Spinach, canned	1 cup	988
Spinach, boiled	1 cup	889
Spinach, raw	1 cup	145
Turnip greens, frozen, boiled	1 cup	851
Turnip greens and turnips, frozen, boiled	1 cup	677
Turnip greens, chopped, boiled	1 cup	529
Turnip greens, canned	1 cup	413
Turnip greens, chopped, raw	1 cup	138
Vegetables, mixed, frozen, boiled	1 cup	43
Vegetables, mixed, canned	1 cup	30
Watercress, chopped, raw	1 cup	85

Adapted from *Foods with Vitamin K – Coumadin*. http://www.coumadin.bmscustomerconnect.com/servlet/servlet.FileDownload?file=00Pi000000bxvTFEAY.

such as cimetidine and omeprazole that inhibit clearance of the R-isomer (CYP1A2 and CYP3A4 > 2C19) produce only a moderate increase in the PT and INR, with dose adjustment rarely needed.[42] Amiodarone inhibits the metabolic clearance of both the S-isomer and R-isomer and potentiates the anticoagulant effect of warfarin.[47] Agents known to induce the metabolism of warfarin include drugs such as barbiturates, rifampicin, and carbamazepine.[48] These drugs increase the metabolic clearance by inducing hepatic mixed oxidase activity and reducing the anticoagulant effect of warfarin in increasing risk of thrombosis without dose adjustment. Although long-term alcohol use has the potential to increase the clearance of warfarin through

TABLE 2.3
Warfarin Drug-Drug Interactions[36–40]

		INTERACTIONS THAT INCREASE PT/INR			
Major Interaction Avoid combination	**Moderate Interaction** Consider alternatives/adjust warfarin dose	**MINOR INTERACTION**			
		Monitor therapy			
Mifepristone When used as an abortifacient Tamoxifen Fibrinolytic agents Alteplase Streptokinase Retaplase Tenecteplase Vorapaxar	Allopurinol Amiodarone Androgens Danazol Oxandrolone Oxymetholone Testosterone Antifungals Fluconazole Miconazole (topical, vaginal) Cimetidine Fenofibrate derivatives Fenofibrate Gemfibrozil 5-Fluorouracil Herbals Fenugreek *Ginkgo biloba* Metronidazole Mifepristone NSAIDs Diclofenac Fenoprofen Ibuprofen Indomethacin Ketoprofen Ketorolac Meloxicam Naproxen Piroxicam Sulindac Phenytoin/fosphenytoin Salicylates Aminosalicylic acid Aspirin Sulfinpyrazone Sulfonamide derivatives Sulfamethoxazole +/– Trimethoprim Sulfisoxazole Tolbutamide Tyrosine kinase Inhibitors Imatinib Sorafenib	Acetaminophen >1.3–2 g/day for multiple consecutive days Anticoagulants Apixaban Bivalirudin Dabigatran Enoxaparin Fondaparinux Heparin Rivaroxaban Antiarrhythmics Dronedarone Propafenone Antifungals Econazole Itraconazole Ketoconazole Miconazole (oral) Posaconazole Voriconazole Antimalarials Proguanil Quinidine Quinine Antineoplastics Capecitabine Etoposide Gemcitabine Ibritumomab Ifosfamide Obinutuzumab Romidepsin Toremifene Ventoclax Vorinostat Bicalutamide Celecoxib Cephalosporin antibiotics Cefazolin Cefotetan Cefoxitin Ceftriaxone Cefepime Cefdinir Cefotaxime Ceftaroline Cephalexin	Chloral hydrate Chondroitin/glucosamine Cobicistat Corticosteroids Hydrocortisone Methylprednisolone Prednisone Disulfiram GLP-1 antagonists Exenatide Lixisenatide Glucagon Green tea HMG-COA inhibitors[a] Fluvastatin Lovastatin Pravastatin Rosuvastatin Simvastatin Ivermectin Levocarnitine Lomitapide Loop diuretics Ethacrynic acid Torsemide Macrolide antibiotics Azithromycin Clarithromycin Erythromycin Miscellaneous antibiotics Chloramphenicol Trimethoprim Mirtazapine Neomycin Omega-3 fatty acids Oritavancin Orlistat Penicillin antibiotics Amoxicillin Ampicillin Oxacillin Penicillin G/V Piperacillin	Pentoxifylline Protease inhibitors Fosamprenavir Saquinavir Tipranavir Proton pump inhibitors[b] Esomeprazole Lansoprazole Omeprazole P2Y12 inhibitors Clopidogrel Prasugrel Ticagrelor Quinolone antibiotics Ciprofloxacin Gemifloxacin Levofloxacin Moxifloxacin Ofloxacin Ranitidine SNRI Desvenlafaxine Duloxetine Levomilnacipran Milnacipran Venlafaxine SSRI Citalopram Escitalopram Fluoxetine Fluvoxamine Paroxetine Sertraline Stimulants, central nervous system Methylphenidate Dexmethylphenidate Sugammadex Sulfonylureas Chlorpropamide Glimepiride Glipizide Glyburide Tetracycline antibiotics Doxycycline Minocycline Tetracycline Tigecycline	Thyroid products Liothyronine Levothyroxine Tolterodine Tramadol Tricyclic antidepressants Tyrosine kinase inhibitors Ceritinib Dasatinib Erlotinib Gefitinib Ibrutinib Nintedanib Vemurafenib Vitamin E Zafirlukast Zileuton

TABLE 2.3
Warfarin Drug-Drug Interactions[36–40]—cont'd

INTERACTIONS THAT DECREASE PT/INR		
Major Interaction	**Moderate Interaction**	**Minor Interaction**
Avoid combination	Consider alternatives/adjust warfarin dose	Monitor therapy
	Antiandrogens	Adalimumab
	Enzalutamide	Aprepitant/fosaprepitant
	Antithyroid agents	Azathioprine
	Methimazole	Bile acid sequestrants
	Propylthiouracil	Colesevelam
	Barbiturates	Cholestyramine
	Amobarbital	Bosentan
	Butabarbital	Coenzyme Q10
	Butalbital	Dabrafenib
	Pentobarbital	Dicloxacillin
	Phenobarbital	Eslicarbazepine
	Secobarbital	Ginseng
	Carbamazepine	Griseofulvin
	Estrogens	Protease inhibitors
	Glutethimide	Darunavir
	Nafcillin	Lopinavir
	Primidone	Ritonavir
	Progesterones	Teriflunomide
	Rifampin	Trazodone
	Sucralfate	6-Mercaptopurine
	St. John's wort	

Interactions That May Increase or Decrease PT/INR

Minor Interaction

Boceprevir
Efavirenz
Leflunomide
Lumacaftor
Metreleptin
Nelfinavir
Telaprevir
Tranilast

[a]Atorvastatin does not appear to alter pharmacodynamic effects of warfarin.
[b]Pantoprazole did not interfere with warfarin pharmacokinetics and anticoagulant effects in a single 26-patient study of 8 days of therapy. Likely due to less inhibitor of CYP219 compared with other PPIs.
INR, international normalized ratio; *PT*, prothrombin time.

a similar mechanism, liver damage can also reduce the metabolism potential of CYP450 enzymes.[48]

Drug interactions also occur through affecting the pharmacodynamics of warfarin. Second- and third-generation cephalosporins inhibit the cyclic interconversion of vitamin K, which can increase the anticoagulant effect of warfarin.[49,50] Thyroxine increases the metabolism of coagulation factors, and salicylate doses greater than 1.5 g daily can increase the anticoagulant effect of warfarin.[33,51] A number of broad-spectrum antibiotics can potentiate the anticoagulant effect of warfarin in critically ill patients who may be deficient in vitamin K by eliminating bacterial flora that assist with vitamin K intake.[52] Drugs such as aspirin, $P2Y_{12}$ inhibitors, and cilostazol provide a pharmacodynamic interaction with warfarin by inhibiting platelets and the coagulation cascade. Other agents such as fibrinolytics induce a significant risk of bleeding and intracranial hemorrhage that is magnified with the concomitant use of warfarin.

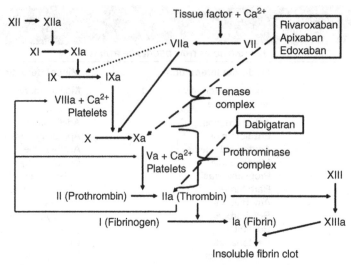

FIG. 2.3 Clotting cascade with targets for direct thrombin inhibitors and direct Xa inhibitors.

DIRECT THROMBIN INHIBITORS
Dabigatran
Pharmacology

Thrombin is an attractive target for anticoagulant drug development. Thrombin is responsible for conversion of fibrin to fibrinogen, activation of factor VIII to be used in the tenase complex, activation of factor V to be used in the prothrombinase complex, and activation of factor XIII for clot stabilization, as well as being a significant agonist for inducting platelet activation (Fig. 2.3).[53] Indirect inhibitors of thrombin, such as unfractionated heparin (UFH) and low molecular weight heparin (LMWH), must first bind to the cofactor antithrombin before binding to and inhibiting the activity of thrombin.[54] Although these indirect inhibitors are able to bind to free soluble thrombin, the size of this anticoagulant-antithrombin complex prohibits for binding to thrombin bound to fibrin or other surfaces, which is still enzymatically active.[54] The direct thrombin inhibitors (DTIs) do not require binding to antithrombin and are able to bind to thrombin directly. Therefore, DTIs are able to inhibit both free and fibrin-bound thrombin and hence inhibit a larger pool of thrombin compared with indirect inhibitors.[55-57] Because DTIs bind directly to the active site of thrombin and minimally to plasma proteins, they produce a predictable anticoagulant response.[57,58] Similar to other DTIs, dabigatran prolongs the thrombin clotting time, PT, activated partial thromboplastin time (aPTT), and ecarin clotting time (ECT).[59] The ECT is the preferred method for measurement of the anticoagulant effects of dabigatran and other DTIs.[59]

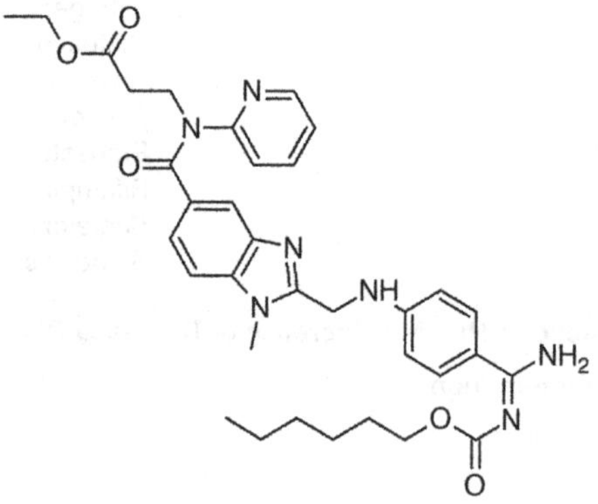

Dabigatran

FIG. 2.4 Chemical structure of dabigatran.

A number of intravenous DTIs, such as argatroban, bivalirudin, and desirudin, have been developed. Approximately 15 years ago, the oral DTI ximelagatran was developed and proven effective at reducing the risk of stroke in patients with atrial fibrillation and in other thrombotic settings.[60,61] Unfortunately, ximelagatran was found to have significant liver toxicity and was not approved for clinical use.[62] Currently, dabigatran, given as dabigatran etexilate, is the only available oral DTI. Dabigatran is a small synthetic molecule that specifically and reversibly inhibits free and fibrin-bound thrombin (Fig. 2.4).[55-57] Dabigatran has minimal binding to other serine proteases such as factor Xa, plasmin, or tissue plasminogen activator.[55] Inhibition of thrombin is achieved by preventing access to the active site of thrombin through formation of a salt bridge between

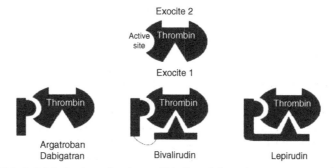

FIG. 2.5 Mechanism of action and binding of direct thrombin inhibitors.[64]

the amidine group of dabigatran and Asp 189 in the active site and through hydrophobic interactions.[55] Dabigatran, similar to melagatran and argatroban, is a univalent inhibitor of thrombin that binds to only the active site of thrombin, whereas other DTIs such as hirudin and desirudin also bind to the substrate (usually fibrinogen) recognition site, also referred to as exosite 1 (Fig. 2.5).[63,64]

Pharmacokinetics

Dabigatran is a highly polar hydrophilic molecule that is not absorbed after oral administration (Fig. 2.4).[65] Therefore, the prodrug dabigatran etexilate was developed to be more lipophilic and less basic to allow for oral absorption in the GI tract.[65–67] This is similar to its precursor melagatran, which had to be administered as ximelagatran for GI absorption. To attain maximal absorption, dabigatran etexilate requires an acidic environment.[58,65,67] To achieve and maintain this acidic environment independent of gastric pH, dabigatran etexilate is formulated as a capsule containing hundreds of 1 mm pellets. Each pellet is composed of a drug-coated tartaric acid core that creates an acidic microenvironment, regardless of variations in individual gastric pH. Although this tartaric acid core is able to achieve a bioavailability of 6%–7%, it is thought it may be the source of the almost 12% incidence of dyspepsia and higher rate of drug discontinuation demonstrated in the phase 3 atrial fibrillation study.[58,65,68,69] Dabigatran dose escalation studies demonstrate that low oral bioavailability is not caused by a saturable first-pass process because plasma concentrations increase in a dose-proportional manner.[68,70] Patients and healthcare professionals should be aware that the capsules should not be altered by chewing, breaking, or opening. Removal of the drug pellets to promote easier swallowing or administration through a feeding tube must be avoided, as this results in a 75% increase in

bioavailability compared with the intact capsule and will increase risk of significant bleeding.[71] It should also be noted that dabigatran etexilate is a hygroscopic molecule that can become unstable in humidity. Therefore, dabigatran etexilate capsules cannot be placed into patient pill boxes and must be stored in their original package, protected from moisture, and used within 4 months of opening.[71]

Once absorbed, dabigatran etexilate is rapidly and completely converted to its active compound, dabigatran. This conversion occurs by ester cleavage by esterase-catalyzed hydrolysis in the enterocytes, portal vein, and liver, leaving minimal prodrug or intermediates detectable in plasma.[65] Peak dabigatran plasma concentrations (C_{max}) are reached within 2 h of administration. After dabigatran reaches its C_{max}, plasma concentrations decline in a biphasic manner, characterized by a rapid distribution phase, resulting in a decrease by >70% during the initial 4–6 h distribution phase, followed by a significantly slower elimination phase.[65] Taking dabigatran with a high-fat, high-calorie meal prolonged the time to reach C_{max} (T_{max}) from 2 to 4 h, although the C_{max} and total drug exposure (area under the curve, [AUC]) remained unchanged. With repeat dosing, the terminal half-life is 12–17 h, the peak and trough concentrations are dose-proportional, and it takes 2–3 days to reach steady-state levels.[65,68] Approximately 35% of circulating dabigatran is protein bound, regardless of concentration.[58] The volume of distribution of dabigatran is approximately 50–70 L, which exceeds the volume of total body water, representing moderate tissue distribution.[65,66]

Dabigatran is not a substrate, inhibitor, or inducer of CYP450 enzymes or known drug transporters, which avoids numerous drug interactions. Moderately severe liver dysfunction (Child-Pugh classification B) appears to have little effect on the pharmacokinetics of dabigatran, with C_{max} being reduced by 15% after a 150 mg dose dabigatran etexilate in 12 affected subjects, when compared with 12 healthy age- and sex-matched control subjects.[72] Other parameters such as T_{max}, the elimination half-life, AUC, volume of distribution, and extent of glucuronidation remained unchanged. No dose adjustments for hepatic dysfunction are determined to be necessary, making it a possible option in these patients. It should be noted that patients with severe hepatic impairment have been excluded from all clinical trials.

Renal excretion is responsible for 80% of the total clearance of dabigatran.[65,66] The remainder of the drug is conjugated with glucuronic acid to form acyl glucuronides, which are predominately excreted via the bile.[65,66] In patients with normal renal function, the average dabigatran C_{max} after a 150 mg dose was 85 ng/mL.[73] The dabigatran C_{max} increased to 109 ng/mL in patients with mild renal impairment, 138 ng/mL in patients with moderate renal impairment, and 205 ng/mL in patients with severe renal impairment. The corresponding increase in AUC was 1.5-, 3.2-, and 6.3-fold higher in subjects with mild, moderate, or severe renal impairment compared with healthy control subjects. The terminal half-life was doubled to 28 h in severe renal impairment, from 14 h in control subjects.[73] The pharmacokinetic properties of dabigatran are summarized in Table 2.4. Dosing recommendations for the use of dabigatran for reducing the risk of stroke in patients with atrial fibrillation are given in Table 2.5.

Drug interactions
Because of the requirement for dabigatran etexilate to have an acidic environment for absorption, drugs that increase gastric pH can lead to reductions in dabigatran exposure. In a crossover study of subjects receiving pantoprazole 40 mg twice daily for 48 h, the gastric pH was increased from 2.2 to 5.9.[74] The C_{max} of dabigatran was reduced by 30% and the AUC was reduced by 20%. These alterations produced small changes in the anticoagulant impact of dabigatran as measured by the ECT and aPTT.[74] In a study with ranitidine, the dabigatran AUC was reduced by 11%–35%. Consequently, the clinical impact of these interactions is likely minimal.[74] Administration of dabigatran 2 h before doses of proton pump inhibitors, H_2 antagonists, or antacids would be recommended if feasible.

Although dabigatran is not influenced by the CYP450 enzyme system, dabigatran etexilate is a substrate with moderate affinity for P-glycoprotein (P-gp) transport system (Fig. 2.6).[75,76] It is important to note that the affinity for P-gp is limited to dabigatran etexilate and not active dabigatran. Therefore, any potential interaction is restricted to affecting drug absorption, and other locations of P-gp such as the liver, kidney, and brain are not affected, with no impact on dabigatran distribution or elimination.[75] Concomitant administration with strong P-gp inducer, rifampin, resulted in both a significant (67%) decrease in dabigatran's AUC and a 66% decrease in C_{max}.[77,78] Therefore, combinations with rifampin or other strong P-gp inducers such as St. John's wort should be avoided, as dabigatran will have reduced effects.

Coadministration of dabigatran with inhibitors of P-gp (ketoconazole, amiodarone, dronedarone, verapamil, quinidine) results in considerable increases

TABLE 2.4
Pharmacologic Properties of the Direct Oral Anticoagulants

	Dabigatran	Rivaroxaban	Apixaban	Edoxaban
Mechanism of action	Direct IIa inhibitor	Direct Xa inhibitor	Direct Xa inhibitor	Direct Xa inhibitor
Bioavailability	3%–7%	66% without food, 80%–100% with food	50%	62%
Onset of anticoagulant activity	1.5 h	2–4 h	2–3 h	1–2 h
Half-life	12–17 h	9–13 h	12 h	9–10 h
Renal clearance	80%	36%	27%	50%
Protein binding	35%	90%	87%	55%
Removed by dialysis	Yes	No	No	No
P-glycoprotein transport	Yes	Yes	Yes	Yes
Hepatic metabolism	None	CYP3A4/5 and CYP2J2	CYP3A4/5	Minimal (4% CYP3A4/5)

in dabigatran C_{max} and AUC.[77,78] Multiple doses of oral ketoconazole produces an increase in dabigatran AUC of 153% and C_{max} of 149%. This combination should be avoided and is contraindicated in Canada and Europe. Coadministration with other P-gp inhibitors, such as amiodarone (increased AUC by 50% and C_{max} by 60%) and clarithromycin (increased AUC by 19% and C_{max} by 15%), results in modest increases in dabigatran and no dose adjustments are necessary. Immediate-release verapamil given 1 h before 150 mg of dabigatran etexilate increases the AUC by 150% and C_{max} by 180%. These increases in AUC and C_{max} are 70% and 90%, respectively, with the extended-release formulation. If verapamil is taken at least 2 h after dabigatran etexilate, the increase in AUC is only 10% and C_{max} is 20%.[77,78] Therefore, no dose adjustments are recommended if used concomitantly with dabigatran; however, it is recommended to administer the dabigatran at least 2 h before these medications.

DIRECT FACTOR XA INHIBITORS
General Pharmacology
Factor Xa sits at the junction between the intrinsic and extrinsic portions of the clotting cascade (Fig. 2.3). During the initiation phase of coagulation, tissue factor–mediated factor VIIa is able to create small amounts of factor Xa, which then converts initial amounts of prothrombin (factor II) to thrombin (factor IIa). This initial creation of thrombin is able to promote its own production through activation of factors V and VIII.

TABLE 2.5
Dosing of Direct Thrombin Inhibitors and Direct Xa Inhibitors in Patients With Atrial Fibrillation

Agent	Standard Dosing	Dose Adjustment[a]	Avoid Use[a]
Dabigatran	150 mg twice daily	75 mg twice daily • CrCl 30–15 mL/min • CrCl 30–50 mL/min with ketoconazole or dronedarone	• CrCl < 15 mL/min • Dialysis • CrCl 30–15 mL/min with amiodarone, verapamil, ketoconazole, dronedarone, diltiazem, and clarithromycin • Rifampin
Rivaroxaban	20 mg once daily with meals	15 mg once daily with meals • CrCl 50–15 mL/min • Dialysis	• Strong CYP3A4 and P-gp inducers (e.g., rifampin, phenytoin, carbamazepine, St. John's wort) • Strong CYP3A4 and P-gp inhibitors (e.g., protease inhibitors, itraconazole, ketoconazole, conivaptan)
Apixaban	5 mg twice daily	2.5 mg twice daily • Two of three criteria: (age ≥ 80 years, weight ≤ 60 mg, or SCr ≥ 1.5 mg/dL) • Use with strong CYP3A4 and P-gp inhibitors (e.g., protease inhibitors, itraconazole, ketoconazole, conivaptan) • Dialysis[b]	• Strong CYP3A4 and P-gp inducers (e.g., rifampin, phenytoin, carbamazepine, St. John's wort) • If on 2.5 mg twice daily, strong CYP3A4 and P-gp inhibitors (e.g., protease inhibitors, itraconazole, ketoconazole, conivaptan)
Edoxaban	60 mg once daily	30 mg once daily • CrCl 15–50 mL/min • Potent P-gp inhibitor (verapamil, dronedarone, or quinidine) • Weight ≤ 60 kg	• CrCl > 95 mL/min • CrCl < 15 mL/min • Dialysis • Rifampin

[a]CrCl in the DOAC trials was calculated using Cockcroft-Gault equation with total body weight.
[b]The apixaban packet label suggests a dose of 5 mg twice daily in patients receiving dialysis who are < 80 years old and weigh > 60 kg. A recent study with multiple days of apixaban administration in patients receiving dialysis demonstrated an approximate twofold increase in C_{max} and area under the curve using 5 mg twice daily and suggested that 2.5 mg twice-daily dose may be more appropriate.
CrCl, creatinine clearance.

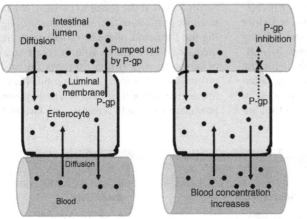
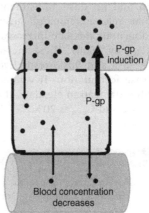

Drug diffuses from intenstinal lumen through luminal membrane into enterocyte. P-gp pumps drug out of cell back into intestinal lumen.

P-gp inhibition

P-gp activity reduced; less drug pumped back into intestine, greater systemic exposure.

P-gp induction

P-gp activity increased; more drug pumped back into intestine, less systemic exposure.

FIG. 2.6 Effect of P-glycoprotein on drug absorption.[76]

The propagation phase of coagulation is promoted by the incorporation of calcium-mediated binding of factor Xa to the platelet surface with factor Va, creating the prothrombinase complex. In this complex, large amounts of prothrombin can be converted to thrombin to promote coagulation. Therefore, factor Xa has become a popular target for inhibition because of its upstream impact on thrombin production.[79,80] Data suggest that inhibition of one molecule of factor Xa can inhibit the later production of hundreds of molecules of thrombin.[81,82] Injectable factor Xa inhibitors, such as UFH, LMWH, and fondaparinux, first must bind to antithrombin to provide their anticoagulant activity. Although these indirect factor Xa inhibitors are able to bind to and inhibit soluble or circulating factor Xa, the size of these complexes prevent them from affecting factor Xa incorporated into the prothrombinase complex or clot-bound factor Xa.[58,83] The oral direct factor Xa inhibitors are able to inhibit factor Xa directly without interacting with antithrombin. Consequentially, the oral direct factor Xa inhibitors are able to bind to and inhibit not only soluble factor Xa, but also clot-bound factor Xa and factor Xa incorporated into the prothrombinase complex, where the majority of thrombin is produced.

Rivaroxaban
Pharmacology

Rivaroxaban is a potent, selective, oxazolidinone-based reversible factor Xa inhibitor with a molecular weight of 436 Da (Fig. 2.7).[58] The inhibition constant (Ki) for FXa in human plasma is 0.4 ± 0.02 nM.[84] Rivaroxaban has 10,000-fold greater selectivity for factor Xa compared with other related serine proteases including thrombin, trypsin, plasmin, factor VIIa, factor IXa, factor XIa, urokinase, and activated protein C.[85] At the molecular level, the action of rivaroxaban is governed by chlorothiophene and morpholinone moieties attached to a central oxazolidinone ring, which bind with high affinity to the S1 and S4 pockets of factor Xa.[86,87] These moieties act through electrostatic interaction with Asp 189 in the S1 pocket of factor Xa. This interaction involves the chlorine substituent of the chlorothiophene moiety, which interacts with the aromatic ring of Tyr228 at the bottom of the S1 pocket.[86,87] This allows rivaroxaban to provide inhibition of free, clot-bound, and prothrombinase-bound factor Xa.[84,88] Inhibition of factor Xa activity by rivaroxaban is increased in a dose-dependent manner. Rivaroxaban induces prolongation of the PT, aPTT, and heparin clotting time and reduces the endogenous thrombin potential, a measure

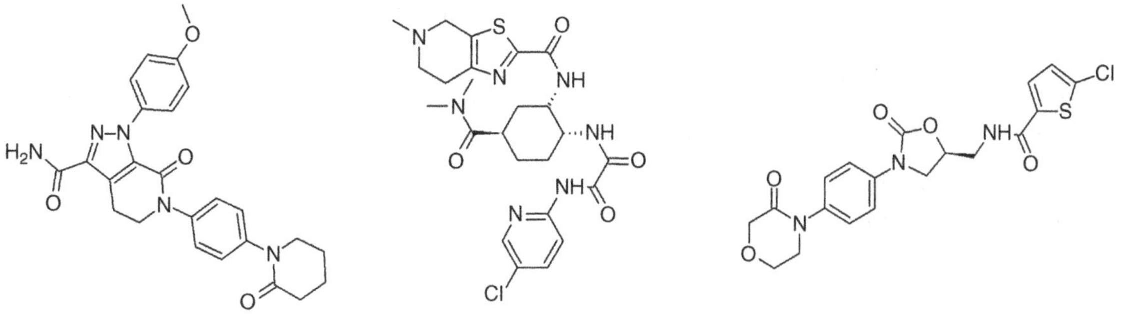

FIG. 2.7 Chemical structure of direct Xa inhibitors.

of thrombin production.[88,89] No direct effects of rivaroxaban on platelets have been demonstrated.[88,90] However, although rivaroxaban does not affect platelet aggregation in platelet-rich plasma, it potently inhibits tissue factor–induced platelet aggregation indirectly, by inhibiting thrombin generation.[91]

Pharmacokinetics

Rivaroxaban is rapidly absorbed, reaching C_{max} in 2–4 h.[58] The drug is provided as a film-coated tablet with a dose-dependent bioavailability. For the 10 mg dose, the bioavailability is estimated to be 80%–100% compared with 66% with the 20 mg dose when given in a fasting state.[92,93] In studies evaluating the impact of administering rivaroxaban in a fasted or fed state, subjects received either two 5 mg tablets (fasted and fed) and four 5 mg tablets (fasted), or one 20 mg tablet (fasted and fed).[93] Results of this study found that there is no influence of a meal on the bioavailability of the 10 mg dose. The presence of food increased the T_{max} for rivaroxaban from 2.75 to 4 h, with increases in the C_{max} of 41% and AUC of 28%, providing a bioavailability of 90%–100%.[92,93] The presence of food was also associated with a reduction in interpatient variability, thus increasing the predictability of rivaroxaban plasma concentrations. These increases in C_{max} and AUC with food are likely because food prolongs residence time in the stomach secondary to reduced gastric motility after a meal and possibly increases the solubility and dissolution.[67] In addition, there was no influence with respect to types of food (a high-fat or high-carbohydrate meal) on the pharmacokinetics of rivaroxaban.[92,93] The AUC and C_{max} are similar when administering whole or crushed rivaroxaban 20 mg tablets with food. Crushed tablets suspended in water, administered via a nasogastric tube, and followed by a liquid meal provide a similar AUC value but an 18% reduction in C_{max}.[94] If administering crushed rivaroxaban, it is important to provide drug release in the stomach for optimal absorption.[95] Rivaroxaban exposure is reduced when the drug is released in the distal small intestine or ascending colon. Medications that alter gastric pH do not modify the pharmacokinetics of rivaroxaban.

Rivaroxaban is highly protein bound (92%–95%), with serum albumin the predominant binding protein, and has a volume of distribution at steady state of approximately 50 L.[58,86] Rivaroxaban has a terminal elimination half-life, of 5–9 h in healthy young subjects and 11–13 in elderly subjects.[96,97] Of the 36% of unchanged rivaroxaban dose eliminated in urine, 30% is eliminated by active renal secretion and 6% by glomerular filtration.[86,98] The majority of rivaroxaban undergoes hepatic metabolism by CYP3A4 and CYP2J2.[99] These two enzymes contribute to a similar extent oxidative degradation of the morpholinone moiety. There is also CYP-independent metabolism, which involves hydrolysis of the amide bonds of rivaroxaban.[94,99] The resulting inactive metabolites are eliminated both renally and via the hepatobiliary route. The pharmacokinetic properties of rivaroxaban are summarized in Table 2.4.

Dosing

Despite a half-life of approximately 12 h, rivaroxaban is dosed once daily for reducing the risk of stroke in patients with atrial fibrillation and for other indications. A number of factors, such as the larger volume of distribution and binding affinity, contribute to once-daily dosing.[58,96,97,100] Also, the rivaroxaban AUC increases dose dependently with both once-daily and twice-daily dosing.[96,97] When comparing the same total daily dose, the C_{max} was higher (~20%) and the C_{trough} was lower (~60%) with once-daily dosing compared with twice-daily dosing, with significant overlap in the confidence intervals between the two.[101] With data demonstrating lower troughs being associated with less bleeding, once-daily dosing would be preferred.[101] In addition, single-dose studies have demonstrated that the inhibitory effects of rivaroxaban at a dose of greater than 5 mg do not return to baseline until after 24 h, which further facilitates its once-daily dosing.[96] Data from a single-dose study in patients on hemodialysis demonstrated a similar C_{max} and AUC for a dose of 15 mg daily compared with subjects with CrCl (creatinine clearance) between 15 and 50 mL/min.[102] This dosing appears in the package label for rivaroxaban.

The pharmacokinetic profile of rivaroxaban in healthy subjects is not substantially affected by age or sex, and therefore no dose adjustments would be necessary.[103] Extremes in weight also do not require dose adjustment.[104] When given with a meal, the C_{max} and T_{max} of rivaroxaban are not altered in subjects weighing ≥ 120 kg, whereas there is a nonsignificant 24% increase in C_{max} when given to those weighing ≤ 50 kg, compared with subjects weighing 70–80 kg.[104] There also appears to be no need for dose adjustment based on patient ethnicity.

Data from a phase I studies demonstrated an increase in rivaroxaban exposure correlated to decreased renal function, as assessed by the Cockcroft-Gault formula using total body weight.[105] In subjects with mild, moderate, or severe renal impairment, the AUC for rivaroxaban was increased by 1.4-, 1.5-, and 1.6-fold, compared with subjects with normal renal function.[104] Simulations in a virtual patient population with atrial fibrillation demonstrate that a rivaroxaban dose of 15 mg once daily in patients with a CrCl of 30–49 mL/min would achieve ACU and C_{max} values similar to those observed with rivaroxaban 20 mg once daily in patients with normal renal function.[101] The pharmacokinetic profile of rivaroxaban is not affected in patients with mild hepatic impairment (Child-Pugh classification A), with a mean 1.2-fold increase in AUC compared with healthy subjects.[106] In patients with moderate hepatic impairment (Child-Pugh classification B), there is an increase in the AUC by 2.3-fold, increase in C_{max} by 1.3-fold, and in increase in the half-life by approximately 2 h, compared with healthy subjects.[106] Dosing of rivaroxaban in patients with atrial fibrillation is described in Table 2.5.

Drug interactions

Rivaroxaban is neither an inducer nor an inhibitor of any CYP450 enzyme.[98] As a substrate for both CYP3A4 and P-gp, concomitant use of rivaroxaban with strong CYP3A4 and P-gp inhibitors would be expected to increase plasma rivaroxaban concentrations.[99,107,108] Administration of rivaroxaban with ketoconazole or ritonavir led to a 2.6- and 2.5-fold increase in mean rivaroxaban AUC and 1.7- and 1.6-fold increase in mean rivaroxaban C_{max}, respectively, with significant increases in pharmacodynamic effects that could result in increased bleeding risk.[107] Consequentially, the use of rivaroxaban with strong inhibitors of both CYP3A4 and P-gp should be avoided.[58] Drugs that strongly inhibit one of either CYP3A4 or P-gp would be expected to have a less of an impact on rivaroxaban pharmacokinetics and pharmacodynamics. Concomitant use of the strong CYP3A4 inhibitor and moderate P-gp inhibitors, clarithromycin and erythromycin, produced small and clinically insignificant increases in rivaroxaban AUC and C_{max}.[76,107] Administration of rivaroxaban with the strong CYP3A4 and P-gp inducer rifampicin produced an approximate 50% decrease in mean rivaroxaban AUC, with parallel decreases in its pharmacodynamic effects.[94,107] This has also been demonstrated with other strong CYP3A4 and P-gp inducers such as carbamazepine, phenobarbital, and phenytoin, with St. John's wort expected to demonstrate similar findings.[94,107] Therefore, these drugs should be avoided in patients receiving rivaroxaban or vice versa.

Apixaban
Pharmacology

Apixaban is an orally active, small-molecule (460 Da), reversible inhibitor of factor Xa.[109,110] Apixaban is a pyrazole derivative, which was based on the compound razaxaban, but with superior potency, selectivity, and oral bioavailability (Fig. 2.7).[58] As with rivaroxaban, apixaban provides its inhibition of factor Xa by binding to two sites on the protein.[109] Apixaban is highly selective for factor Xa, with no impact on activated protein C, factor IXa, factor VIIa, or thrombin and no alteration in platelet aggregation.[110,111] Apixaban inhibits FXa with a Ki of 0.08 nmol/L.[110] As with other oral direct Xa inhibitors, apixaban inhibits factor Xa incorporated in the prothrombinase complex, clot-bound factor Xa, or free/soluble factor Xa.[58] Apixaban inhibits thrombin generation in vitro, increasing the lag time to peak thrombin concentration and reducing the maximum thrombin generation rate and the peak thrombin concentration.[112,113] Apixaban exhibits linear pharmacokinetics and produces concentration-dependent increases in clotting assays, PT, and aPTT, with a direct linear relationship with anti-Xa activity and apixaban plasma concentrations.[112,113]

Pharmacokinetics

Apixaban is rapidly absorbed, reaching C_{max} approximately 1–3 h after oral administration.[114] Apixaban has an oral bioavailability of approximately 50% and is absorbed in the stomach and small intestine.[114] Subjects provided a high-fat, high-calorie meal did not demonstrate differences in apixaban C_{max}, AUC, or half-life compared with subjects in a fasting state.[58] Therefore, apixaban can be administered with or without food. Apixaban has a half-life of 9–14 h (mean 12.7 h) and achieves steady-state concentrations within 3 days.[114] After achieving C_{max}, apixaban plasma concentrations demonstrate an initial rapid decline and then a more gradual terminal phase. Apixaban has a small volume of distribution of approximately 21 L and is 87% protein bound.[112,114] The limited volume of distribution is likely due to limited extravascular tissue distribution and not the result of extensive plasma protein binding.

After oral administration, unchanged apixaban is the major component in human plasma with no active circulating metabolites. Apixaban is eliminated by multiple routes, with approximately 50% excreted by the hepatobiliary route unchanged in the feces and approximately 25% excreted renally unchanged in the urine.[114] Apixaban is metabolized via O-demethylation and hydroxylation mainly by CYP3A4/5 with minor contributions from CYP1A2 and CYP2J2.[115] Apixaban should be avoided in patients with hepatic disease associated with coagulopathy and in those with severe hepatic impairment because of the lack of data from their exclusion in clinical trials. The pharmacokinetic properties of apixaban are summarized in Table 2.4.

Dosing

Lower peak-to-trough concentration ratios are observed with twice-daily compared with once-daily dosing requirements.[58] Pharmacokinetic data have demonstrated that apixaban 5 mg twice daily produces higher median trough plasma concentrations (107 ng/mL) compared with 10 mg once daily (80.5 ng/mL) with a similar AUC.[116] In addition, there were twice as many venous thromboembolism events with 10 mg once daily compared with 5 mg twice daily.[116] These data, along with the small volume of distribution, contribute to apixaban being dosed twice daily.

Caution is recommended in patients with mild (Child-Pugh classification A) or moderate hepatic impairment (Child-Pugh classification B); however, no dose adjustments are recommended.[117] Renal impairment has no effect on the C_{max} of apixaban.[114] Conversely, the AUC increases as renal function

deteriorates.[114] Compared with patients with normal renal function, subjects with mild, moderate, and severe renal impairment demonstrate an increase in apixaban AUC of 16%, 29%, and 44%, respectively.[71] Patients with a serum creatinine of greater than 2.5 mg/dL or a CrCl of less than 25 mL/min were excluded from the phase 3 atrial fibrillation trial.[118] Based on these data, no dosage adjustment is necessary for patients with mild or moderate renal impairment. Data from a single-dose study in patients on hemodialysis demonstrated a similar C_{max} and AUC for a dose of 5 mg daily twice daily compared with subjects with CrCl between 15 and 50 mL/min as long as they were also younger than 80 years and weighed more than 60 kg.[119] This dosing appears in the package label for apixaban. More recent data with repeated does of apixaban in patients on hemodialysis had demonstrated an approximate 2-fold increase in AUC and 1.8-fold increase in C_{max}.[120] These data suggest that the 5 mg twice-daily dose of apixaban in these patients should be avoided, and a dose of 2.5 mg twice daily may be more appropriate.

Dose adjustments are not recommended based on extreme body weight, age, or ethnicity.[71,121] Both single- and multiple-dose studies demonstrate that the pharmacokinetics and pharmacodynamics of apixaban in Japanese and Chinese subjects are similar to those in white subjects. However, study results demonstrate that increased weights of >120 kg are associated with an approximately 30% lower AUC, and weights of <50 kg are associated with an approximate 30% higher apixaban AUC.[122] There is also a 32% increase in the AUC of apixaban detected in the elderly compared with younger subjects.[123] These findings influenced the dosing recommendations for apixaban used in the phase 3 atrial fibrillation trial.[118] Dosing recommendations for the use of apixaban in patients with atrial fibrillation are described in Table 2.5.

Drug interactions

Apixaban has the potential to interact with several medications, considering it is metabolized through CYP450 and is a P-gp substrate.[115] Nevertheless, because over 70% of the administered dose of apixaban is excreted as unchanged parent drug, the overall metabolic potential for a drug-drug interaction with apixaban is reduced.[114] Apixaban is not an inducer or inhibitor of CYP450 enzymes or P-gp.[115]

Concomitant use of strong CYP3A4 inhibitors and P-gp inhibitors, such as ketoconazole, itraconazole, ritonavir, and clarithromycin, requires a 50% reduction in dose for patients using the 10 or 5 mg twice-daily dose.[124] These agents are contraindicated in patients already receiving 2.5 mg twice daily of apixaban. A study with oral ketoconazole once daily led to a 2-fold increase in the mean AUC and 1.6-fold increase in C_{max} of apixaban.[125] Medications moderately inhibiting CYP3A4 or P-gp are expected to have less of an impact on apixaban plasma concentrations. In a study with diltiazem, a moderate CYP3A4 inhibitor and weak P-gp inhibitor produced a 1.5-fold increase in mean AUC, suggesting that medications that inhibit both pathways must be evaluated for use.[125] Concomitant administration with rifampin, a potent CYP3A4 inducer and potent P-gp inducer, produced a 54% decrease in the mean AUC and a 42% decrease in C_{max} of apixaban.[126] These reductions in apixaban exposure may translate into decreased efficacy, and this combination should be avoided. The concomitant use of apixaban with other potent CYP3A4 and P-gp inducers, such as St. John's wort or the aromatic antiseizure medications phenytoin, carbamazepine, and phenobarbital, may produce significant decreases in apixaban exposure.[115]

Edoxaban
Pharmacology
Similar to rivaroxaban and apixaban, edoxaban is an orally active, small-molecule (548 Da), reversible factor Xa inhibitor (Fig. 2.7).[127,128] As with the other direct oral factor Xa inhibitors, edoxaban exhibits a 10,000-fold greater selectivity for factor Xa compared with other serine proteins such as factor VIIa, t-PA, plasmin, or trypsin.[128] Administered as edoxaban tosylate, the compound competitively inhibits free factor Xa directly without the need for antithrombin and factor Xa incorporated in the prothrombinase complex. The concentration-dependent inhibition of factor Xa leads to reduced thrombin generation and thrombin-induced platelet aggregation. Edoxaban inhibited factor Xa with Ki values of 0.561 nM for free factor Xa and 2.98 nM for prothrombinase.[128] Edoxaban exhibits linear pharmacokinetics and produces concentration-dependent increases in the PT, INR, and aPTT.[129,130] However, changes in these laboratory assays with edoxaban tend to be unpredictable and highly variable, reducing their use as a monitoring tool in clinical practice.[130]

Pharmacokinetics
Edoxaban achieves a rapid C_{max} in approximately 1–2 h after administration and achieves steady-state concentrations within 3 days.[129,131] Edoxaban has an estimated oral bioavailability of 62% that is not affected by food, with absorption occurring predominantly in the proximal small intestine.[132,133] Therefore, edoxaban can be administered with or without regard of food.[133] The bioavailability of edoxaban is consistent at doses from 10 to 30 mg but decreases by 6.7% for every 30 mg increase in dose, which is likely due to a decreased dissolution rate.[134] Edoxaban has a half-life of 10–14 h and a larger volume of distribution than any other DOAC at approximately 107 L, which aids in once-daily dosing.[129] Edoxaban is approximately 55% protein bound, and free drug remains mostly as the parent compound in the plasma.[129]

More than 70% of edoxaban is eliminated as unchanged drug.[131] The major metabolite, referred to as M-4, is created through hydrolysis by carboxylesterase-1 in human liver microsomes and in the cytosol.[127,131] Although the M-4 metabolite does have anticoagulant activity, it does not contribute to the pharmacologic activity of edoxaban because it is present at less than 10% of total edoxaban exposure and is more highly protein bound (80%).[131,135] Hepatic metabolism by the CYP450 system, mainly CYP3A4, accounts for metabolism of less than 4% of the total edoxaban dose, making drug interactions with this enzyme system clinically insignificant.[131,136] In healthy subjects, approximately 60% of edoxaban is eliminated via the feces and 35% in the urine.[131] Mild to moderate hepatic impairment does not meaningfully change the C_{max} or AUC of edoxaban, which is consistent with the limited hepatic involvement in edoxaban metabolism and clearance.[137] Conversely, the pharmacokinetic profile of edoxaban is altered in patients with renal impairment. Edoxaban elimination occurs in the kidneys at a rate higher than glomerular filtration, which suggests active secretion is also involved.[131] The edoxaban AUC increased by 32%, 74%, and 72% in patients with mild, moderate, and severe renal insufficiency compared with subjects with normal renal function.[127,138] Patients receiving peritoneal dialysis experienced a 93% increase in edoxaban AUC.[139] The pharmacokinetic properties of edoxaban are summarized in Table 2.4.

Dosing
Despite having a half-life of 10–14 h, edoxaban is dosed once daily for reducing the risk of stroke in patients with atrial fibrillation and for other indications. The large volume of distribution and binding affinity contribute to once-daily dosing.[100,129] Edoxaban has demonstrated the ability to have sustained anticoagulant effect for 24 h when measuring anti-Xa activity, and prothrombin fragments 1 + 2, as well as an increased thrombin generation lag time.[140] Once-daily dosing was also chosen based on results from modeling data from a phase 2 study.[141] In this analysis, the most

significant predictor for bleeding was the period during which intrinsic factor Xa activity was maintained at 15% or less.[142,143] During this study, there was more bleeding with the dose of 30 mg twice daily compared with those receiving 60 mg once daily. The predictive threshold for intrinsic factor Xa activity was maintained for 18.8 h with the 30 mg twice-daily dose, compared with 13.7 h for the 60 mg once-daily dose.[141-143] Efficacy was not different between the doses.

Dose adjustment is not necessary in patients with mild to moderate hepatic impairment, whereas patients with severe hepatic impairment were not included in the phase 3 trial.[137,144] Because of the accumulation, patients with a CrCl between 15 and 50 mL/min should have their dose reduced from 60 mg daily to 30 mg daily.[143] Decreasing body weight is associated with increasing edoxaban exposure. Consequentially, patients weighing 60 kg or less should receive the dose of 30 mg daily instead of 60 mg daily.[143,145] Dosing of edoxaban in patients with atrial fibrillation is described in Table 2.5.

Drug interactions

The majority of edoxaban pharmacokinetic drug interactions result from inhibition or induction of the P-gp efflux transporter, which is responsible for intestinal transport (Fig. 2.6).[76,136] Edoxaban taken with quinidine demonstrates an increase in edoxaban C_{max} of 85% and AUS of 77%.[132,146] Coadministration with dronedarone resulted in a C_{max} and AUC increase of 46% and 85%, respectively.[146] This drug interaction also increased the 24-h edoxaban concentration by 158%. Additionally, verapamil increased the edoxaban C_{max} by 53%, the AUC by 53%, and the 24-h edoxaban concentration by 29%.[146] As per the phase 3 clinical trial, patients receiving quinidine, dronedarone, or verapamil should receive the reduced dose of 30 mg daily instead of 60 mg daily.[144] It should be noted that patients receiving azole antifungal agents, such as ketoconazole, or protease inhibitors were excluded from the phase 3 trial because of concerns about increased edoxaban exposure.[144,147] Conversely, the use of rifampin, a P-gp inducer, resulted in a significant 34% reduction in the edoxaban AUC.[148] Therefore, the combination of rifampin and edoxaban should be avoided.

DISCLOSURE STATEMENT

Dr. Dobesh has served as a consultant for Boehringer Ingelheim, The Pfizer/BMS Alliance, Janssen Pharmaceuticals, Daiichi Sankyo Inc, and Portola Pharmaceuticals. Dr. Stacy has served as a consultant for Janssen Pharmaceuticals.

REFERENCES

1. Nelsestuen GL, Zytkovicz TH, Howard JB. The mode of action of vitamin K. Identification of gamma-carboxyglutamic acid as a component of prothrombin. *J Biol Chem*. 1974;249:6347–6350.
2. Whitlon DS, Sadowski JA, Suttie JW. Mechanism of coumarin action: significance of vitamin K epoxide reductase inhibition. *Biochemistry*. 1978;17:1371–1377.
3. Choonara IA, Malia RG, Haynes BP, et al. The relationship between inhibition of vitamin K1 2,3-epoxide reductase and reduction of clotting factor activity with warfarin. *Br J Clin Pharmacol*. 1988;25:1–7.
4. Stafford DW. The vitamin K cycle. *J Thromb Haemost*. 2005;3:1873–1878.
5. Friedman PA, Rosenberg RD, Hauschka PV, et al. A spectrum of partially carboxylated prothrombins in the plasmas of coumarin treated patients. *Biochem Biophys Acta*. 1977;494:271–276.
6. Nelsestuen GL. Role of g-carboxyglutamic acid: an unusual transition required for calcium-dependent binding of prothrombin to phospholipid. *J Biol Chem*. 1976;251:5648–5656.
7. Prendergast FG, Mann KG. Differentiation of metal ion induced transitions of prothrombin fragment 1. *J Biol Chem*. 1977;252:840–850.
8. Borowski M, Furie BC, Bauminger S, et al. Prothrombin requires two sequential metal-dependent conformational transitions to bind phospholipid. *J Biol Chem*. 1986;261:14969–14975.
9. Becker R. The importance of factor Xa regulatory pathways in vascular thromboresistance: focus on protein Z. *J Thromb Thrombolysis*. 2005;19:135–137.
10. Breckenridge A. Oral anticoagulant drugs: pharmacokinetic aspects. *Semin Hematol*. 1978;15:19–26.
11. Kelly JG, O'Malley K. Clinical pharmacokinetics of oral anticoagulants. *Clin Pharmacokinet*. 1979;4:1–15.
12. O'Reilly RA. Vitamin K and the oral anticoagulant drugs. *Annu Rev Med*. 1976;27:245–261.
13. Miners JO, Birkett DJ. Cytochrome P4502C9: an enzyme of major importance in human drug metabolism. *Br J Clin Pharmacol*. 1998;45:525–538.
14. Godbillon J, Richard J, Gerardin A, Meinertz T, Kasper W, Jähnchen E. Pharmacokinetics of the enantiomers of acenocoumarol in man. *Br J Clin Pharmacol*. 1981;12:621–629.
15. Haustein KO. Pharmacokinetic and pharmacodynamic properties of oral anticoagulants, especially phenprocoumon. *Semin Thromb Hemost*. 1999;25:5–11.
16. Mentré F, Pousset F, Comets E, et al. Population pharmacokinetic-pharmacodynamic analysis of fluindione in patients. *Clin Pharmacol Ther*. 1998;63:64–78.
17. Johnson JA, Gong L, Whirl-Carrillo M, et al. Clinical pharmacogenetics implementation consortium guidelines for CYP2C9 and VKORC1 genotypes and warfarin dosing. *Clin Pharmacol Ther*. 2011;90:625–629.
18. Scordo MG, Pengo V, Spina E, Dahl ML, Gusella M, Padrini R. Influence of CYP2C9 and CYP2C19 genetic

polymorphisms on warfarin maintenance dose and metabolic clearance. *Clin Pharmacol Ther.* 2002;72:702–710.

19. Lindh JD, Holm L, Andersson ML, Rane A. Influence of CYP2C9 genotype on warfarin dose requirements—a systematic review and meta-analysis. *Eur J Clin Pharmacol.* 2009;65:365–375.

20. Loebstein R, Yonath H, Peleg D, et al. Individual variability in sensitivity to warfarin: nature or nurture. *Clin Pharmacol Ther.* 2001;70:159–164.

21. Marsh S, King CR, Porche-Sorbet RM, Scott-Horton TJ, Eby CS. Population variation in VKORC1 haplotype structure. *J Thromb Haemost.* 2006;4:473–474.

22. Li T, Chang CY, Jin DY, Lin PJ, Khvorova A, Stafford DW. Identification of the gene for vitamin K epoxide reductase. *Nature.* 2004;427:541–544.

23. Rieder MJ, Reiner AP, Gage BF, et al. Effect of VKORC1 haplotypes on transcriptional regulation and warfarin dose. *N Engl J Med.* 2005;352:2285–2293.

24. Geisen C, Watzka M, Sittinger K, et al. VKORC1 haplotypes and their impact on the inter-individual and interethnic variability of oral anticoagulation. *Thromb Haemost.* 2005;94:773–779.

25. Sconce EA, Khan TI, Wynne HA, et al. The impact of CYP2C9 and VKORC1 genetic polymorphism and patient characteristics upon warfarin dose requirements: proposal for a new dosing regimen. *Blood.* 2005;106:2329–2333.

26. Harrington DJ, Underwood S, Morse C, Shearer MJ, Tuddenham EGD, Mumford AD. Pharmacodynamic resistance to warfarin associated with a Val66Met substitution in vitamin K epoxide reductase complex subunit 1. *Thromb Haemost.* 2005;93:23–26.

27. O'Reilly RA, Rytand DA. "Resistance" to warfarin due to unrecognized vitamin K supplementation. *N Engl J Med.* 1980;303:160–161.

28. Suttie JW, Mummah-Schendel LL, Shah DV, Lyle BJ, Greger JL. Vitamin K deficiency from dietary vitamin K restriction in humans. *Am J Clin Nutr.* 1988;47:475–480.

29. Fasco MJ, Hildebrandt EF, Suttie JW. Evidence that warfarin anticoagulant action involves two distinct reductase activities. *J Biol Chem.* 1982;257:11210–11212.

30. *Foods with Vitamin K – Coumadin.* http://www.coumadin.bmscustomerconnect.com/servlet/servlet.FileDownload?file=00Pi000000bxvTFEAY.

31. Mammen EF. Coagulation abnormalities in liver disease. *Hematol Oncol Clin North Am.* 1992;6:1247–1257.

32. Richards RK. Influence of fever upon the action of 3,3- methylene bis-(4- hydroxoycoumarin). *Science.* 1943;97:313–316.

33. Owens JC, Neely WB, Owen WR. Effect of sodium dextrothyroxine in patients receiving anticoagulants. *N Engl J Med.* 1962;266:76–79.

34. Self TH, Reaves AB, Oliphant CS, Sands C. Does heart failure exacerbation increase response to warfarin? A critical review of the literature. *Curr Med Res Opin.* 2006;22:2089–2094.

35. Dreisbach AW, Japa S, Gebrekal AB, et al. Cytochrome P4502C9 activity in end-stage renal disease. *Clin Pharmacol Ther.* 2003;73:475–477.

36. *Coumadin [Package Insert].* Princeton, NJ: Bristol-Myers Squibb Company; 2011.

37. *Warfarin Sodium – Oral. Drug Facts and Comparisons.* 2017 ed. St. Louis, MO: Wolters Kluwer; 2017:225–231.

38. Hansten PD, Horn JR. *Drug Interactions Analysis and Management.* St. Louis, MO: Wolters Kluwer Health; 2014.

39. Warfarin interactions. In: *Clinical Pharmacology.* Tampa, FL: Elsevier/Gold Standard. https://www-clinicalkey-com.library1.unmc.edu/pharmacology/monograph/650?sec=moninte. Updated periodically.

40. Warfarin drug interactions. In: *Lexi-drugs Online.* Hudson, Ohio: Lexi-Comp, Inc. https://online-lexi-com.library1.unmc.edu/lco/action/doc/retrieve/docid/patch_f/7879#f_interactions. Updated periodically.

41. Anthony M, Romero K, Malone DC, Hines LE, Higgins L, Woosley RL. Warfarin interactions with substances listed in drug information compendia and in the FDA-approved label for warfarin sodium. *Clin Pharmacol Ther.* 2009;86:425–429.

42. Wittkowsky AK. Drug interactions update: drugs, herbs, and oral anticoagulation. *J Thromb Thrombolysis.* 2001;12:67–71.

43. Breckenridge A, Orme M, Wesseling H, Lewis RJ, Gibbons R. Pharmacokinetics and pharmacodynamics of the enantiomers of warfarin in man. *Clin Pharmacol Ther.* 1974;15:424–430.

44. O'Reilly RA. Studies on the optical enantiomorphs of warfarin in man. *Clin Pharmacol Ther.* 1974;16:348–354.

45. O'Reilly RA. The stereoselective interaction of warfarin and metronidazole in man. *N Engl J Med.* 1976;295:354–357.

46. O'Reilly RA. Stereoselective interaction of trimethoprim-sulfamethoxazole with the separated enantiomorphs of racemic warfarin in man. *N Engl J Med.* 1980;302:33–35.

47. O'Reilly RA, Trager WF, Rettie AE, Goulart DA. Interaction of amiodarone with racemic warfarin and its separated enantiomorphs in humans. *Clin Pharmacol Ther.* 1987;42:290–294.

48. Cropp JS, Bussey HI. A review of enzyme induction of warfarin metabolism with recommendations for patient management. *Pharmacotherapy.* 1997;17:917–928.

49. Bechtold H, Andrassy K, Jähnchen E, et al. Evidence for impaired hepatic vitamin K1 metabolism in patients treated with N-methyl-thiotetrazole cephalosporins. *Thromb Haemost.* 1984;51:358–361.

50. Weitekamp MR, Aber RC. Prolonged bleeding times and bleeding diathesis associated with moxalactam administration. *JAMA.* 1983;249:69–71.

51. Rothschild BM. Hematologic perturbations associated with salicylate. *Clin Pharmacol Ther.* 1979;26:145–152.

52. Udall JA. Human sources and absorption of vitamin K in relation to anticoagulation stability. *JAMA.* 1965;194:127–129.

53. Bauer KA. New anticoagulants: anti IIa vs. anti Xa – is one better? *J Thromb Thrombolysis.* 2006;21:67–72.

54. Weitz JI, Hudoba M, Massel D, Maraganore J, Hirsh J. Clot-bound thrombin is protected from inhibition by heparin-antithrombin III but is susceptible to inactivation by antithrombin III-independent inhibitors. *J Clin Invest.* 1990;86:385–391.

55. Hauel NH, Nar H, Priepke H, Ries U, Stassen JM, Wienen W. Structure-based design of novel potent nonpeptide thrombin inhibitors. *J Med Chem.* 2002;45:1757–1766.

56. Wienen W, Stassen JM, Priepke H, Ries UJ, Hauel N. In-vitro profile and ex-vivo anticoagulant activity of the direct thrombin inhibitor dabigatran and its orally active prodrug, dabigatran etexilate. *Thromb Haemost.* 2007;98:155–162.

57. Hankey GJ, Eikelboom JW. Dabigatran etexilate: a new oral thrombin inhibitor. *Circulation.* 2011;123:1436–1450.

58. Eriksson BI, Quinlan DJ, Weitz JI. Comparative pharmacodynamics and pharmacokinetics of oral direct thrombin and factor Xa inhibitors in development. *Clin Pharmacokinet.* 2009;48:1–22.

59. Dobesh PP, Terry KJ. Measuring or monitoring of novel anticoagulants: which test to request? *Curr Emerg Hosp Med Rep.* 2013;1:208–216.

60. Albers GW, Diener HC, Frison L, et al., SPORTIF Executive Steering Committee for the SPORTIF V Investigators. Ximelagatran vs warfarin stroke prevention in patients with nonvalvular atrial fibrillation: a randomized trial. *JAMA.* 2005;293:690–698.

61. Schulman S, Wåhlander K, Lundström T, Clason SB, Eriksson H, THRIVE III Investigators. Secondary prevention of venous thromboembolism with the oral direct thrombin inhibitor ximelagatran. *N Engl J Med.* 2003;349:1713–1721.

62. Boudes PF. The challenges of new drugs benefits and risks analysis: lessons from the ximelagatran FDA Cardiovascular Advisory Committee. *Contemp Clin Trials.* 2006;27:432–440.

63. Ageno W, Gallus AS, Wittkowsky A, Crowther M, Hylek EM, Palareti G. Oral anticoagulation therapy: antithrombotic therapy and prevention of thrombosis, 9th ed: American College of Chest Physicians Evidence-Based Clinical Practice Guidelines. *Chest.* 2012;141(suppl):e44S–e88S.

64. *Mechanism of Action of Univalent and Bivalent DTIs.* https://www.researchgate.net/figure/259629896_fig5_Figure-3-Mechanism-of-action-of-univalent-and-bivalent-DTIs-48-DTIs-direct-thrombin.

65. Stangier J. Clinical pharmacokinetics and pharmacodynamics of the oral direct thrombin inhibitor dabigatran etexilate. *Clin Pharmacokinet.* 2008;47:285–295.

66. Eisert WG, Hauel N, Stangier J, Wienen W, Clemens A, van Ryn J. Dabigatran: an oral novel potent reversible nonpeptide inhibitor of thrombin. *Arterioscler Thromb Vasc Biol.* 2010;30:1885–1889.

67. Golub AL, Frost RW, Betlach CJ, Gonzalez MA. Physiologic considerations in drug absorption from the gastrointestinal tract. *J Allergy Clin Immunol.* 1986;78:689–694.

68. Stangier J, Rathgen K, Stähle H, Gansser D, Roth W. The pharmacokinetics, pharmacodynamics and tolerability of dabigatran etexilate, a new oral direct thrombin inhibitor, in healthy male subjects. *Br J Clin Pharmacol.* 2007;64:292–303.

69. Connolly SJ, Ezekowitz MD, Yusuf S, et al., RE-LY Steering Committee and Investigators. Dabigatran versus warfarin in patients with atrial fibrillation. *N Engl J Med.* 2009; 361:1139–1151.

70. Blech S, Ebner T, Ludwig-Schwellinger E, Stangier J, Roth W. The metabolism and disposition of the oral direct thrombin inhibitor, dabigatran, in humans. *Drug Metab Dispos.* 2008;36:386–399.

71. Cabral KP. Pharmacology of the new target-specific oral anticoagulants. *J Thromb Thrombolysis.* 2013;36:133–140.

72. Stangier J, Stähle H, Rathgen K, Roth W, Shakeri-Nejad K. Pharmacokinetics and pharmacodynamics of dabigatran etexilate, an oral direct thrombin inhibitor, are not affected by moderate hepatic impairment. *J Clin Pharmacol.* 2008;48:1411–1419.

73. Stangier J, Rathgen K, Stähle H, Mazur D. Influence of renal impairment on the pharmacokinetics and pharmacodynamics of oral dabigatran etexilate: an open-label, parallel-group, single-centre study. *Clin Pharmacokinet.* 2010;49:259–268.

74. Stangier J, Stähle H, Rathgen K, Fuhr R. Pharmacokinetics and pharmacodynamics of the direct oral thrombin inhibitor dabigatran in healthy elderly subjects. *Clin Pharmacokinet.* 2008;47:47–59.

75. Lin JH, Yamazaki M. Role of P-glycoprotein in pharmacokinetics: clinical implications. *Clin Pharmacokinet.* 2003;42:59–98.

76. Kaatz S, Mahan CE. Stroke prevention in patients with atrial fibrillation and renal dysfunction. *Stroke.* 2014;45:2497–2505.

77. Walenga JM, Adiguzel C. Drug and dietary interactions of the new and emerging oral anticoagulants. *Int J Clin Pract.* 2010;64:956–967.

78. Nutescu E, Chuatrisorn I, Hellenbart E. Drug and dietary interactions of warfarin and novel oral anticoagulants: an update. *J Thromb Thrombolysis.* 2011;31:326–343.

79. Alexander JH, Singh KP. Inhibition of factor Xa: a potential target for the development of new anticoagulants. *Am J Cardiovasc Drugs.* 2005;5:279–290.

80. Rai R, Sprengeler PA, Elrod KC, Young WB. Perspectives on factor Xa inhibition. *Curr Med Chem.* 2001;8:101–119.

81. Harenberg J, Wurzner B, Zimmermann R, et al. Bioavailability and antagonization of the low molecular weight heparin CY216 in man. *Thromb Res.* 1986;44: 549–554.

82. Cade JF, Buchanon MR, Boneu B, et al. A comparison of the antithrombotic and hemorrhagic effects of low molecular weight heparin fractions: the influence of the method of preparation. *Thromb Res.* 1984;35:613–625.

83. Rezaie AR. Prothrombin protects factor Xa in the prothrombinase complex from inhibition by the heparin-antithrombin complex. *Blood.* 2001;97:2308–2313.

84. Gerotziafas GT, Elalamy I, Depasse F, Perzborn E, Samama MM. In vitro inhibition of thrombin generation, after tissue factor pathway activation, by the oral, direct factor Xa inhibitor rivaroxaban. *J Thromb Haemost.* 2007;5:886–888.

85. Graff J, von Hentig N, Misselwitz F, et al. Effects of the oral, direct factor Xa inhibitor rivaroxaban on platelet-induced thrombin generation and prothrombinase activity. *J Clin Pharmacol.* 2007;47:1398–1407.

86. Perzborn E, Roehrig S, Straub A, Kubitza D, Mueck W, Laux V. Rivaroxaban: a new oral factor Xa inhibitor. *Arterioscler Thromb Vasc Biol.* 2010;30:376–381.

87. Laux V, Perzborn E, Kubitza D, et al. Preclinical and clinical characteristics of rivaroxaban: a novel, oral, direct factor Xa inhibitor. *Semin Thromb Hemost.* 2007;33:515–523.

88. Perzborn E, Strassburger J, Wilmen A, et al. In vitro and in vivo studies of the novel antithrombotic agent BAY 59-7939—an oral, direct Factor Xa inhibitor. *J Thromb Haemost.* 2005;3:514–521.

89. Samama MM, Martinoli JL, LeFlem L, et al. Assessment of laboratory assays to measure rivaroxaban—an oral, direct factor Xa inhibitor. *Thromb Haemost.* 2010;103:815–825.

90. Kubitza D, Becka M, Mueck W, Zuehlsdorf M. Safety, tolerability, pharmacodynamics, and pharmacokinetics of rivaroxaban—an oral, direct factor Xa inhibitor—are not affected by aspirin. *J Clin Pharmacol.* 2006;46:981–990.

91. Perzborn E, Kubitza D, Misselwitz F. Rivaroxaban. A novel, oral, direct factor Xa inhibitor in clinical development for the prevention and treatment of thromboembolic disorders. *Hämostaseologie.* 2007;27:282–289.

92. Kubitza D, Becka M, Zuehlsdorf M, Mueck W. Effect of food, an antacid, and the H$_2$ antagonist ranitidine on the absorption of BAY 59-7939 (rivaroxaban), an oral direct factor Xa inhibitor, in healthy subjects. *J Clin Pharmacol.* 2006;46:549–558.

93. Stampfuss J, Kubitza D, Becka M, Mueck W. The effect of food on the absorption and pharmacokinetics of rivaroxaban. *Int J Clin Pharmacol Ther.* 2013;51:549–561.

94. Mueck W, Stampfuss J, Kubitza D, Becka M. Clinical pharmacokinetic and pharmacodynamic profile of rivaroxaban. *Clin Pharmacokinet.* 2014;53:1–16.

95. DeWald TA, Becker RC. The pharmacology of novel oral anticoagulants. *J Thromb Thrombolysis.* 2014;37:217–233.

96. Kubitza D, Becka M, Voith B, Zuehlsdorf M, Wensing G. Safety, pharmacodynamics, and pharmacokinetics of single doses of BAY 59-7939, an oral, direct factor Xa inhibitor. *Clin Pharmacol Ther.* 2005;78:412–421.

97. Kubitza D, Becka M, Wensing G, Voith B, Zuehlsdorf M. Safety, pharmacodynamics, and pharmacokinetics of BAY 59-7939—an oral, direct Factor Xa inhibitor—after multiple dosing in healthy male subjects. *Eur J Clin Pharmacol.* 2005;61:873–880.

98. Weinz C, Schwarz T, Kubitza D, et al. Metabolism and excretion of rivaroxaban, an oral direct factor Xa inhibitor, in rats, dogs, and humans. *Drug Metab Dispos.* 2009;37:1056–1064.

99. Lang D, Freudenberger C, Weinz C. In vitro metabolism of rivaroxaban, an oral, direct factor Xa inhibitor, in liver microsomes and hepatocytes of rats, dogs, and humans. *Drug Metab Dispos.* 2009;37:1046–1055.

100. Dobesh PP, John F. Reducing the risk of stroke in patients with nonvalvular atrial fibrillation with direct oral anticoagulants. Is one of these not like the others? *J Atr Fibrillation.* 2016;9:66–74.

101. Mueck W, Lensing AWA, Agnelli G, Decousus H, Prandoni P, Misselwitz F. Rivaroxaban: population pharmacokinetic analyses in patients treated for acute deep-vein thrombosis and exposure simulations in patients with atrial fibrillation treated for stroke prevention. *Clin Pharmacokinet.* 2011;50:675–686.

102. Dias C, Moore KT, Murphy J, et al. Pharmacokinetics, pharmacodynamics, and safety of single-dose rivaroxaban in chronic hemodialysis. *Am J Nephrol.* 2016;43:229–236.

103. Kubitza D, Becka M, Roth A, et al. The influence of age and gender on the pharmacokinetics and pharmacodynamics of rivaroxaban – an oral, direct factor Xa inhibitor. *J Clin Pharmacol.* 2013;53:249–255.

104. Kubitza D, Becka M, Zuehlsdorf M, et al. Body weight has limited influence on the safety, tolerability, pharmacokinetics, or pharmacodynamics of rivaroxaban (BAY 59-7939) in healthy subjects. *J Clin Pharmacol.* 2007;47:218–226.

105. Kubitza D, Becka M, Mueck W, et al. Effects of renal impairment on the pharmacokinetics, pharmacodynamics and safety of rivaroxaban, an oral, direct factor Xa inhibitor. *Br J Clin Pharmacol.* 2010;70:703–712.

106. Kubitza D, Roth A, Becka M, et al. Effect of hepatic impairment on the pharmacokinetics and pharmacodynamics of a single dose of rivaroxaban – an oral, direct Factor Xa inhibitor. *Br J Clin Pharmacol.* 2013;76:89–98.

107. Mueck W, Kubitza D, Becka M. Co-administration of rivaroxaban with drugs that share its elimination pathways: pharmacokinetic effects in healthy subjects. *Br J Clin Pharmacol.* 2013;76:455–466.

108. Gnoth MJ, Buetehorn U, Muenster U, et al. In vitro and in vivo P-glycoprotein transport characteristics of rivaroxaban. *J Pharmacol Exp Ther.* 2011;338:372–380.

109. Wong PC, Pinto DJ, Zhang D. Preclinical discovery of apixaban, a direct and orally bioavailable factor Xa inhibitor. *J Thromb Thrombolysis.* 2011;31:478–492.

110. Pinto DJ, Orwat MJ, Koch S, et al. Discovery of 1-(4-methoxyphenyl)-7-oxo-6-(4-(2-oxopiperidin-1-yl)phenyl)-4,5,6,7-tetrahydro-1H-pyrazolo[3,4-c]pyridine-3-carboxamide (apixaban, BMS-562247), a highly potent, selective, efficacious, and orally bioavailable inhibitor of blood coagulation factor Xa. *J Med Chem.* 2007;50:5339–5356.

111. Wong PC, Jiang X. Apixaban, a direct factor Xa inhibitor, inhibits tissue-factor induced human platelet aggregation in vitro: comparison with direct inhibitors of factor VIIa, XIa and thrombin. *Thromb Haemost.* 2010;104:302–310.

112. He K, Luettgen JM, Zhang D, et al. Preclinical pharmacokinetics and pharmacodynamics of apixaban, a potent and selective factor Xa inhibitor. *Eur J Drug Metab Pharm.* 2011;36:129–139.

113. Wong PC, Crain EJ, Xin B, et al. Apixaban, an oral, direct and highly selective factor Xa inhibitor: in vitro, antithrombotic and antihemostatic studies. *J Thromb Haemost.* 2008;6:820–829.

114. Raghavan N, Frost CE, Yu Z, et al. Apixaban metabolism and pharmacokinetics after oral administration to humans. *Drug Metab Dispos.* 2009;37:74–81.

115. Wang L, Zhang D, Raghavan N, et al. In vitro assessment of metabolic drug-drug interaction potential of apixaban through cytochrome P450 phenotyping, inhibition, and induction studies. *Drug Metab Dispos.* 2010;38:448–458.

116. Leil TA, Feng Y, Zhang L, Paccaly A, Mohan P, Pfister M. Quantification of apixaban's therapeutic utility in prevention of venous thromboembolism: selection of phase III trial dose. *Clin Pharmacol Ther.* 2010;88:375–382.

117. Frost CE, Yu Z, Wang, et al. Single-dose safety and pharmacokinetics of apixaban in subjects with mild or moderate hepatic impairment. *Clin Pharmacol Ther.* 2009;85(suppl 1):S34. [Abstract].

118. Granger CB, Alexander JH, McMurray JJV, et al., ARISTOTLE Committees and Investigators. Apixaban versus warfarin in patients with atrial fibrillation. *N Engl J Med.* 2011;365:981–992.

119. Wang X, Tirucherai G, Marbury TC, et al. Pharmacokinetics, pharmacodynamics, and safety of apixaban in subjects with end-stage renal disease on hemodialysis. *J Clin Pharmacol.* 2016;56:628–636.

120. Mavrakanas TA, Samer CF, Nessim SJ, Frisch G, Lipman ML. Apixaban pharmacokinetics at steady state in hemodialysis patients. *J Am Soc Nephrol.* 2017;28:2241–2248.

121. Scaglione F. New oral anticoagulants: comparative pharmacology with vitamin K antagonists. *Clin Pharmacokinet.* 2013;52:69–82.

122. Upreti VV, Wang J, Barrett YC, et al. Effect of extremes of body weight on the pharmacokinetics, pharmacodynamics, safety and tolerability of apixaban in healthy subjects. *Br J Clin Pharmacol.* 2013;76:908–916.

123. Frost CE, Song Y, Shenker A, et al. Effects of age and sex on the single-dose pharmacokinetics and pharmacodynamics of apixaban. *Clin Pharmacokinet.* 2015;54:651–662.

124. Bristol-Myers Squibb Company. *Eliquis: Prescribing Information;* 2016. https://packageinserts.bms.com/pi/pi_eliquis.pdf.

125. Frost CE, Byon W, Song Y, et al. Effect of ketoconazole and diltiazem on the pharmacokinetics of apixaban, an oral direct factor Xa inhibitor. *Br J Clin Pharmacol.* 2015;79:838–846.

126. Vakkalagadda B, Frost C, Byon W, et al. Effect of rifampin on the pharmacokinetics of apixaban, an oral direct inhibitor of factor Xa. *Am J Cardiovasc Drugs.* 2016;16:119–127.

127. Parasrampuria DA, Truitt KE. Pharmacokinetics and pharmacodynamics of edoxaban, a non-vitamin K antagonist oral anticoagulant that inhibits clotting factor Xa. *Clin Pharmacokinet.* 2016;55:641–655.

128. Furugohri T, Isobe K, Honda Y, et al. DU-176b, a potent and orally active factor Xa inhibitor: in vitro and in vivo pharmacological profiles. *J Thromb Haemost.* 2008;6:1542–1549.

129. Ogata K, Mendell-Harary J, Tachibana M, et al. Clinical safety, tolerability, pharmacokinetics, and pharmacodynamics of the novel factor Xa inhibitor edoxaban in healthy volunteers. *J Clin Pharmacol.* 2010;50(7):743–753.

130. Cuker A, Husseinzadeh H. Laboratory measurement of the anticoagulant activity of edoxaban: a systematic review. *J Thromb Thrombolysis.* 2015;39:288–294.

131. Bathala MS, Masumoto H, Oguma T, He L, Lowrie C, Mendell J. Pharmacokinetics, biotransformation, and mass balance of edoxaban, a selective, direct factor Xa inhibitor, in humans. *Drug Metab Dispos.* 2012;40(12):2250–2255.

132. Matsushima N, Lee F, Sato T, Weiss D, Mendell J. Bioavailability and safety of the factor Xa inhibitor edoxaban and the effects of quinidine in healthy subjects. *Clin Pharm Drug Dev.* 2013;2:358–366.

133. Mendell J, Tachibana M, Shi M, et al. Effects of food on the pharmacokinetics of edoxaban, an oral direct factor Xa inhibitor, in healthy volunteers. *J Clin Pharmacol.* 2011;51:687–694.

134. Yin OQ, Miller R. Population pharmacokinetics and dose-exposure proportionality of edoxaban in healthy volunteers. *Clin Drug Investig.* 2014;34:743–752.

135. Jönsson S, Simonsson US, Miller R, Karlsson MO. Population pharmacokinetics of edoxaban and its main metabolite in a dedicated renal impairment study. *J Clin Pharmacol.* 2015;55:1268–1279.

136. Mikkaichi T, Yoshigae Y, Masumoto H, et al. Edoxaban transport via P-glycoprotein is a key factor for the drug's disposition. *Drug Metab Dispos.* 2014;42:520–528.

137. Mendell J, Johnson L, Chen S. An open-label, phase I study to evaluate the effects of hepatic impairment on edoxaban pharmacokinetics and pharmacodynamics. *J Clin Pharmacol.* 2015;55:1395–1405.

138. Fanikos J, Burnett AE, Mahan CE, Dobesh PP. Renal function considerations for stroke prevention in atrial fibrillation. *Am J Med.* 2017;130:1015–1023.

139. Parasrampuria DA, Marbury T, Matsushima N, et al. Pharmacokinetics, safety, and tolerability of edoxaban in end-stage renal disease subjects undergoing haemodialysis. *Thromb Haemost.* 2015;113:719–727.

140. Wolzt M, Samama MM, Kapiotis S, Ogata K, Mendell J, Kunitada S. Effect of edoxaban on markers of coagulation in venous and shed blood compared with fondaparinux. *Thromb Haemost.* 2011;105:1080–1090.

141. Weitz JI, Connolly SJ, Patel I, et al. Randomised, parallel-group, multicentre, multinational phase 2 study comparing edoxaban, an oral factor Xa inhibitor, with warfarin for stroke prevention in patients with atrial fibrillation. *Thromb Haemost.* 2010;104:633–641.

142. Song S, Dang D, Halim AB, Miller R. Population pharmacokinetic – pharmacodynamic modeling analysis of intrinsic FXa and bleeding from edoxaban treatment. *J Clin Pharmacol*. 2014;54:910–916.

143. Salazar DE, Mendell J, Kastrissios H, et al. Modeling and simulations of edoxaban exposure and response relationships in patients with atrial fibrillation. *Thromb Haemost*. 2012;107:925–936.

144. Giugliano RP, Ruff CT, Braunwald E, et al. Edoxaban versus warfarin in patients with atrial fibrillation. *N Engl J Med*. 2013;369:2093–2104.

145. Yamashita T, Koretsune Y, Yasaka M, et al. Randomized, multicenter, warfarin-controlled phase II study of edoxaban in Japanese patients with non-valvular atrial fibrillation. *Circ J*. 2012;76:1840–1847.

146. Mendell J, Zahir H, Matsushima N, et al. Drug-drug interaction studies of cardiovascular drugs involving P-glycoprotein, an efflux transporter, on the pharmacokinetics of edoxaban, an oral factor Xa inhibitor. *Am J Cardiovasc Drugs*. 2013;13:331–342.

147. Parasrampuria DA, Mendell J, Shi M, Matsushima N, Zahir H, Truitt K. Edoxaban drug-drug interactions with ketoconazole, erythromycin, and cyclosporine. *Br J Clin Pharmacol*. 2016;82:1591–1600.

148. Mendell J, Chen S, He L, Desai M, Parasramupria DA. The effect of rifampin on the pharmacokinetics of edoxaban in healthy adults. *Clin Drug Investig*. 2015;35:447–453.

CHAPTER 3

Anticoagulation Drug Trials for Stroke Prevention in Atrial Fibrillation

DAVID A. MANLY, MD • CHRISTOPHER B. GRANGER, MD

INTRODUCTION

Atrial fibrillation (AF) is the most common sustained cardiac arrhythmia and significantly increases the risk of stroke and other thromboembolic events.[1] Vitamin K antagonists (VKAs) have long been used to reduce stroke (and mortality) associated with AF. Numerous trials in the 1990s demonstrated the effectiveness of VKAs to reduce stroke. However, variability and unpredictability in the anticoagulant effect requires careful monitoring and adjustment, and bleeding complications including intracranial hemorrhage limit its clinical use. Indeed, multiple studies have demonstrated that patients with AF are woefully undertreated, and even when treated, studies show the mean time in therapeutic range for the majority of patients is only around 50%.[2-8]

The last 10 years have seen significant advancements and additions to the armamentarium for stroke prevention for patients with AF. These advancements have come from the success of several large trials demonstrating both the safety and efficacy of non-VKA oral anticoagulants (NOACs) in the prevention of stroke and systemic embolism. These drugs work through selective inhibition of a coagulation factor: either factor Xa (rivaroxaban, apixaban, edoxaban) or thrombin (dabigatran).

This chapter reviews anticoagulation drug trials in AF.

ASPIRIN AND OTHER ANTIPLATELET AGENTS

Current data do not support the use of aspirin for the prevention of thromboembolic events in patients with AF and high stroke risk (CHA_2DS_2-VASc score of 2 or more). This recommendation comes from numerous studies demonstrating marginal benefits of aspirin over control as well as VKA superiority over antiplatelet agents in the prevention of stroke or systemic embolism (Vitamin K Antagonists section). The most recent international guidelines from the European Society of Cardiology provide a level III strength of evidence A (do not use due to harm) for aspirin to prevent stroke in AF.[9] The older US guidelines recommend that aspirin may be considered (Class IIB recommendation) for patients with AF and low stroke risk (CHA_2DS_2-Vasc score of 1).[10]

The recommendations for aspirin use in AF come predominately from seven trials conducted in the late 1980s and early 1990s, which studied the safety and efficacy of aspirin monotherapy versus placebo or no therapy on the outcome of stroke prevention in patients with AF.[11-17] Doses of aspirin in these trials ranged from 50 to 1300 mg daily, and no trial showed a significant reduction in stroke, with one exception, SPAF-I. The SPAF-I trial demonstrated a 42% significant reduction in stroke with 325 mg of aspirin a day, but the trial was stopped early, excluded most patients older than 75 years, and the stroke reduction effect was driven by an implausible reduction in one of two strata, patients eligible for oral anticoagulation.[12] A metaanalysis of these seven trials found that aspirin monotherapy (at an average dose of approximately 220 mg daily) is marginally effective at reducing stroke in patients with AF (see Fig. 3.1), because of the SPAF-1 results.[18] The relative risk (RR) reduction for aspirin versus placebo or no treatment was 19% (95% confidence interval [CI], −1 to 35%); however, given the above limitations, many interpret the overall data as showing no strong evidence for any benefit from aspirin in stroke prevention.[19]

Two recent large randomized trials evaluated the efficacy of dual antiplatelet therapy with aspirin and clopidogrel in patients with AF. The ACTIVE-W (Atrial Fibrillation Clopidogrel Trial with Irbesartan for Prevention of Vascular Events) trial compared the combination of aspirin and clopidogrel with warfarin, while the ACTIVE-A trial compared the combination of aspirin and clopidogrel with aspirin monotherapy in patients who were deemed "unsuitable" for VKA.[20,21] The combination of aspirin (75–100 mg daily) and

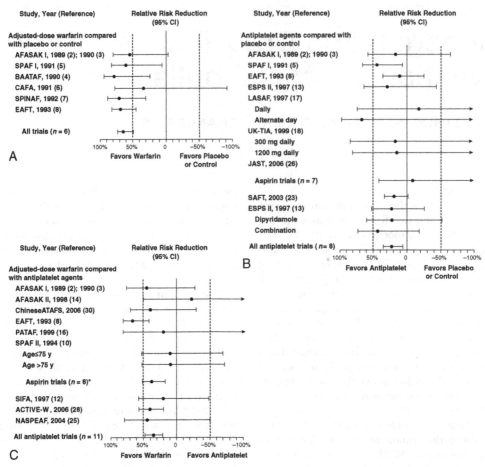

FIG. 3.1 Antithrombotic therapy for stroke prevention in patients with nonvalvular atrial fibrillation (AF). (A) Adjusted-dose warfarin compared with placebo or no treatment in six randomized trials. (B) Antiplatelet agents compared with placebo or no treatment in eight randomized trials. In SAFT, aspirin was combined with low, inefficacious dosages of warfarin. In ESPS II, *combination* refers to aspirin plus dipyridamole. (C) Adjusted-dose warfarin compared with antiplatelet agents in 11 randomized trials. Nonaspirin antiplatelet agents were indobufen (SIFA), clopidogrel plus aspirin (ACTIVE-W), and triflusal (NASPEAF). Horizontal lines represent 95% CIs around point estimates. (Adapted from Hart RG, Pearce LA, Aguilar MI. Meta-analysis: antithrombotic therapy to prevent stroke in patients who have nonvalvular atrial fibrillation. *Ann Intern Med.* 2007;146(12):857–867.)

clopidogrel (75 mg daily) was found to be superior to aspirin alone (28% RR reduction in stroke; 95% CI, 17%–38%; $P < .0002$), however, at the expense of significantly increased bleeding (2%/year with the addition of clopidogrel vs. 1.3% with aspirin monotherapy; RR 1.57; 95% CI, 1.29–1.92; $P < .001$).[20] Although the modest effect of preventing stroke in the context of an increase in bleeding does not support the use of dual antiplatelet therapy for stroke prevention, it does provide evidence of some stroke prevention for patients who otherwise need dual antiplatelet therapy.

The ACTIVE-W trial compared warfarin (goal INR [international normalized ratio] 2.0-3.0) with the combination of aspirin (75-100 mg daily) and clopidogrel (75 mg daily) in patients with AF and a mean $CHADS_2$ score of 2. The trial was terminated early as the combination of aspirin and clopidogrel proved inferior to warfarin. There was a significantly higher rate of stroke (RR 1.72; 95% CI, 1.24-2.37; $P = .001$) and systemic embolism (RR 4.66; 95% CI, 1.58-13.8; $P = .005$) in the aspirin and clopidogrel arm without a significant difference in major bleeding between the two groups (2.42%/year with clopidogrel plus aspirin vs. 2.21%/year with warfarin, RR 1.1; 95% CI 0.83-1.45; $P = .53$).[21,22] The RR reduction for stroke in patients treated with warfarin compared with combination aspirin and clopidogrel was 40% (95% CI, 18%–56%, $P < .001$).

The AVERROES trial directly compared aspirin (81–325 mg once daily, with two-thirds enrolled receiving 81 mg daily) versus apixaban (5 mg twice daily) in patients deemed unsuitable for warfarin therapy. This trial was terminated early because of clear superiority of apixaban over aspirin for the prevention of stroke in patients with AF. Importantly, major bleeding between aspirin and apixaban was similar, with numerically fewer patients with intracranial hemorrhage in the apixaban arm.[23,24] AVERROES provided further rationale to avoid using aspirin for stroke prevention, as apixaban is far more effective with comparable safety.

VITAMIN K ANTAGONISTS

VKAs have long been the standard of care for thromboembolic protection in AF. Pooled data from recent randomized trials estimate the average yearly risk of stroke or systemic embolism in patients with AF treated with warfarin to be around 1.66%, with the risk of thromboembolic events in VKA-treated patients rising with increasing $CHADS_2$ score (0.89%/year for low risk, 1.45%/year for intermediate risk, and 2.5%/year for high risk).[25] Patients enrolled in trials, however, tend to have lower risk than unselected patient populations. Despite the numerous pharmacologic drawbacks, including a narrow therapeutic window, multiple dietary and drug interactions, and the need for monitoring and occasional dose-adjustments, VKAs have been shown to significantly reduce the rate of stroke, systemic embolism, and death in patients with AF. Although the use of the VKA for stroke prevention in AF in high-income countries is decreasing in the NOAC era, there is still compelling data for its efficacy and safety.

Six prior trials have evaluated the efficacy of VKA against placebo or no treatment: AFASAK-I, SPAF-I, BAATAF, CAFA, SPINAF, and EAFT.[11–13,26–28] A 2007 metaanalysis of these trials demonstrated that when compared with placebo or no treatment, adjusted-dose warfarin (average achieved INR was 2.0–2.9) resulted in a 64% RR reduction for ischemic and hemorrhagic stroke.[18] The average stroke rate among patients assigned to the placebo or control groups was 4.5%/year in the primary prevention trials and 12%/year in patients with prior stroke or transient ischemic attack (TIA). With the addition of warfarin, there was an absolute risk reduction of 2.7%/year (number needed to treat [NNT] = 37) for the primary prevention of stroke in patients with AF and an absolute risk reduction of 8.4%/year (NNT = 12) for the secondary prevention of stroke or TIA in patients with AF. Importantly, when stratifying for stroke severity, VKAs were also effective in reducing both disabling and nondisabling strokes. This finding has been supported by a Swedish observational study that evaluated patients who presented with acute stroke and AF. Patients already on VKA therapy not only had less severe strokes, but also had a lower 30-day mortality.[29]

VKAs have also been shown to be superior to antiplatelet agents in patients with AF (Fig. 3.1). A metaanalysis of eight adjusted-dose warfarin versus aspirin trials demonstrated a 38% RR reduction (95% CI, 18–52) in stroke or systemic embolism in patients treated with VKA.[18] The absolute risk reduction of VKA versus aspirin in the primary prevention group was 0.7%/year (NNT = 142) and an astounding 7%/year (NNT = 14) in the secondary prevention group. When this analysis was further expanded to include three other nonaspirin antiplatelet trials, the RR reduction remained steady around 37% (95% CI, 23–48). When warfarin was directly compared with the combination of aspirin and clopidogrel in the ACTIVE-W trial, the trial was terminated early because of the clear superiority of warfarin without appreciable differences in bleeding.[21]

In terms of safety with VKA, the incidence of major bleeding occurs at a rate of 1.40%–3.40%/year in contemporary trials of patients treated for AF. The annual rate of intracerebral hemorrhage is estimated around 0.33%–0.80%/year. Numerous risk scores (ATRIA, RIETE, HAS-BLED) have been formulated to assess bleeding risk in the computation of benefit versus harm.[30–32] However, concern over bleeding risk remains to be the greatest barrier to appropriate thromboembolic protection in patients with AF, especially in older patients. Thus, the European Guidelines recommend no longer using bleeding risk scores to decide who should be and who should not be treated with anticoagulants.[9] It is well known that geriatric patients have both increased stroke and bleeding risks. The BAFTA (Birmingham Atrial Fibrillation Treatment of the Aged) study evaluated warfarin (INR goal 2–3) versus aspirin (75 mg daily) in patients older than 75 years with a mean age of enrollment of 81.5 years.[33] Warfarin was superior to aspirin in stroke prevention (1.8%/year with warfarin vs. 3.8%/year with aspirin, $P = .003$; RR reduction 0.48%; absolute yearly risk reduction 2%) without a significant increase in extracranial bleeding (1.4%/year for warfarin vs. 1.6%/year for aspirin, $P = .67$) or in the composite of all major bleeding (1.9%/year for warfarin vs. 2.0%/year for aspirin, $P = .09$). The trial was underpowered to detect a difference in major central nervous system bleeding.

NON–VITAMIN K ANTAGONIST ORAL ANTICOAGULANTS TRIALS

The impetus to develop the NOACs was to have drugs that were as good as VKAs for stroke prevention but easier to use. Thus, clinical trials began in the 2000s to show that NOACs were at least as good as warfarin at preventing stroke, using "noninferiority" designs to show that the new drugs preserved, with a high level of confidence, at least half of the benefit of warfarin based on the historical warfarin trials.[34] Each of the large trials testing a NOAC versus warfarin demonstrated non-inferiority for stroke prevention, leading to worldwide regularity approval and incorporation into clinical practice guidelines. The 2014 AHA/ACC/HRS Guideline for the Management of Patients With Atrial Fibrillation assigned apixaban, dabigatran, and rivaroxaban as Class IB recommendation to prevent thromboembolic events in patients with AF and a CHA_2DS_2-VASc of 2 or greater.[10] The European Society of Cardiology 2016 guideline recommends all four of the NOACs—dabigatran, rivaroxaban, apixaban, and edoxaban—over VKAs for AF as a Class I recommendation.[9]

RE-LY (Randomized Evaluation of Long-Term Anticoagulation Therapy) was the first major randomized trial to investigate the safety and efficacy of a NOAC in patients with AF.[35] RE-LY was constructed as a noninferiority trial of dabigatran, which is an oral prodrug with rapid serum conversion to a direct, competitive inhibitor of thrombin. It was prescribed as either 110 or 150 mg twice daily versus open label adjusted-dose warfarin. Exclusion criteria for this trial were the presence of a severe heart-valve disorder, stroke within 14 days or severe stroke within 6 months before screening, a condition that increased the risk of hemorrhage, a creatinine clearance (CrCl) of less than 30 mL/min, active liver disease, and pregnancy. Patients were followed up an average of 2 years. Patients in the warfarin group maintained a therapeutic INR (2.0–3.0) a mean of 64% of the time. The mean CHADS$_2$ score for patients in the warfarin group was 2.1 versus 2.1 and 2.2 in the 110 mg dabigatran and 150 mg dabigatran group, respectively. Patients in the warfarin arm met the primary outcome of stroke or systemic embolism at 1.69%/year compared with 1.53%/year in the group that received 110 mg of dabigatran (RR with dabigatran, 0.91; 95% CI, 0.74–1.11; $P<.001$ for noninferiority) and 1.11%/year in the group that received 150 mg of dabigatran (RR, 0.66; 95% CI, 0.53–0.82; $P<.001$ for superiority). Major bleeding was defined in this trial as a reduction in the hemoglobin level of at least 20 g/L, transfusion of at least 2 units of blood, or symptomatic bleeding in a critical area or organ. Major bleeding

occurred significantly less in the 110 mg dabigatran group than in warfarin group (2.71%/year vs. 3.36%/year, $P=.003$). There was no significant difference in major bleeds in the 150 mg dabigatran group versus warfarin group (3.11%/year vs. 3.36%/year, $P=.31$). Mortality was evaluated as a secondary outcome and was unchanged between the 110 mg dabigatran and warfarin group (3.75%/year vs. 4.13%/year, $P=.13$); however, there was a trend toward lower mortality (and a significant reduction in cardiovascular mortality) in the 150 mg dabigatran group (total mortality 3.64%/year vs. 4.13%/year for warfarin, $P=.051$).

ROCKET-AF (Rivaroxaban Once Daily Oral Direct Factor Xa Inhibition Compared With Vitamin K Antagonism for Prevention of Stroke and Embolism Trial in Atrial Fibrillation) evaluated the safety and efficacy of rivaroxaban 20 mg daily (or 15 mg daily in patients with a CrCl of 30–49 mL/min) versus warfarin in patients with AF.[36] Rivaroxaban is a direct factor Xa inhibitor. Exclusion criteria for this trial were hemodynamically significant mitral stenosis (MS), prosthetic heart valve, stroke within 14 days or severe stroke within 3 months before screening, a condition that increased the risk of hemorrhage, a need for anticoagulation other than AF, a CrCl of less than 30 mL/min, significant liver disease, and pregnancy.[36] ROCKET-AF differed from RE-LY in that it was a double-blinded trial where sham INR values were used in the rivaroxaban group. The median follow-up period was 590 days for the per-protocol population and 707 days for the intention-to-treat population. The mean CHADS$_2$ score was 3.5. Patients in the warfarin group maintained a therapeutic INR a mean of 55% of the time. The primary end point of stroke or systemic embolism occurred in 188 patients in the rivaroxaban group (1.7%/year) and 241 in the warfarin group (2.2%/year) in the per-protocol population (hazard ratio [HR] in the rivaroxaban group, 0.79; 95% CI, 0.66–0.96; $P<.001$ for noninferiority). When all randomized patients of the intention-to-treat population were included, primary events occurred in 269 patients in the rivaroxaban group (2.1%/year) and 306 patients in the warfarin group (2.4%/year) (HR, 0.88; 95% CI, 0.74–1.03; $P<.001$ for noninferiority; $P=.12$ for superiority). Rates of major and clinically relevant nonmajor bleeding events were similar between the rivaroxaban and warfarin groups (14.9% and 14.5%/year, respectively; HR in the rivaroxaban group, 1.03; 95% CI, 0.96–1.11; $P=.44$). Major bleeding events were comparable between the two drugs (rivaroxaban at 3.6%/year vs. warfarin at 3.4%/year, $P=.58$). Rivaroxaban had a significantly decreased rate of intracranial hemorrhage (0.5% vs. 0.7%/year; $P=.02$) and fatal bleeding (0.2% vs. 0.5%/year; $P = .003$), however, an increased rate of major bleeding from the gastrointestinal tract (3.2%/year vs. 2.2%, $P < .001$).

J-ROCKET-AF (Japanese Rivaroxaban Once daily oral direct factor Xa inhibition Compared with vitamin K antagonism for prevention of stroke and Embolism Trial in Atrial Fibrillation) was a randomized, double-blind phase III trial of rivaroxaban in Japanese patients with AF.[37] Despite being a global trial, ROCKET-AF did not enroll in Japan. The reason for the lack of inclusion in the larger global rivaroxaban study (ROCKET-AF) was that pharmacokinetic modeling suggested that the steady-state concentration of a 15 mg rivaroxaban dose in Japanese patients would be equivalent to the 20 mg rivaroxaban dose in Caucasian patients. Additionally, Japanese guidelines recommend lower anticoagulation targets for warfarin, which would obviously affect analysis of the warfarin control arm. This was a double-dummy trial in which both arms of the study received a placebo (warfarin placebo in the active treatment arm of rivaroxaban 15 mg daily or rivaroxaban placebo in the warfarin control arm; note that patients with a CrCl 30–49 mL/min received 10 mg rivaroxaban daily). Warfarin was dose-adjusted to a target INR of 2.0–3.0 in patients 69 years and younger, or a reduced INR of 1.6–2.6 in patients aged 70 years or older, which is consistent with Japanese guidelines. Patients were followed up for 30 months. The mean $CHADS_2$ score was 3.27 in the rivaroxaban group and 3.22 in the warfarin group. Rivaroxaban was found to be noninferior to warfarin. The primary efficacy outcome (composite of stroke and systemic embolism) was met in 11/637 patients in the rivaroxaban arm (1.26%/year) compared with 22/637 patients in the warfarin arm (2.61%/year; HR 0.49, CI 0.24–1.0, $P = .05$). There was no difference in the primary safety outcome (composite of major bleeding and clinically relevant nonmajor bleeding) between rivaroxaban and warfarin, 18.04%/year for rivaroxaban versus 16.42%/year for warfarin (HR 1.11, CI 0.87–1.42).

The ARISTOTLE trial (Apixaban for Reduction in Stroke and Other Thromboembolic Events in Atrial Fibrillation) evaluated the safety and efficacy of 5 mg twice-daily, fixed dose of apixaban (or reduced dose of 2.5 mg twice daily for patients meeting two or more of the following criteria: an age of ≥80 years, a body weight ≤ 60 kg, or a serum creatinine level of ≥1.5 mg/dL) versus dose-adjusted warfarin in patients with AF.[38] Exclusion criteria in this trial were AF due to a reversible cause, moderate or severe MS, conditions other than AF that required anticoagulation (e.g., a prosthetic heart valve), stroke within the previous 7 days, a need for aspirin at a dose of >165 mg a day or for both aspirin and clopidogrel, and severe renal insufficiency (serum creatinine level of >2.5 mg/dL or calculated CrCl of <25 mL/min). The mean $CHADS_2$ score was 2.1 for both groups. Patients in the warfarin group had a therapeutic INR (2.0–3.0) an average of 62% of the time. The primary end point of stroke or systemic embolism occurred in 212 patients in the apixaban group (1.27%/year) as compared with 265 patients in the warfarin group (1.60%/year) (HR in the apixaban group, 0.79; CI 0.66–0.95; $P < .001$ for noninferiority and $P = .01$ for superiority). The primary safety outcome of major bleeding occurred less frequently in the apixaban group (2.13%/year in the apixaban group, as compared with 3.09%/year in the warfarin group; HR 0.69; 95% CI, 0.60–0.80; $P < .001$). Notably, the rate of intracranial hemorrhage was significantly less with apixaban, occurring at a frequency of 0.33%/year as compared with 0.80%/year for warfarin (HR 0.42, CI 0.30–0.58, $P < .001$). The rate of death from any cause was also significantly lower in the apixaban group at 3.52%/year compared with 3.94%/year in the warfarin group (HR 0.89; CI 0.80–0.99; $P = .047$).

Apixaban was also compared with aspirin in the AVERROES trial (Apixaban Versus Acetylsalicylic Acid to Prevent Stroke in AF Patients Who Have Failed or Are Unsuitable for Vitamin K Antagonist Treatment).[23] This was a double-blind, double-dummy study of apixaban 5 mg twice daily versus aspirin 81–324 mg daily in 5599 patients who were considered unsuitable for warfarin therapy. Patients were considered unsuitable for VKA if they had a prior adverse event (although exclusion criteria for serious bleed in last 6 months or high bleeding risk), poor anticoagulant control, requirement for other treatments that may interact with VKA, or the patient was unable or unwilling to adhere to dose or INR monitoring instructions. Patients taking open-label aspirin were encouraged to discontinue it. The mean $CHADS_2$ score was 2, with approximately 36% of patients within the moderate risk strata for stroke ($CHADS_2$ or CHA_2DS_2-VASc score of 1). The majority of patients in this study received 81–162 mg of aspirin in the aspirin control arm (64% received 81 mg aspirin daily, 27% received 162 mg aspirin daily). The study was prematurely terminated at a mean follow-up of 1 year because of the clear superiority of apixaban to prevent stroke or systemic embolism compared with aspirin. The rate of stroke or systemic embolism occurred at a rate of 1.6%/year in the apixaban group versus 3.7%/year in the aspirin group (HR with apixaban, 0.45, 95% CI, 0.32–0.62; $P < .001$). The rate of ischemic stroke was significantly decreased, occurring 1.1%/year with apixaban and 3.0%/year with aspirin (HR with apixaban, 0.37; 95% CI, 0.25–0.55; $P < .001$).

Because of early termination, the study was underpowered to detect a difference in intracerebral hemorrhage or cardiovascular death. Patients in the apixaban group did benefit from a reduction in the rate of hospitalization for cardiovascular causes (12.6%/year for apixaban vs. 15.9%/year with aspirin, $P<.001$). There was no significant difference in major bleeding (1.4%/year with apixaban vs. 1.2%/year with aspirin, HR with apixaban, 1.13; 95% CI, 0.74–1.75; $P=.57$); however, minor bleeding is more common with apixaban (HR with apixaban, 1.24; 95% CI, 1.00–1.53; $P=.05$). Perhaps one of the most significant outcomes of this study, designed for patients unable to comply with VKA therapy, was the adherence to the study medication. At 2 years, permanent discontinuation of apixaban was 12% lower than aspirin, related to the fewer serious adverse events in the apixaban group compared with the aspirin control group (22% vs. 27% respectively, $P<.001$). This trial suggested that NOACs might fill a gap in the use of anticoagulants for the prevention of thromboembolic events in patients with AF, as nearly 40% of the patients included in this study listed "refusal to take VKA" as a reason for inclusion.

The most recent randomized trial to evaluate the safety and efficacy of a NOAC versus warfarin in patients with AF was ENGAGE-AF-TIMI 48 (Effective Anticoagulation with Factor Xa Next Generation in Atrial Fibrillation–Thrombolysis in Myocardial Infarction 48).[39] Edoxaban is an oral, reversible, direct factor Xa inhibitor that can be administered as once-daily dosing. This trial evaluated once-daily edoxaban at two dose regimens, 60 mg (high dose) or 30 mg (low dose), with adjusted-dose warfarin at goal INR 2.0–3.0. The dose of edoxaban in either group would be cut down to half (to 30 mg or 15 mg respectively) if any of the following conditions were met: CrCl 30–50 mL/min, body weight < 60 kg, or concomitant use of verapamil, quinidine, or dronedarone. Key exclusion criteria were similar to those in other NOAC megatrials: AF due to a reversible disorder; an estimated CrCl of less than 30 mL/min; a high risk of bleeding; use of dual antiplatelet therapy; moderate-to-severe MS; other indications for anticoagulation therapy; acute coronary syndromes, coronary revascularization, or stroke within 30 days before randomization. The mean CHADS$_2$ score was 2.8 in all three groups. Patients in the warfarin group had a therapeutic INR (2.0–3.0) an average of 68% of the time. The primary end point of stroke or systemic embolism occurred in 232 patients in the warfarin group (1.50%/year), as compared with 182 patients in the high-dose edoxaban group (1.18%/year; HR vs. warfarin, 0.79; 97.5% CI, 0.63–0.99; $P<.001$ for noninferiority, $P=.02$ for superiority) and 253 patients in the low-dose edoxaban group (1.61%/year; HR vs. warfarin, 1.07; 97.5% CI, 0.87–1.31; $P=.005$ for

noninferiority, $P=.44$ for superiority). Ischemic stroke was significantly higher with low-dose edoxaban than with warfarin; consequently, that dose is not approved for stroke prevention. Major bleeding, as defined by the International Society of Thrombosis and Haemostasis, occurred 3.43%/year with warfarin compared with 2.75%/year with high-dose edoxaban (HR, 0.80; 95% CI, 0.71–0.91; $P<.001$) and 1.61% with low-dose edoxaban (HR, 0.47; 95% CI, 0.41–0.55; $P<.001$). Warfarin therapy had a higher rate of intracranial bleeding, 0.85%/year, compared with 0.39%/year with high-dose edoxaban and 0.26%/year with low-dose edoxaban ($P<.001$ for the comparison of warfarin with each dose of edoxaban). Gastrointestinal bleeding was highest in the high-dose edoxaban group (1.51%/year), followed by warfarin at 1.23%/year, and then low-dose edoxaban at 0.82%/year. The rates of major bleeding plus clinically relevant nonmajor bleeding were also lower in both doses of edoxaban as compared with warfarin (11.10%/year with high-dose edoxaban vs. 7.97%/year with low-dose edoxaban vs. 13.02%/year with warfarin). Both high-dose and low-dose edoxaban treatment groups had a reduction in the annualized rate of cardiovascular death (includes bleeding) compared with warfarin group (3.17% with warfarin vs. 2.74% with high-dose edoxaban [HR, 0.86; 95% CI, 0.77–0.97; $P=.01$] and 2.71% with low-dose edoxaban [HR, 0.85; 95% CI, 0.76–0.96; $P=.008$]). When the high-dose and low-dose edoxaban regimens were compared with each other, the primary efficacy end point of stroke and systemic embolism was lower in the high-dose edoxaban group ($P<.001$). This outcome was driven by a significant reduction in the incidence of ischemic stroke of 29% with high-dose edoxaban (236 vs. 333 events), which more than offset the lower incidence of hemorrhagic stroke in the low-dose edoxaban group. The FDA, but not other national regulatory bodies, has labeling that indicates that edoxaban should not be used in patients with a CrCl > 95 mL/min, as there was an apparent increased ischemic stroke risk in this subpopulation compared with warfarin group.

A metaanalysis of RE-LY, ROCKET-AF, ARISTOTLE, and ENGAGE-AF-TIMI 48 demonstrated a favorable risk-benefit profile of the NOACs compared with warfarin.[40] Including patients treated with doses of NOACs approved in the United States, there was a significantly lower risk of stroke or systemic embolism with NOACs, a more than 50% reduction in intracranial hemorrhage, and a statistically significant 10% reduction in all-cause mortality.

Table 3.1 compares the patient-level characteristics between the four trials. The number of women and age of enrollment were relatively similar between

TABLE 3.1
Baseline Characteristics of the Intention-to-Treat Populations in the NOAC Trials

	RE-LY			ROCKET-AF		ARISTOTLE		ENGAGE-AF-TIMI 48			COMBINED	
	Dabigatran 150 mg (n=6076)	Dabigatran 110 mg (n=6015)	Warfarin (n=6022)	Rivaroxaban (n=7131)	Warfarin (n=7133)	Apixaban (n=9120)	Warfarin (n=9081)	Edoxaban 60 mg (n=7035)	Edoxaban 30 mg (n=7034)	Warfarin (n=7036)	NOAC (n=42,411)	Warfarin (n=29,272)
Age (years)	71.5 (8.8)	71.4 (8.6)	71.6 (8.6)	73 (65–78)	73 (65–78)	70 (63–76)	70 (63–76)	72 (64–68)	72 (64–78)	72 (64–78)	71.6	71.5
≥75 years	40%	38%	39%	43%	43%	31%	31%	41%	40%	40%	38%	38%
Women	37%	36%	37%	40%	40%	36%	35%	39%	39%	38%	38%	37%
ATRIAL FIBRILLATION TYPE												
Persistent or permanent	67%	68%	66%	81%	81%	85%	84%	75%	74%	75%	76%	77%
Paroxysmal	33%	32%	34%	18%	18%	15%	16%	25%	26%	25%	24%	22%
CHADS$_2$[a]	2.2 (1.2)	2.1 (1.1)	2.1 (1.1)	3.5 (0.94)	3.5 (0.95)	2.1 (1.1)	2.1 (1.1)	2.8 (0.97)	2.8 (0.97)	2.8 (0.98)	2.6 (1.0)	2.6 (1.0)
0–1	32%	33%	31%	0	0	34%	34%	<1%	<1%	<1%	17%	17%
2	35%	35%	37%	13%	13%	36%	36%	46%	47%	47%	35%	33%
3–6	33%	33%	32%	87%	87%	30%	30%	54%	53%	53%	43%	50%
Previous stroke or TIA[a]	20%	20%	20%	55%	55%	19%	18%	28%	29%	28%	29%	30%
Heart failure[b]	32%	32%	32%	63%	62%	36%	35%	58%	57%	58%	46%	47%
Diabetes	23%	23%	23%	40%	40%	25%	25%	36%	36%	36%	31%	31%
Hypertension	79%	79%	79%	90%	91%	87%	88%	94%	94%	94%	88%	88%
Prior myocardial infarction	17%	17%	16%	17%	18%	15%	14%	11%	12%	12%	15%	15%

Continued

TABLE 3.1

Baseline Characteristics of the Intention-to-Treat Populations in the NOAC Trials—cont'd

	RE-LY			ROCKET-AF		ARISTOTLE		ENGAGE-AF-TIMI 48			COMBINED	
	Dabigatran 150 mg (n = 6076)	Dabigatran 110 mg (n = 6015)	Warfarin (n = 6022)	Rivaroxaban (n = 7131)	Warfarin (n = 7133)	Apixaban (n = 9120)	Warfarin (n = 9081)	Edoxaban 60 mg (n = 7035)	Edoxaban 30 mg (n = 7034)	Warfarin (n = 7036)	NOAC (n = 42,411)	Warfarin (n = 29,272)
CREATININE CLEARANCE[c]												
<50 mL/min	19%	19%	19%	21%	21%	17%	17%	20%	19%	19%	19%	19%
50–80 mL/min	48%	49%	49%	47%	48%	42%	42%	43%	44%	44%	45%	45%
>80 mL/min	32%	32%	32%	32%	31%	41%	41%	38%	38%	37%	36%	36%
Previous VKA use[d]	50%	50%	49%	62%	63%	57%	57%	59%	59%	59%	57%	57%
Aspirin at baseline	39%	40%	41%	36%	37%	31%	31%	29%	29%	30%	34%	34%
Median follow-up (years)[e]	20	20	20	1.9	1.9	1.8	1.8	2.8	2.8	2.8	2.2	2.2
Individual median TTR	NA	NA	NA	NA	58 (43–71)	NA	66 (52–77)	NA	NA	68 (57–77)	NA	65 (51–76)

Data are mean (SD), median (IQR), or percent, unless otherwise indicated. *AF*, atrial fibrillation; *CHADS$_2$*, stroke risk factor scoring system in which one point is given for history of congestive heart failure, hypertension, age ≥ 75 years, and diabetes, and two points are given for history of stroke or transient ischemic attack; *NA*, not available; *NOAC*, non–vitamin K oral anticoagulant oral anticoagulant; *TIA*, transient ischemic attack; *TTR*, time in therapeutic range; *VKA*, vitamin K antagonist.

[a]ROCKET-AF and ARISTOTLE included systemic embolism as criterion of stroke risk factor.

[b]ROCKET-AF included, as evidence for the heart failure risk factor, left ventricular ejection fraction <35%; ARISTOTLE included as risk factor of heart failure left ventricular ejection fraction <40%.

[c]RE-LY: <50, 50–79, ≥80 mL/min; ARISTOTLE: ≤50, >50–80, >80 mL/min.

[d]RE-LY, ARISTOTLE, and ENGAGE-AF-TIMI: 48 defined as patients who used VKAs for ≥60 days; ROCKET-AF patients who used VKAs for 6 weeks at time of screening.

[e]IQRs not available.

Adapted from Ruff CT, Giugliano RP, Braunwald E, et al. Comparison of the efficacy and safety of new oral anticoagulants with warfarin in patients with atrial fibrillation: a meta-analysis of randomized trials. *Lancet*. 2014;383:955–962.

trials. Notable differences were the underlying risk of stroke (as suggested by the mean CHADS$_2$ score), history of prior stroke or TIA, and the presence of systolic heart failure. Across the four phase III landmark trials, 42,411 patients received NOACs, whereas 29,272 patients were enrolled in the warfarin control arms. Patients allocated to receive a "high-dose" NOAC had a significant reduction in the composite of stroke and systemic embolism (19% reduction compared with warfarin, driven primarily by a significant reduction in intracranial hemorrhage; Fig. 3.2), as well as a significant reduction in all-cause mortality (Fig. 3.3). The rates of ischemic strokes and myocardial infarction were similar between those patients receiving a NOAC and warfarin. Patients receiving warfarin had significantly less gastrointestinal bleeding (Fig. 3.4). The low-dose NOAC regimens (dabigatran 110 mg and edoxaban 30 mg) had similar efficacy to warfarin in overall stroke prevention, but with an increase in ischemic stroke.

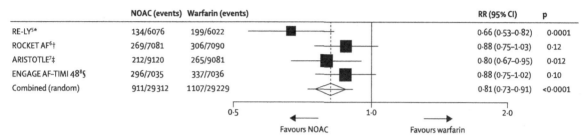

FIG. 3.2 Stroke and systemic embolism in the NOAC trials. (Adapted from Ruff CT, Giugliano RP, Braunwald E, et al. Comparison of the efficacy and safety of new oral anticoagulants with warfarin in patients with atrial fibrillation: a meta-analysis of randomized trials. *Lancet.* 2014;383:955–962.)

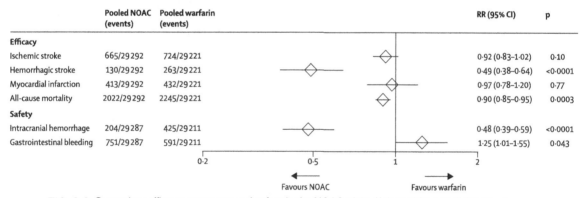

FIG. 3.3 Secondary efficacy outcomes and safety in the NOAC trials. (Adapted from Ruff CT, Giugliano RP, Braunwald E, et al. Comparison of the efficacy and safety of new oral anticoagulants with warfarin in patients with atrial fibrillation: a meta-analysis of randomized trials. *Lancet.* 2014;383:955–962.)

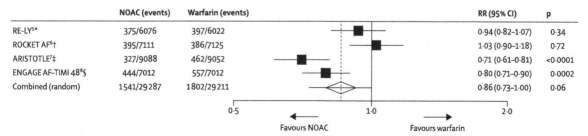

FIG. 3.4 Major bleeding in the NOAC trials. (Adapted from Ruff CT, Giugliano RP, Braunwald E, et al. Comparison of the efficacy and safety of new oral anticoagulants with warfarin in patients with atrial fibrillation: a meta-analysis of randomized trials. *Lancet.* 2014;383:955–962.)

There have been many analyses and publications regarding subgroup populations from the NOAC versus warfarin trials. In general, the effects of the NOACs versus warfarin have been consistent across subgroups. This includes the high-risk populations of the elderly, the frail with high fall risk, and patients with moderate renal insufficiency (although patients with a CrCl of <30 mL/min were generally excluded from the trials).

RHEUMATIC ATRIAL FIBRILLATION

The risk of stroke or systemic embolism is increased in patients with AF and MS as compared with patients with nonrheumatic AF.[41] This difference is thought to be secondary to left atrial remodeling, fibrosis, and calcification in the setting of chronic pressure overload, which predisposes to stasis and endocardial injury.[42] VKAs have long been prescribed to prevent thromboembolic events in patients with rheumatic AF and in patients who have undergone valve replacement. Early studies on the natural history of rheumatic MS suggested that as many as 30% of patients experienced an embolic event during the course of the disease, most commonly in the form of a stroke.[43,44]

Because of the high thrombotic risk associated with rheumatic AF, the majority of NOAC clinical trials excluded patients with rheumatic MS and those patients who had valve replacement with a mechanical prosthesis. Only one trial has studied the clinical efficacy and safety of a NOAC against warfarin in patients with a mechanical heart valve. The RE-ALIGN trial (Randomized, Phase II Study to Evaluate the Safety and Pharmacokinetics of Oral Dabigatran Etexilate in Patients After Heart Valve Replacement) evaluated dabigatran at doses of 150, 220, and 300 mg twice daily (to achieve a serum trough level of at least 50 ng/mL) in patients with mechanical heart valves at the aortic and/or mitral position.[45] The study was terminated early because of an excess of thromboembolic and bleeding events in the dabigatran group. Consequently, use of a NOAC for stroke prevention in patients with a mechanical prosthesis has a Class III warning for harm from the ACC/AHA/HRS 2014 guidelines.[10]

Each of the trials comparing NOACs with warfarin included patients with various degrees of valvular heart disease. The ARISTOTLE trial included around 26% of patients with a history of moderate or severe valvular heart disease or prior valve surgery. Patients with valvular heart disease were noted to have higher rates of stroke or systemic embolism (3.2% vs. 2.4% respectively; HR, 1.34; 95% CI, 1.10–1.62; P=.003) and an increased risk of death (9.1% vs. 6.2%; HR, 1.48; 95% CI, 1.32–1.67;

P<.001) as compared with those without valvular heart disease.[46] The efficacy and safety of apixaban versus warfarin is consistent among patients with and without valvular heart disease. Similarly, the effects of rivaroxaban versus warfarin were consistent in the 14.1% of patients in ROCKET-AF with "significant valvular heart disease."[47] Dabigatran was similarly as safe and effective as warfarin in the RE-LY trial irrespective of the presence of valvular heart disease that was present in 22% of enrolled patients.[48] In the ENGAGE-AF trial, edoxaban had similar safety and efficacy versus warfarin in patients with and without valvular heart disease and in patients with bioprosthetic heart valves.[49,50] The common nature of valvular heart disease in the trials evaluating NOACs, and the consistent findings of the effects, has led the European guidelines to abandon the term "nonvalvular" AF as a confusing misnomer.[9]

UNANSWERED QUESTIONS AND FUTURE TRIALS

Drug development over the past 10 years has dramatically changed the pharmacologic landscape for stroke prevention in AF. When compared with warfarin, NOACs have demonstrated at least comparable efficacy with a more favorable safety profile, while obviating some of the pharmacologic barriers inherent to VKA dosing and monitoring. As the drug development search for reversal agents continues (idarucizumab is commercially available for dabigatran reversal),[51] it is evident that major bleeding with NOACs in clinical trials is comparable or better than warfarin, and intracranial hemorrhage is much less likely. Despite all the advancements and trials that have been completed, there is still much to be answered about anticoagulation management in AF. Numerous trials are ongoing to further delineate the safety and efficacy of NOACs in various patient populations with AF, such as acute coronary syndromes with percutaneous coronary intervention (AUGUSTUS)[52] and end-stage renal disease (RENAL-AF).[53] In addition, because of their ease of administration and more favorable safety profile, a trial is ongoing to determine the threshold for anticoagulation in patients with device-detected (pacemaker/defibrillator) asymptomatic AF (ARTESiA).[54]

REFERENCES

1. Colilla S, Crow A, Petkun W, Singer DE, Simon T, Liu X. Estimates of current and future incidence and prevalence of atrial fibrillation in the U.S. adult population. *Am J Cardiol*. 2013;112:1142–1147.

2. Glazer NL, Dublin S, Smith NL, et al. Newly detected atrial fibrillation and compliance with antithrombotic guidelines. *Arch Intern Med.* 2007;167:246–252.

3. Lewis WR, Fonarow GC, LaBresh KA, et al. Differential use of warfarin for secondary stroke prevention in patients with various types of atrial fibrillation. *Am J Cardiol.* 2009;103:227–231.

4. Ogilvie IM, Newton N, Welner SA, et al. Underuse of oral anticoagulants in atrial fibrillation: a systematic review. *Am J Med.* 2010;123:638–645.

5. Waldo AL, Becker RC, Tapson VF, et al. Hospitalized patients with atrial fibrillation and a high risk of stroke are not being provided with adequate anticoagulation. *J Am Coll Cardiol.* 2005;46:1729–1736.

6. Zimetbaum PJ, Thosani A, Yu HT, et al. Are atrial fibrillation patients receiving warfarin in accordance with stroke risk? *Am J Med.* 2010;123:446–453.

7. van Walraven C, Jennings A, Oake N, et al. Effect of study setting on anticoagulation control: a systematic review and metaregression. *Chest.* 2006;129:1155–1166.

8. Baker WL, Cios DA, Sander SD, et al. Meta-analysis to assess the quality of warfarin control in atrial fibrillation patients in the United States. *J Manag Care Pharm.* 2009;15:244–252.

9. Kirchhof P, Benussi S, Kotecha D, et al. 2016 ESC Guidelines for the management of atrial fibrillation developed in collaboration with EACTS. *Eur Heart J.* 2016;37:2893–2962.

10. January CT, Wann LS, Alpert JS, et al. 2014 AHA/ACC/HRS guideline for the management of patients with atrial fibrillation: executive summary: a report of the American College of Cardiology/American Heart Association Task Force on practice guidelines and the Heart Rhythm Society. *Circulation.* 2014;130:2071–2104.

11. Petersen P, Boysen G, Godtfredsen J, Andersen ED, Andersen B. Placebo- controlled, randomised trial of warfarin and aspirin for prevention of thromboembolic complications in chronic atrial fibrillation. The Copenhagen AFASAK study. *Lancet.* 1989;1:175–179.

12. Stroke Prevention in Atrial Fibrillation Study. Final results. *Circulation.* 1991;84:527–539.

13. Secondary prevention in non-rheumatic atrial fibrillation after transient ischaemic attack or minor stroke. EAFT (European Atrial Fibrillation Trial) Study Group. *Lancet.* 1993;342:1255–1262.

14. Diener HC, Lowenthal A. Antiplatelet therapy to prevent stroke: risk of brain hemorrhage and efficacy in atrial fibrillation. *J Neurol Sci.* 1997;153:112.

15. Benavente O, Hart R, Koudstaal P, Laupacis A, McBride R. Antiplatelet therapy for preventing stroke in patients with atrial fibrillation and no previous history of stroke or transient ischemic attacks. In: Warlow C, Van Gijn J, Sandercock P, eds. *Stroke Module of the Cochrane Database of Systematic Reviews.* Oxford, UK: The Cochrane Collaboration; 1999.

16. Posada IS, Barriales V. Alternate-day dosing of aspirin in atrial fibrillation. LASAF Pilot Study Group. *Am Heart J.* 1999;138:137–143.

17. Japan Atrial Fibrillation Stroke Trial Group. Low-dose aspirin for prevention of stroke in low-risk patients with atrial fibrillation: Japan Atrial Fibrillation Stroke Trial. *Stroke.* 2006;37:447–451.

18. Hart RG, Pearce LA, Aguilar MI. Meta-analysis: antithrombotic therapy to prevent stroke in patients who have nonvalvular atrial fibrillation. *Ann Intern Med.* 2007;146(12):857–867.

19. Freedman BS, Gersh BJ, Lip GY. Misperceptions of aspirin efficacy and safety may perpetuate anticoagulant underutilization in atrial fibrillation. *Eur Heart J.* 2015;36:653–656.

20. Connolly SJ, Pogue J, Hart RG, et al. Effect of clopidogrel added to aspirin in patients with atrial fibrillation. *N Engl J Med.* 2009;360:2066–2078.

21. Connolly S, Pogue J, Hart R, et al. Clopidogrel plus aspirin versus oral anticoagulation for atrial fibrillation in the Atrial Fibrillation Clopidogrel Trial with Irbesartan for prevention of Vascular Events (ACTIVE W): a randomised controlled trial. *Lancet.* 2006;367:1903–1912.

22. Connolly SJ, Eikelboom JW, Ng J, et al. Net clinical benefit of adding clopidogrel to aspirin therapy in patients with atrial fibrillation for whom vitamin K antagonists are unsuitable. *Ann Intern Med.* 2011;155(9):579.

23. Connolly SJ, Eikelboom J, Joyner C, et al. Apixaban in patients with atrial fibrillation. *N Engl J Med.* 2011;364:806–817.

24. Flaker GC, Eikelboom JW, Shestakovska O, et al. *Stroke.* 2012;43:3291–3297.

25. Agarwal S, Hachamovitch M, Menon V. Current trial-associated outcomes with warfarin in prevention of stroke in patients with nonvalvular atrial fibrillation a meta-analysis. *Arch Intern Med.* 2012;172(8):623–631.

26. The Boston Area Anticoagulation Trial for Atrial Fibrillation Investigators, Singer DE, Hughes RA, et al. The effect of low-dose warfarin on the risk of stroke in patients with nonrheumatic atrial fibrillation. *N Engl J Med.* 1990;323:1505–1511.

27. Connolly SJ, Laupacis A, Gent M, Roberts RS, Cairns JA, Joyner C. Canadian Atrial Fibrillation Anticoagulation (CAFA) Study. *J Am Coll Cardiol.* 1991;18:349–355.

28. Ezekowitz MD, Bridgers SL, James KE, et al. Warfarin in the prevention of stroke associated with nonrheumatic atrial fibrillation. Veterans Affairs Stroke Prevention in Nonrheumatic Atrial Fibrillation Investigators. *N Engl J Med.* 1992;327:1406–1412.

29. Johnsen SP, Svendsen ML, Hansen ML, Brandes A, Mehnert F, Husted SE. Preadmission oral anticoagulant treatment and clinical outcome among patients hospitalized with acute stroke and atrial fibrillation: a nationwide study. *Stroke.* 2014;45(1):168–175.

30. Fang MC, Go AS, Chang Y, et al. A new risk scheme to predict warfarin-associated hemorrhage: the ATRIA (Anticoagulation and Risk Factors in Atrial Fibrillation) Study. *J Am Coll Cardiol.* 2011;58:395–401.

31. Ruiz-Gimenez N, Suarez C, Gonzalez R, et al. Predictive variables for major bleeding events in patients presenting with documented acute venous thromboembolism: findings from the RIETE Registry. *Thromb Haemost.* 2008;100:26–31.

32. Pisters R, Lane DA, Nieuwlaat R, et al. A novel user-friendly score (HAS-BLED) to assess 1-year risk of major bleeding in patients with atrial fibrillation: the Euro Heart Survey. *Chest.* 2010;138:1093–1100.

33. Mant J, Hobbs FD, Fletcher K, et al. Warfarin versus aspirin for stroke prevention in an elderly community population with atrial fibrillation (the Birmingham Atrial Fibrillation Treatment of the Aged Study, BAFTA): a randomised controlled trial. *Lancet.* 2007;370:493–503.

34. Jackson K, Gersh BJ, Stockbridge N, et al. Antithrombotic drug development for atrial fibrillation: proceedings, Washington, DC, July 25-27, 2005. *Am Heart J.* 2008;155:829–840.

35. Connolly SJ, Ezekowitz MD, Yusuf S, et al. Dabigatran versus warfarin in patients with atrial fibrillation. *N Engl J Med.* 2009;361:1139–1151.

36. Patel MR, Mahaffey KW, Garg J, et al. Rivaroxaban versus warfarin in nonvalvular atrial fibrillation. *N Engl J Med.* 2011;365:883–891.

37. Hori M, Matsumoto M, Tanahashi N, et al. Rivaroxaban vs. warfarin in Japanese patients with atrial fibrillation – the J-ROCKET AF study. *Circ J.* 2012;76(9):2104–2111. Epub 2012 Jun 5.

38. Granger CB, Alexander JH, McMurray JJ, et al. Apixaban versus warfarin in patients with atrial fibrillation. *N Engl J Med.* 2011;365:981–992.

39. Giugliano RP, Ruff CT, Braunwald E, et al. Edoxaban versus warfarin in patients with atrial fibrillation. *N Engl J Med.* 2013;369:2093–2104.

40. Ruff CT, Giugliano RP, Braunwald E, et al. Comparison of the efficacy and safety of new oral anticoagulants with warfarin in patients with atrial fibrillation: a meta-analysis of randomized trials. *Lancet.* 2014;383:955–962.

41. Wolf PA, Dawber TR, Thomas Jr HE, Kannel WB. Epidemiologic assessment of chronic atrial fibrillation and risk of stroke: the Framingham study. *Neurology.* 1978;28:973–977.

42. Shrestha NK, Moreno FL, Narciso FV, Torres L, Calleja HB. Two-dimensional echocardiographic diagnosis of left-atrial thrombus in rheumatic heart disease. A clinicopathologic study. *Circulation.* 1983;67(2):341–347.

43. Rowe JC, Bland EF, Sprague HB, White PD. The course of mitral stenosis without surgery: ten- and twenty-year perspectives. *Ann Intern Med.* 1960;52:741.

44. Coulshed N, Epstein EJ, McKendrick CS, Galloway RW, Walker E. Systemic embolism in mitral valve disease. *Br Heart J.* 1970;32(1):26.

45. Van de Werf F, Brueckmann M, Connolly SJ, et al. A comparison of dabigatran etexilate with warfarin in patients with mechanical heart valves: the Randomized, phase II study to Evaluate the sAfety and pharmacokinetics of oraL dabIGatran etexilate in patients after heart valve replacemeNt (RE-ALIGN). *Am Heart J.* 2012;163:931–937.

46. Avezum A, Lopes RD, Schulte PJ, et al. Apixaban in comparison with warfarin in patients with atrial fibrillation and valvular heart disease: findings from the apixaban for reduction in stroke and other thromboembolic events in atrial fibrillation (ARISTOTLE) trial. *Circulation.* 2015;132(8):624.

47. Breithardt G, Baumgartner H, Berkowitz SD, et al. Clinical characteristics and outcomes with rivaroxaban versus warfarin in patients with non-valvular atrial fibrillation but underlying native mitral and aortic valve disease participating in the ROCKET AF trial. *Eur Heart J.* 2014;35: 3377–3385.

48. Ezekowitz MD, Nagarakanti R, Noack H, et al. Comparison of dabigatran and warfarin in patients with atrial fibrillation and valvular heart disease: the RE-LY trial (randomized evaluation of long-term anticoagulant therapy). *Circulation.* 2016;134:589–598.

49. De Caterina R, Renda G, Carnicelli AP, et al. Valvular heart disease patients on edoxaban or warfarin in the ENGAGE AF-TIMI 48 trial. *J Am Coll Cardiol.* 2017;69:1372–1382.

50. Carnicelli AP, De Caterina R, Halperin JL, et al. Edoxaban for the prevention of thromboembolism in patients with atrial fibrillation and bioprosthetic valves. *Circulation.* 2017;135:1273–1275.

51. Pollack Jr CV, Reilly PA, van Ryn J, et al. Idarucizumab for dabigatran reversal – full cohort analysis. *N Engl J Med.* 2017;377(5):431–441. https://doi.org/10.1056/NEJMoa1707278. Epub 2017 Jul 11.

52. *An Open-label, 2 × 2 Factorial, Randomized Controlled, Clinical Trial to Evaluate the Safety of Apixaban vs. Vitamin K Antagonist and Aspirin vs. Aspirin Placebo in Patients with Atrial Fibrillation and Acute Coronary Syndrome or Percutaneous Coronary Intervention (AUGUSTUS).* Retrieved from: https://clinicaltrials.gov/ct2/show/NCT02415400 [Identification No. NCT02415400].

53. *Trial to Evaluate Anticoagulation Therapy in Hemodialysis Patients with Atrial Fibrillation (RENAL-AF).* Retrieved from: https://clinicaltrials.gov/ct2/show/NCT02942407 [Identification No. NCT02942407].

54. *Apixaban for the Reduction of Thrombo-embolism in Patients with Device-detected Sub-clinical Atrial Fibrillation (ARTESiA).* Retrieved from: https://clinicaltrials.gov/ct2/show/NCT01938248 [Identification No. NCT01938248].

Risk Stratification in Atrial Fibrillation

FARHAN SHAHID, MBBS, BSC • MIKHAIL DZESHKA, MD • EDUARD
SHANTSILA, MD, PHD • GREGORY Y.H. LIP, MD, FRCP, FACC, FESC

INTRODUCTION

Atrial fibrillation (AF) confers an increased risk of stroke, which has a greater morbidity and mortality risk than non-AF-related stroke.[1,2] Hence, stroke prevention in this population is a pivotal point in the management of AF. Up until recently, patients in need of stroke prevention were offered vitamin K antagonists (VKAs; e.g., warfarin). Over recent years, the landscape of oral anticoagulation (OAC) has dramatically changed to the point that there are now four alternative agents to warfarin, that is, the non-VKA oral anticoagulants (NOACs).[3] The comparable efficacy, lower risk of intracerebral hemorrhage (ICH), and convenience of the NOACs compared with well-managed warfarin have led to the update of clinical guidelines to emphasize the importance of early detection in management of patients diagnosed with AF. Specifically, NOACs are now recommended as a first-choice therapy in OAC-naïve patients, and switching to NOAC may be considered in those with low time in therapeutic range (TTR) despite good adherence or patient willing.[4]

However, the risk of stroke from AF is not homogenous and takes into account a number of risk factors, all of which are heterogeneous in their contribution to stroke risk in AF. These risk factors have been used to formulate risk stratification schemes, which are proposed to help assess stroke risk in patients with AF.[5] Such risk assessment strategies have been based on a consensus of opinion or clinical trials with the analysis of the nonwarfarin cohorts and various cohort studies to assess thromboembolic risk. The resulting schemas vary greatly in their complexity and number of risk factors.[6]

CHADS₂

The CHADS$_2$ (congestive heart failure, hypertension, age > 75 years, diabetes [all 1 point each]; previous stroke [2 points]) score is a simple scoring system using five common stroke risk factors, derived from the combination of two separate risk schemas based on the historical trials of SPAF (the Atrial Fibrillation Investigators

[AFI] and the SPAF-1 trial) and subsequently validated in a registry of hospitalized nonvalvular AF patients.[7]

In the collaborative analysis, AFI aimed to assess thromboembolic risk in AF patients who did not receive OAC and pooled the data from several trials, including Atrial Fibrillation, Aspirin, Anticoagulation Study from Copenhagen, Denmark (AFASAK); the Stroke Prevention in Atrial Fibrillation (SPAF) study; the Boston Area Anticoagulation Trial in Atrial Fibrillation (BAATAF); the Canadian Atrial Fibrillation Anticoagulation study; and the Veterans Affairs Stroke Prevention in Non-rheumatic Atrial Fibrillation (SPINAF) study who did not receive OAC.[8] Stroke risk factors identified in individual studies differed between each other, and therefore they were tested in a pooled cohort. In this analysis, independent risk factors for stroke were increasing age for each decade of life, history of hypertension, diabetes, and previous stroke or transient ischemic attack (TIA).[8]

A second SPAF analysis identified risk factors for stroke in patients treated with aspirin. Features putting patients at increased risk were identified and included women older than 75 years and those of either gender with systolic hypertension (>160 mmHg), prior thromboembolism, and impaired left ventricular function.[9] Gage et al. then amalgamated the two schemes and created the CHADS$_2$ score by modifying several features (*prior cerebral ischemia, history of hypertension, age > 75 years, recent* CHF, diabetes) and validated that these features corresponded to higher risk in a National Registry of Atrial Fibrillation consisting of 1733 Medicare beneficiaries aged 65–95 years with nonrheumatic AF not given warfarin at hospital discharge.[7]

The CHADS$_2$ score was recommended in the 2012 American College of Chest Physicians[10] as a tool to identify patients at higher risk for stroke who should be considered for anticoagulation. In original validation studies, "low-risk" patients were classed as having a CHADS$_2$ score of 0, moderate-risk patients as having a CHADS$_2$ score 1–2, and high-risk patients as having a CHADS$_2$ score > 2.[11] Such a categorization put >60% of patients into the "moderate-risk" category and may result in inappropriate decision with respect to stroke prevention, i.e., choice between OAC and aspirin. The assignment of either aspirin or OAC as treatment for moderate-risk patients suggested that either therapy was equivalent, which has been shown not to be the case, with a poor net clinical benefit of aspirin when compared with OAC in the prevention of AF-related stroke.[12] In addition, patients with previous stroke would score 2 and would be categorized as "moderate risk," even though previous stroke is a risk factor that conveys one of the highest risks of subsequent stroke. Given these shortcomings, more recent categorizations of $CHADS_2$ have redefined "moderate risk" as $CHADS_2$ score 1 and "high risk" as $CHADS_2$ score ≥ 2.[13]

Like most clinical risk scoring systems, various validation studies have found a modest predictive value of the $CHADS_2$ score with c-statistics approximately 0.6. Since the introduction of the $CHADS_2$ score, there has been the emergence of new data, which had not been extensively validated previously. Female sex, ages 65–74 years, and vascular disease are now recognized as good predictors of stroke in the AF population.[14] Indeed, the $CHADS_2$ score identifies "low-risk" patients less reliably, and even those with a $CHADS_2$ score of 0 can have a stroke rate as high as 3.2%/year.[15]

CHA_2DS_2VASc

Given the subsequent evidence that additional factors contribute to increased stroke risk in patients with AF, the European Society of Cardiology guidelines incorporated the "CHA_2DS_2VASc score" as the preferred schema to assess stroke risk. To date, this is the commonest risk stratification schema. One advantage of CHA_2DS_2VASc over the $CHADS_2$ score is the better ability to identify patients at truly low risk (i.e., CHA_2DS_2VASc score of 0 in males and 1 in females) of AF-related stroke, without contributing to increased complexity of use.[16,17] Scores range from 0 to 9 and emphasize the importance of "major risk factors" including age ≥ 75 years, which scores 2 points as part of the updated schema, and previous stroke or TIA, which also is given 2 points. Vascular disease is also incorporated into the scoring system and includes myocardial infarction, aortic plaque, and peripheral vascular disease. Female sex was given acknowledgment as being a higher risk factor for AF-related stroke than male gender.[14] With CHA_2DS_2VASc, one point is given to previously established risk factors (systolic heart failure, hypertension, diabetes, ages 65–74 years). Renal impairment is not part of the CHA_2DS_2VASc score and has not been shown to add independent prognostic information for AF-related stroke.[18]

The CHA_2DS_2VASc score was first described in 1996 and termed the Birmingham schema algorithm.[19] This risk stratification tool was distributed locally and regionally and used to encourage general practitioners to identify AF patients at "high risk" of stroke. In the United Kingdom, the National Institute for Health and Care Excellence adopted this approach in its 2006 guidelines for stroke risk assessment of AF patients.[20,21]

The CHA_2DS_2VASc score was shown to improve risk stratification compared with the $CHADS_2$ score and other risk stratification schema in a 2010 analysis involving 1084 patients in the Euro Heart Survey for AF.[19] The CHA_2DS_2VASc showed acceptable predictability for high-risk patients but was particularly good in identifying low-risk patients (those with a stroke risk of <1%/year with a CHA_2DS_2VASc score = 0 in males or 1 in females), thus avoiding incorrect placement of patients into the moderate-risk group.[22,23] Indeed, a large Danish cohort study (73,538 patients) found clear benefit of the CHA_2DS_2VASc score over the $CHADS_2$ in predicting stroke and thromboembolism, especially among those previously categorized as low risk with the older score.[24] Broadly, similar observations have been found from other studies.[16,25]

R_2CHADS_2 SCORE

Studies dating back 20 years have provided evidence of the adverse prognosis of renal dysfunction in animal stroke models.[26] Recent human "real-world" prospective studies have shown that patients with an acute stroke and a severely reduced estimated glomerular filtration rate (eGFR) have higher mortality in comparison with those with moderate renal dysfunction.[27] An eGFR below 60 mL/min/1.73 m^2 is associated with a significant adverse prognosis with regard to stroke and death over a 2-year period ($P < .05$).[28] Furthermore, renal impairment was independently associated with higher risk of death in AF patients.

The R_2CHADS_2 score was defined by adding two points for renal impairment to the $CHADS_2$ score, being derived from a subanalysis of the ROCKET AF trial.[29] In this highly selected anticoagulated trial cohort, those with moderate renal dysfunction were found to be at higher risk of AF-related stroke. However, patients with an eGFR < 30 mL/min were excluded from the ROCKET AF trial and thus conclusions regarding the impact of severe renal dysfunction cannot be drawn from this subanalysis. Further validation in a Swedish AF cohort study have not shown any additive value of one or two points for chronic kidney disease when added to the $CHADS_2$ or CHA_2DS_2VASc scores.[30]

QSTROKE SCORE

The QStroke score is a complex weighted formula with 17 variables and separate calculations for males and females. It was derived to calculate the risk of stroke in both AF and non-AF patients. Included in this scoring system were current variables derived from the QRISK2, Framingham, and the CHA_2DS_2VASc scores.[31] Patient demographics from 451 general practices throughout England and Wales, totaling 3.5 million patients, were used to calculate this algorithm.

Validation of this scoring system included 1.9 million patients aged between 25 and 84 years with a total of 38,404 strokes experienced during the study duration. Among patients with AF, the QStroke score showed a statistically improved performance over the CHA_2DS_2VASc and $CHADS_2$ scores (although marginal), and the c-statistics for all three scores were still approximately 0.6.[31] Of note, patients with a history of stroke or TIA were excluded in the derivation of this scoring system, despite this being one of the strongest predictors of subsequent stroke.[19]

ATRIA STROKE SCORE

Before the introduction of both the $CHADS_2$ and CHA_2DS_2VASc scores, the AnTicoagulation and Risk factors In AF (ATRIA) cohort was established.[32] The ATRIA score was first derived and subsequently validated using data from the ATRIA cohort with follow-up only in patients who had an ongoing healthcare plan.[32,33] This score encompasses a point score range of 0–12 or 7–15 depending on whether there was a history of previous stroke, that is, different assigned points applied to a primary or secondary prevention cohort. The complexity of the ATRIA scoring system does not allow for simple and quick decision-making in clinical settings. Since its original paper, various large studies have found the CHA_2DS_2VASc to outperform the ATRIA score in predicting stroke risk.[34,35]

In a recent large Swedish cohort study including 152,153 patients with AF who were never on warfarin, a comparison of the predictive values of ATRIA, $CHADS_2$, and CHA_2DS_2VASc risk scores showed that the c-statistic for the ATRIA score was statistically significantly higher than that of the CHA_2DS_2VASc score. However, when categorical scores were optimized (i.e., instead of originally published cut-points of 0–5 points for low risk, 6 points for moderate risk, and 7–15 points for high risk, they were adjusted to fit local population incidence of ischemic stroke of <1%/year for low risk, 1%–2%/year for moderate risk, and ≥2%/year for high risk), there was no longer any advantage

of the ATRIA score.[17] In addition, the cohort studied was restricted to patients who did not use anticoagulant therapy during the follow-up period, which results in "conditioning on the future" and biasing outcomes toward lower event rates by excluding the (high-risk) subjects who needed to be started on OAC over the follow-up period.[36]

DO BIOMARKERS IMPROVE RISK ASSESSMENT FOR ATRIAL FIBRILLATION–RELATED STROKE?

The addition of biomarkers ("biologic markers"), whether blood, urine, or imaging (cardiac or cerebral), has been proposed as a means of improving stroke risk stratification in AF patients.[37,38] Biomarkers will always improve on the predictive capability of clinical risk scores, at least statistically.

Among biomarkers that were shown to be associated with heightened stroke risk in AF and therefore might be incorporated into stroke risk scores to improve their prediction ability, there are markers of inflammation (C-reactive protein and scope of cytokines), coagulation activity (D-dimer), cardiovascular stress (natriuretic peptides, growth differentiation factor 15), myocardial injury (troponins), myocardial fibrosis (galectin 3, soluble ST2), endothelial dysfunction (Von Willebrand factor), and renal dysfunction (creatinine, cystatin C).[39]

Biomarkers have long been used for diagnostic purposes and to guide therapy of cardiovascular conditions (e.g., heart failure). However, with the introduction of contemporary high-sensitivity laboratory assays, which have made detection of circulating biomarkers possible at lower thresholds, biomarkers are now widely implicated in management of stable diseases, associated with presumably lower cardiomyocytes damage, myocardial wall stress, and heart dysfunction.

Of the range of tested biomarkers, the highest evidence in AF was obtained for cardiac troponins and natriuretic peptides by their utilization in large AF cohorts of phase 3 stroke prevention trials on NOACs. In the RE-LY trial, patients with troponin I concentration below 10 ng/L (nondetectable) had significantly lower rate of stroke (0.84%/year) compared with those with detectable troponin I level with 10 ng/L increment. The highest stroke and systemic embolism rate of 2.09%/year was observed in patients with troponin I above 40 ng/L (hazards ratio [HR] 1.99, 95% confidence interval [CI] 1.17–3.39).[40] Consistent findings were obtained in the Apixaban for Reduction in Stroke and Other Thromboembolic Events in Atrial

Fibrillation (ARISTOTLE) trial cohort, in which both troponin I and T were detected even at lower concentration, and an increase in biomarkers within normal range was predictive of stroke, major bleeding, and cardiovascular and total mortality.[41,42]

Brain natriuretic peptide (BNP) and its amino terminal precursor (NT-proBNP) were also tested for refinement of stroke prediction in AF. In the RE-LY cohort, only patients with NT-proBNP level higher than 1402 ng/L had higher risk of stroke and systemic embolism (2.3%/year), where NT-proBNP less than 387 ng/L served as reference (0.92%/year; HR 2.40, 95% CI 1.41–4.07).[40] In the ARISTOTLE trial cohort, annual rates of cardiac death ranged from 0.86% in lower quartile to 4.14% in upper quartile (HR 2.50, 95% CI 1.81–3.45).[43]

Both troponins and natriuretic peptides provided improved prognostic discrimination for stroke risk when added to CHADS$_2$ and CHA$_2$DS$_2$-VASc score, but net reclassification improvement was particularly apparent for the risk of cardiovascular death.[40–43] The latter may point out that either high normal troponin levels or increasing natriuretic peptide levels reflects those pathological changes in myocardium, which are due to coronary heart disease, heart failure, aging, etc., i.e., risk factors already present in clinical stroke risk scores, rather than adding truly independent predictive information for thromboembolism. Measurement of biomarkers therefore may be attractive in AF because they are capable of detection of myocardial stress or injury at subclinical or early clinical stages. This was realized with derivation and validation of ABC stroke risk score.[37] However, before wide use of biomarkers in routine clinical practice, one should consider the following.

Biomarkers provide more accurate risk assessment but at the expense of being less simple and practical for "quick" decision-making in busy clinics or wards. Furthermore, there would be added expense and delay in getting such results. In addition, logic would dictate that event rates for a particular CHA$_2$DS$_2$VASc score or biomarker level would also vary by population and study setting.

More recent validations of biomarkers for risk stratification have been conducted in highly selected anticoagulated trial cohorts, and the true additive value of a biomarker to stroke risk needs be derived from AF cohorts with no antithrombotic therapy.[37] In addition, many biomarkers may have important interlaboratory or intralaboratory assay variability, and some may have a diurnal variation or be influenced by concomitant drug therapies. Lastly, some biomarkers are also

predictive of stroke, bleeding, and death, and the nonspecialist clinician dealing with the AF patient would have to juggle all these endpoints, counsel the patient, and make therapeutic decisions accordingly.

Therefore, for busy clinicians seeing an AF patient, would one see a recently diagnosed, anticoagulation-naive AF patient and measure some 10–20 biomarkers (at huge expense and delay), and then bring the patient back weeks later to inform him/her of his/her AF-related stroke risk? Notwithstanding that even a single stroke risk factor matters and that CHA$_2$DS$_2$VASc reliably identifies low-risk AF patients with event rates < 1%/year (considered the stroke threshold for initiating OAC, especially with the NOACs), the practical approach for everyday clinical practice would be to initially identify low risk quickly and simply (i.e., a CHA$_2$DS$_2$-VASc score of 0 in males, or 1 in females), as these patients do not need any antithrombotic therapy.

Of course, management of cardiovascular patients is continuously improving, and mobile applications have a role in current progress. They simplify keeping records and calculations, aiding risk assessment and clinical decisions. Incorporation of more patient's data to get more precise endpoint estimates in future may be even more attractive. Whether more precise estimates of risk stratification will change management remains to be seen.

THE ABC-STROKE SCORE

The ABC score refers to age, biomarkers (NT-proBNP and high-sensitivity troponins), and clinical history. This scoring system was internally validated in 14,701 nonvalvular AF patients and externally validated in 1400 patients with AF over a median follow-up of 3.4 years. When compared with the "gold standard" CHA$_2$DS$_2$VASc score, the ABC score performed favorably, with c-indices of 0.66, $P < .001$ in the externally validated cohort.[37] Although one can argue the ABC score is easier to remember, it is not a simple 1- to 2-point scoring system and depends on the availability of biomarker tests that may not be available in all hospitals and may be subject to assay and diurnal variability.

The strengths of the ABC-stroke score study include the large derivation and validation cohort sizes, with good calibration, as the prediction of events was similar in both cohorts. The major limitation of this study is that all the patients in RE-LY and half the patients in ARISTOTLE (upon which this score was validated) were on anticoagulants. Therefore, when trying to apply this score to an anticoagulant-naïve population will it be

TABLE 4.1
Comparison of Risk Assessment Schemas in Patients Being Considered for Thromboprohylaxis in Atrial Fibrillation–Related Stroke

Risk Factor	CHADS$_2$	CHA$_2$DS$_2$VASc	R$_2$CHADS$_2$	QStroke	ATRIA	ABC
Age (years)	≥75	65–74; ≥75	≥75	25–84	≥65	44–90
Female	✗	✓	✗	✓	✓	✗
Previous stroke/TE events	✓	✓	✓	✗	✓	✓
Hypertension	✓	✓	✓	✓	✓	✗
Heart failure	✓	✓	✓	✓	✓	✗
Diabetes	✓	✓	✓	✓	✓	✗
Vascular disease	✗	✓	✗	✓	✗	✗
eGFR < 60 mL/min/1.73 m^2	✗	✗	✓	✗	✗	✗
Moderate/severe CKD	✗	✗	✗	✗	✓	✗
Atrial fibrillation	✗	✗	✗	✓	✗	✗
Proteinuria	✗	✗	✗	✗	✓	✗
Troponin I (ng/L)	✗	✗	✗	✗	✗	✓
NT-proBNP (ng/L)	✗	✗	✗	✗	✗	✓

✓ indicates inclusion of the parameter; ✗ means exclusion of the parameter.
The QStroke score includes additional risk factors of ethnicity, deprivation score, smoking status, total cholesterol:HDL ratio, body mass index, family history of coronary disease, rheumatoid arthritis, valvular heart disease.
CKD, chronic kidney disease; *eGFR*, estimated glomerular filtration rate; *TE*, thromboembolism.

accurate? Furthermore, biomarkers are not a static measure and change with time; therefore, frequent blood tests to measure biomarkers may be warranted.

Table 4.1 summarizes the risk factors involved in calculating stroke risk in the major risk stratification models, and Fig. 4.1 represents a guide to help in the risk stratification and management of patients with AF with regard to OAC. The SAMe-TT$_2$R$_2$ (sex female, age < 60 years, medical history [more than two comorbidities], treatment [interacting drugs, e.g., amiodarone for rhythm control], tobacco use [doubled], race [doubled]) score is incorporated into this table. Although not used to risk stratify likelihood of stroke in AF patients, the SAMe-TT$_2$R$_2$ scoring system was derived and validated to identify patients who would be both suitable but maybe more importantly not suitable for warfarin and hence benefit from NOAC therapy as first-line treatment.[44]

Despite numerous risk factors being linked to stroke risk in AF, their incorporation into stroke risk models must be balanced against practical use and the net benefit in predicting stroke risk in busy hospital settings. To date the commonest risk stratification schema used for AF patients to assess stroke risk is the CHA$_2$DS$_2$VASc score, which best suits current approach to prevent stroke and systemic embolism in AF, i.e., exclude truly low-risk patients and offer OAC to the rest of them.

ASSESSMENT OF BLEEDING RISK IN PATIENTS WITH ATRIAL FIBRILLATION

Bleeding risk assessment is another important component in the assessment of patients with AF who are being considered for OAC. Like stroke risk, bleeding risk assessment in AF patients has been the subject of much misinterpretation on its purpose and use.[45] Bleeding risk factors are often modifiable, and the appropriate (and responsible) use of a bleeding risk score is to identify bleeding risk factors and correct those that are reversible. Where electronic health records are provided, automated "alert flags" can be assigned to patients potentially at risk of bleeding for more regular review, treatment, and follow-up.[45] Recent guidelines have focused on highlighting the reversible bleeding risk factors, as well as the nonreversible bleeding risk factors and biomarkers associated with increased bleeding. Of note is that the same biomarkers associated with bleeding are also associated with increased stroke, cardiovascular events, and mortality.[4,22]

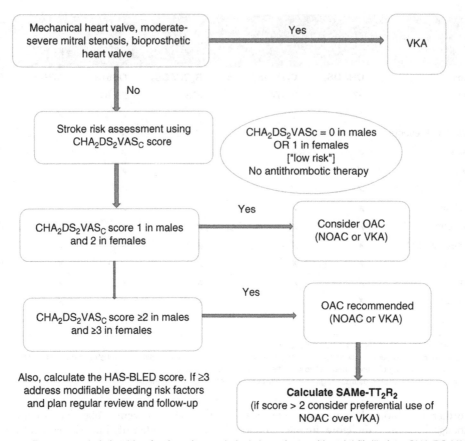

FIG. 4.1 Recommended algorithm for thromboprophylaxis in patients with atrial fibrillation. *CHA₂DS₂VASc score*, congestive heart failure, hypertension, age, diabetes, previous stroke/TIA, vascular disease; *NOAC*, non-VKA oral anticoagulant; *SAMe-TT₂R₂*, sex, age, medical history, treatment with interacting drugs, tobacco use, race; *VKA*, vitamin K antagonist.

Annual bleeding rates are between 1.3% and 7.2% in patients taking warfarin.[46] Patients with AF in whom OAC is appropriate may benefit from assessment of bleeding risk to maximize interventions to reduce this risk. Many of the risk factors associated with AF-related stroke also overlap with OAC-associated bleeding risk, but some of the latter risk factors are reversible. Thus, a balance must be achieved between providing appropriate stroke thromboprophylaxis while taking measures to minimize the incidence of bleeding. Several scores have been proposed to aid assessment of bleeding risk.[47–49]

HAS-BLED

The HAS-BLED (hypertension systolic blood pressure > 160 mmHg, abnormal liver/renal function [with creatinine 200 μmol/L], stroke, bleeding history or predisposition, labile international normalized ratio [INR; in range < 60% of the time], elderly [>65 years], and concomitant drugs/alcohol) score for assessment of bleeding risk in patients being considered for OAC is recommended by various guidelines.[4,49] The HAS-BLED score is a simple score that is the most widely validated in AF and non-AF populations, as well as in patients on no antithrombotic therapy, aspirin, or OAC and is, thus, applicable to patients at all stages of the patient management pathway.

The HAS-BLED score was developed and validated in 2010 using the Euro Heart Survey population.[49] The HAS-BLED score demonstrates a good predictive ability in this cohort with a c-statistic of 0.72, with excellent prediction of bleeding risk on antiplatelet therapy (c-statistic of 0.91) or no antithrombotic therapy (c-statistic of 0.85). Further validation studies have shown the HAS-BLED score to be an effective predictor of bleeding in warfarin-naïve patients and in those receiving warfarin plus aspirin or nonwarfarin anticoagulants.[50] The HAS-BLED has also been validated to predict bleeding in non-AF cohorts, including those with venous thromboembolism,[51] bridging therapy,[52] and acute coronary syndrome undergoing percutaneous coronary interventions.[53] Of note, it was shown to be predictive of ICH, the most feared complication of OAC.[54]

Many of the potentially reversible bleeding risk factors are contained within the HAS-BLED score; therefore, a high HAS-BLED score is not an excuse to withhold OAC, but rather helps identify correctable risk factors.[22,55,56] Recent studies have shown how other "new" bleeding risk scores would significantly underperform in VKA-treated patients, by not considering the quality of anticoagulation control (e.g., TTR), which is a parameter within the HAS-BLED score (the L or "labile INR" criterion).[54,57] This is important as VKA remains the most widely used OAC worldwide.

With HAS-BLED, patients are categorized into low-moderate risk with a score of 0–2 and high risk with a score$\geq$3. In a previous metaanalysis, the HAS-BLED score outperformed the HEMORR$_2$HAGES and ATRIA bleeding scores, with superior net reclassification improvements, most evident in low- and high-risk groups.[58] Similar findings have been found where the HAS-BLED score was more sensitive in predicting bleeding risk than both the HEMORR$_2$HAGES and ATRIA scores, with the added major benefit due to ease of use in everyday clinical practice.[59]

The superiority of the HAS-BLED score over other bleeding risk schemas is partially explained by the incorporation of the TTR, a criterion, which is only relevant to VKA users. Other bleeding risk scores (HEMORR$_2$HAGES, ATRIA, ORBIT—older age [$\geq$75 years], reduced hemoglobin/hematocrit/history of anemia, bleeding history, insufficient kidney function, and treatment with antiplatelet) fail to acknowledge the strong association with poor TTR and major bleeding[60] and may result in suboptimal bleeding risk assessment among patients on VKA therapy.

HEMORR$_2$HAGES

Another bleeding risk score is the HEMORR$_2$HAGES (hepatic or renal disease, ethanol abuse, malignancy, older age>75 years, reduced platelet count, rebleeding risk, uncontrolled hypertension, anemia, genetic factors—CYP2C9 single nucleotide polymorphisms, excessive falls risk, previous stroke/TIA).

The HEMORR$_2$HAGES risk score was the first bleeding risk score derived and validated in AF patients.

However, because of the complexity of information required to make accurate bleeding risk assessment, its use has become infrequent with the arrival of simpler bleeding risk scores. Genetic testing is rarely used and not widely available in all healthcare systems, and blood tests for anemia and platelet count must be available before assessment, which is not always the case. Furthermore, important factors such as use of concomitant medications and antiplatelet therapy are not considered with this bleeding risk score. Validation through the National Registry of Atrial Fibrillation showed better prediction than older risk scores (c-statistic of 0.67).[47]

The ATRIA bleeding score (anemia with hemoglobin <13 g/dL in males and <12 g/dL in females, severe renal disease with glomerular filtration rate<30 mL/min or dialysis dependent, age>75 years, prior bleeding, and hypertension) has been proposed as another alternative.[47,48]

The ATRIA bleeding risk score was first presented in 2010 and covered many of the risk factors already present in the HAS-BLED scoring system.[61] This complex weighted schema allocates three points for anemia, three points for severe renal disease, two points for age>75 years, and one point for either previous bleeding or hypertension. Thus, 5–10 points are deemed high bleeding risk. Validation cohorts have shown this score was superior in predicting bleeding events to the HEMORR2HAGES score, with a c-statistics of 0.74, with highest predictability in higher-risk groups of 5.8%.

However, the composition and risk factors used in the ATRIA score are less specified compared with other scoring systems. For example, a history of hypertension rather than uncontrolled hypertension is used. Concomitant use of aspirin and labile INRs if on warfarin (both being strongly related to bleeding risks) are also omitted from the score. A further study also found that of the 127 adjudicated major bleeding events, 21.3% of events occurred in the "low-risk" HAS-BLED category, compared with 96.6% for ATRIA. Adding "labile INR" to the ATRIA score has been shown to significantly improve its predictive ability for bleeding risks.[54]

ORBIT

The ORBIT score allocates one point for older age, two points for reduced hemoglobin/hematocrit/anemia, two points for bleeding history, one point for renal impairment, and finally one point for treatment with antiplatelet drugs.[62] Data for ORBIT were derived from an industry-sponsored observational registry and validated using the (anticoagulated) ROCKET AF trial cohort. The ROCKET AF trial recruited only high-risk patients with AF (i.e., $CHA_2DS_2VASc \geq 2$), and patients with severe renal impairment were omitted from the trial. In addition, warfarin-treated patients in the ROCKET AF trial had poor TTR (mean 55%), with the ORBIT-AF study using only patients who remained on warfarin as part of the derivation cohort. In a previous analysis, 87.4% of major bleeding events occurred in the "low-risk" category for ORBIT, and adding a "labile INR" criterion improved the predictive value of this score among VKA-treated patients.[54] Similar observations were noted in a post hoc analysis of 2293 patients with AF on OAC derived from the AMADEUS trial (Evaluating the Use of SR34006 Compared With Warfarin or Acenocoumarol in Patients With Atrial Fibrillation), where the HAS-BLED score outperformed the ATRIA and ORBIT schemas in predicting clinically relevant bleeding, and addition of TTR to both the ATRIA and ORBIT scores improved the predictive ability measured using c-statistics ($P = .001$ and $P = .002$, respectively).[57]

ABC BLEEDING SCORE

As with the ABC stroke risk score, the complexity of the bleeding score is a major limitation in the day-to-day use of this schema. The ABC bleeding score was validated in a large cohort of patients involved in the ARISTOTLE trial. Biomarker data were available for 14,537 ARISTOTLE participants, and major bleeding occurred in 662 subjects.[63]

In derivation of the ABC bleeding risk score, the strongest predictors of major bleeding among ARISTOTLE participants were growth differentiation factor 15 (GDF-15), hemoglobin, cardiac troponin T (cTnT-hs), age, and history of a bleed. These five variables were subsequently included in the ABC bleeding risk–prediction model, and its ability to predict major bleeding was compared with that of the HAS-BLED score and the newer ORBIT score.

The ABC bleeding risk score showed a c-index of 0.68, whereas HAS-BLED achieved a c-index of 0.61 and the ORBIT, a c-index of 0.65.[63] Although clinically and scientifically appealing, availability of such markers is neither efficient nor always available when rapid clinical decisions must be made regarding bleeding risk and its management in patients.

In summary, bleeding risk assessment is an important part of the clinical decision-making process. Given that, in vast majority of cases, benefits of OAC for stroke prevention outweigh risk of major bleeding, even elevated bleeding risk score has not been used as a reason to withhold OAC. Table 4.2 summarizes the key features included in the main bleeding risk assessment

tools. To date, the HAS-BLED score is the simplest, best validated, and clinical practice–centered tool to manage bleeding risk.

Simple yet methodical approach is best, such that the decision-making process for busy clinicians is helped by keeping concepts simple and practical. AF is so common, and the default should be to offer stroke prevention to all AF patients unless deemed to be at low risk. Risk stratification, either stroke or bleeding, is also not a "one-off" assessment but a dynamic process, reflecting the elderly AF population with a high rate of hospitalizations, comorbidities, and polypharmacy. Thus, risk assessment should not be performed once, e.g., before OAC initiation, but on a regular basis.

CENTRAL NERVOUS SYSTEM IMAGING TO REFINE STROKE AND BLEEDING RISK ASSESSMENT

With the higher availability of neuroimaging techniques such as magnetic resonance (MRI), increasing evidence for the presence of various brain lesions, often not associated with clinical presentation of ischemic events (i.e., ischemic stroke or TIA) or hemorrhagic events (i.e., hemorrhagic stroke, ICH), has emerged.

Among the spectrum of lesions, cerebral microinfarcts or silent brain infarctions (SBIs) represent a common finding with an estimated 40% prevalence of MRI-diagnosed lesions in stroke-free AF patients.[64] Of note, prevalence of SBI in elderly people without AF, as evidenced in the Rotterdam Scan Study cohort, is twofold lower.[65] They can be located subcortically or cortically, with the latter being considered amenable for accelerated cognitive decline in AF patients.[66] Mechanisms of SBI development include small vessel disease (e.g., atherosclerosis and cerebral amyloid angiopathy), cerebral hypoperfusion, and microembolism, which are likely to act synergistically, but microembolism is considered as the leading contributor in AF.[67]

AF was associated with higher probability of SBI (odds ratio [OR] 2.62, 95% CI 1.81–3.80) independently of paroxysmal or nonparoxysmal AF pattern in patients without stroke history.[64] In those with a history of stroke or TIA compared with their counterparts without detected arrhythmia, risk was even higher (OR 4.8, 95% CI 1.5–14.9).[68]

Apart from cognitive decline, SBI confers increased stroke risk independently of other established stroke risk factors, e.g., age, sex, hypertension, diabetes mellitus, AF, intima-media thickness, smoking, and history of TIA.[65] Metaanalysis has shown such an association to be uniform in various subgroups, i.e., stroke-free

CHAPTER 4   Risk Stratification in Atrial Fibrillation   **55**

TABLE 4.2
Comparison of risk factors used in assessment of bleeding risk in AF patients requiring OAC. The HAS BLED score uses an age >65 for elderly, whereas this is ≥75 in the ATRIA schema and >75 for HEMORR$_2$HAGES. (Reversible factors are highlighted in italics and underlined).

Risk Factor	Has Bled	Hemorr2Hages	Atria	Orbit	ABC
Hypertension	✓	✓	✓	✗	✗
Abnormal Liver/Renal function	✓	✓	✓	✓	✗
Stroke	✓	✓	✗	✗	✗
Bleeding/Rebleeding risk	✓	✓	✓	✓	✓
Liable INR	✓	✗	✗	✗	✗
Elderly	✓	✓	✓	✓	✓
Concomitant drugs/alcohol	✓	✓	✗	✓	✗
Malignancy	✗	✓	✗	✗	✗
Reduced PLT count/function	✗	✓	✗	✗	✗
Anaemia	✗	✓	✓	✓	✓
High falls risk	✗	✓	✗	✗	✗
Genetic factors	✗	✓	✗	✗	
cTnT-hs	✗	✗	✗	✗	✓
GDF-15	✗	✗	✗	✗	✓

individuals from general population (HR 2.06, 95% CI 1.64–2.59) and patients with a history of stroke (HR 2.00, 95% CI 1.08–3.71).[69] Unfortunately, AF patients represented only a minority of the study population; hence extrapolation of these findings should be treated with caution. In AF patients, two times higher incidence of symptomatic stroke was reported in Korean cohort during 5.5-year follow-up in those patients who did have silent stroke based on MRI at baseline (5.6% vs. 2.7%/year; HR 1.79, 95% CI 1.09–2.93).[70]

However, on a background of limited evidence, screening for SBIs and their implication to guide OAC as stroke prevention therapy cannot be supported at present time.[67] Albeit many studies confirm a prognostic role of SBI, the data are derived from heterogeneous populations with application of differing study designs and therefore were not always consistent. Bias from technical aspects of MRI should also be considered.[67] Furthermore, despite claims for the independent prognostic value of imaging markers, they share many risk factors, e.g., age, hypertension, kidney dysfunction,[70,71] and therefore their additive role in stroke risk assessment might be redundant. Given that even single stroke risk factor carries excess of stroke risk, i.e., above 1%/year, and necessitates OAC as the only effective means of prevention, intentional or odd detection of SBI via

neuroimaging will not affect decision-making in AF patients, because they are unlikely to be of low stroke risk based on clinical assessment with the CHA$_2$DS$_2$-VASc score to exclude them from OAC.[72] On the other hand, where SBIs are detected in low-risk patients, no sufficient evidence is available thus far to initiate OAC. The same applies for another type of ischemic lesions—white matter hyperintensities or leukoaraiosis, which are mostly attributable to small vessel disease, and their prevalence and prognostic significance have been even less addressed in AF patients.[67]

Cerebral microbleeds (CMBs) are another common finding in neuroimaging that correspond to small foci of hemosiderin accumulation because of capillary-derived hemorrhage or small artery leakage. Anatomically, CMBs can appear in the cortex and are attributable to amyloid angiopathy, whereas subcortical CMBs are considered to be a consequence of hypertensive angiopathy.[73] Similarly to SBIs, prevalence of CMBs increases with age.[74] In the Rotterdam Scan Study, CMBs ranged from 6.5% in patients aged 45–50 years to 35.7% in those aged 80 years and older. At least one CMB was detected in 15.3% of study participants.[75]

CMBs are more prevalent in patients with AF,[74,76] but association of AF and CMB might merely reflect shared vascular risk factors, e.g., age and hypertension.[67]

Perhaps, because of overlap of risk factors for ischemic and bleeding events, CMBs were found to be predictive of ischemic lesions (e.g., SBI and white matter hyperintensities on MRI as well as stroke recurrence),[76,77] and association of the presence and number of CMBs with CHA_2DS_2-VASc score was yielded.[78] However, CMBs attracted more attention as a marker of bleeding risk.[79] Indeed more CMBs were shown in patients on OAC,[74] and they were found to have predictive role for ICH (relative risk [RR] 7.7, 95% CI 4.1–14.7).[80] Of note, single CMB might be benign in terms of ICH development, whereas multiple CMBs were associated with higher incidence of future ICH (RR 8.0, 95% CI 3.2–20.0).[80]

Is there a need to perform MRI for CMB assessment and subsequent adjustment of stroke prevention therapy in AF patients? Current data are limited and therefore do not advocate this.[79] There were suggestions made to tailor OAC based on the number and location of CMB; for example, according to one algorithm, neurologic consultation, repeated MRI scans, and nonvitamin K oral anticoagulants were suggested in case of "high risk," defined as lobar cortical CMB, or five and more subcortical CMBs; and OAC discontinuation in case of CMB progression on repeated MRI.[73]

Notwithstanding higher risk of ICH when CMBs are detected, OAC for stroke prevention always brings positive net clinical benefit, where low stroke risk is not a case, which increases with higher stroke and bleeding risk.[81] Reinitiation of anticoagulation after a bleeding event, including ICH, is often clinically justified.[4] In the recent metaanalysis that included 5306 ICH cases, reinitiation of OAC was associated with significantly lower risk of thromboembolic complications (RR 0.34, 95% CI 0.25–0.45) with no elevation in risk of recurrent ICH.[82]

Therefore, routine incorporation of neuroimaging in AF management path as well as imaging-detected asymptomatic SBI and CMB in stroke and bleeding risk assessment in AF patients is lacking sufficient evidence thus far; it will require additional costs and unlikely improve stroke risk prevention compared with current practice.

DOES EVERYONE WITH ATRIAL FIBRILLATION NEED STROKE RISK ASSESSMENT?

Previous large-scale registry analysis identified a vast underutilization of OAC in "high-risk" patients who were admitted with a stroke over a 4-year period. In 29% of the patients admitted with an acute stroke deemed secondary to AF, only 40% were on OAC in

the form of warfarin. Furthermore, 75% of patients taking warfarin were found to have a subtherapeutic INR (<2.0) on admission. Only 18% were on appropriate antithrombotic therapy with INR in acceptable range.[83]

Further systemic reviews have highlighted the underuse of appropriate OAC in AF patients, especially in those regarded as high-risk from AF-related stroke.[84] The hesitancy by physicians to prescribe OAC for patients who would clearly benefit from such prophylaxis is not entirely understood. This reluctance has also been found when studying patients' opinions toward OAC and bleeding risk.[85] One such hypothesis is that there is an overestimation of bleeding risk of patients with AF, and this acts as a deterrent from anticoagulation. This particularly holds true for the elderly population, where aspirin is wrongly thought of as a safer alternative for stroke prophylaxis.[12] Since the introduction of NOACs, the "tipping point," i.e., point at which benefits from stroke prevention with OAC are balanced with hazards of hemorrhagic complications, for initiating anticoagulation is at a stroke risk of 0.9% above which the net clinical benefit is in favor of OAC rather than not.[86] For warfarin, the tipping point threshold is 1.7%,[86] although this may even be lower with high TTRs.[87] Further recent studies have shown better persistence with the use of NOACs versus warfarin.[88]

THE ELDERLY

As stroke risk increases with age, the absolute benefit of OAC increases with age, and while bleeding risk also increases with age, this increase was not only slight, but rates were greater in elderly patients taking aspirin than in those taking OAC.[89]

Indeed, OAC is often replaced by the antiplatelet therapy aspirin in the elderly because of fears of ICH.[90] Those clinicians who swap antithrombotic therapy for AF in favor of antiplatelet drugs refer to metaanalysis of Hart et al.[91] that demonstrated 22% reduction in risk of stroke with aspirin compared with placebo. Of note, when this analysis was narrowed to the aspirin-only trials, nonsignificant 19% stroke risk reduction was observed.[91] Furthermore, 22% stroke risk reduction was driven by single arm of Stroke Prevention in Atrial Fibrillation 1 (SPAF-1) trial with aspirin 325 mg, and effect of aspirin was heterogeneous.[91]

Aspirin failed to reduce risk of stroke in the elderly population aged 75 years or over in the BAFTA (Birmingham Atrial Fibrillation Treatment of the Aged) study. The combined endpoint of major stroke, arterial embolism, or other ICH was significantly lower in warfarin arm (1.8% vs. 3.8%; RR 0.48, 95% CI 0.28–0.80) driven by strike reduction while there was broadly similar incidence of ICH in aspirin (1.6%) and warfarin (1.4%).[92] OAC is clearly superior to antiplatelet therapy with an RR reduction of 38% (18%–52%).[91] Thus, when deciding on the appropriate use of OAC in patients, the risk of bleeding should not be used as a contraindication as well as the use of aspirin cannot be justified on the perception that it provides suitable stroke prophylaxis with a more favorable bleeding risk, as the evidence does not support this.

Falls are another risk factor for major bleeding, including ICH, in anticoagulated patients, resulting in misperception that patient will benefit from OAC suspension.[93] Similarly to AF, prevalence of falls increases with population aging. Yearly, approximately 30%–40% of adults aged 65 years or older experience at least one fall. Cognitive, gait, strength, balance, sensory deficit, acute illness, medications, alcohol, all can contribute to falls.[94,95] However, even without apparent risk factors for falls, 10% of people aged 75 years or older in community-dwelling may experience fall.[94]

Undoubtedly, falls contribute significantly into morbidity and disability and affect patient's quality of life. In the large real-world cohort of patients with AF on OAC (Loire Valley Atrial Fibrillation Project), history of falls was independently associated with stroke/thromboembolism (HR 5.19; 95% CI 2.1–12.6), major bleeding (HR 3.32, 95% CI 1.23–8.91), and all-cause mortality (HR 3.69, 95% CI 1.52–8.95).[96]

Analysis performed among Medicare beneficiaries with AF on OAC who were documented to have high fall risk in their records yielded significantly higher risk of ICH compared with other patients (2.8% vs. 1.1%/100 patient-years; HR 1.9, 95% CI 1.3–2.9).[93] Given that patients at high risk of falls also had multiple stroke risk factors, net clinical benefit would be in favor of OAC.[93,96] It was estimated that 295 falls should happen during a year, only then risk of falls-related ICH will outweigh OAC benefits in terms of stroke prevention.[97] Unfortunately, the number of patients at high risk of falls discharged on warfarin was significantly lower than in other patients.[93,96]

Thus, perception of high risk of falls has not to be a reason to withhold OAC, as in most cases the magnitude of gain from stroke prevention far outweighs the small increase in serious bleeding.[97] Many falls are preventable. Therefore, fall risk assessment and management, e.g., with timed up-and-go test, the 30-s chair stand test, and the 4-stage balance test, are included in the STEADI (Stopping Elderly Accidents, Deaths, and Injuries) tool kit to aid first of all primary care providers to manage elderly patients.[94]

PAROXYSMAL ATRIAL FIBRILLATION AND STROKE RISK

Current guidelines emphasize the presence of stroke risk factors rather than type of AF as a reason for thromboprophylaxis. Observational data suggest that stroke risk is accentuated irrespective of AF subtype in the presence of stroke risk factors.[98,99] Nonetheless, impact of AF burden as a combination of AF pattern (i.e., paroxysmal, persistent, and permanent), duration of AF history from the first onset, number and duration of AF paroxysms on patient's stroke risk was addressed in many studies.

Indeed, studies performed thus far showed inconsistent results. The annual stroke rate was similar in patients with intermittent (3.2%) and sustained (3.3%) AF in pooled cohort of Stroke Prevention in Atrial Fibrillation I, II, and III trials.[100] No difference between paroxysmal and nonparoxysmal types of AF with respect to rate of stroke or systemic embolism was observed in ACTIVE W (Atrial Fibrillation Clopidogrel Trial With Irbesartan for Prevention of Vascular Events) trial,[101] Stockholm Cohort of Atrial Fibrillation,[102] RE-LY (Randomized Evaluation of Long-Term Anticoagulation Therapy) trial,[103] and GISSI-AF (Gruppo Italiano per lo Studio della Sopravvivenza nell'Infarto Miocardico–Atrial Fibrillation) trial.[104]

However, there is growing body of evidence that nonparoxysmal patterns of AF, particularly permanent AF, confer higher risk of stroke and systemic embolism compared with paroxysmal AF. For example, the European Atrial Fibrillation Trial with a follow-up of 594 patients-years found AF duration > 1 year was an independent risk factor for secondary stroke.[105] A post hoc analysis of data from the Atrial Fibrillation Clopidogrel Trial with Irbesartan for prevention of vascular events (ACTIVE-A) and Apixaban versus Acetylsalicylic Acid to Prevent Stroke in Atrial Fibrillation Patients Who Have Failed or Are Unsuitable for Vitamin K Antagonist Treatment (AVERROES) trials also suggested that the pattern of AF was a strong independent predictor of stroke risk, second only to previous TIA or stroke.[106] Here, permanent AF had an annual stroke risk of 4.2% compared with 2.1% with PAF and 3.0% with persistent AF, equating to an HR of 1.83 for permanent AF versus PAF and 1.44 for persistent AF versus PAF.

A subanalysis of the Rivaroxaban Once daily Oral Direct Factor Xa Inhibition Compared With Vitamin K Antagonism for Prevention of Stroke and Embolism Trial in Atrial Fibrillation (ROCKET AF) trial also found that anticoagulated patients with persistent AF (11,548 patients) were at higher risk of stroke versus those with

PAF (2514 patients).[107] Patients with persistent AF had higher rates of stroke and all-cause mortality (adjusted rates for stroke 2.18 vs. 1.73 events/100 patients-years, $P = .048$).

Prespecified analysis of ARISTOTLE trial according to AF type yielded significantly higher rate of stroke or systemic embolism in patients with persistent or permanent AF than in patients with paroxysmal AF (1.52% vs. 0.98%; HR 0.70, 95% CI 0.51–0.93) with a trend toward higher mortality.[108] Consistently, in the ENGAGE AF-TIMI 48 trial (Effective Anticoagulation With Factor Xa Next Generation in Atrial Fibrillation–Thrombolysis in Myocardial Infarction 48), the primary outcome of stroke or systemic embolism occurred less commonly in patients with paroxysmal AF (1.49%/year) compared with persistent (1.83%/year; HR 0.79, 95% CI 0.66–0.90) and permanent AF (1.95%/year; HR 0.78, 95% CI 0.67–0.93) with a significant reduction in mortality.[109]

Other studies did not reveal differences in stroke risk between AF types but found worse prognosis in nonparoxysmal AF. That was the case in the Euro Heart Survey on Atrial Fibrillation, where stroke rate did not differ between AF types, but total and cardiovascular mortality was higher in permanent AF.[110] Higher mortality was also reported in patients with permanent AF compared with paroxysmal AF who survived stroke (17.8% vs. 11.6%, respectively) in the FibStroke study.[111] Hohnloser et al.[112] performed post hoc analysis of the AVERROES (Apixaban vs. Acetylsalicylic Acid to Prevent Stroke in Atrial Fibrillation Patients Who Have Failed or Are Unsuitable for Vitamin K Antagonist Treatment) trial and found significantly higher rate of heart failure–related hospitalizations in patients with permanent AF, compared with paroxysmal or persistent AF, that translated also into higher mortality in the former group.[112] Similar findings were derived in the observational MOVE (MOrbiditätsdaten von Vorhofflimmer-Patienten Evaluieren) cohort.[113]

Confounding of AF type may be more evident in patients with less stroke risk factors. That was observed in the analysis of SPORTIF (Stroke Prevention using ORal Thrombin Inhibitor in atrial Fibrillation) III and V cohorts, where patients with paroxysmal AF overall experienced less strokes or systemic embolic events than those with persistent AF, but in high-risk subgroup there was no statistically significant difference according to AF type.[114]

However, caution is advised, as marked heterogeneity exists between the studies, with variability in OAC use. Furthermore, PAF patients tend to be younger and have less comorbidity, and statistical adjustment cannot completely account for all biologic variables.[101,103,107,115]

Whether permanent AF is associated with worse prognosis or not, one has to remember that stroke risk as assessed with CHA_2DS_2VASc score is associated with probability of future adverse events than AF itself because all patients classified within paroxysmal AF class may be inherently heterogeneous in terms of clinical characteristics.[116] Hence, defining AF as paroxysmal should not be considered as a single criterion to rule out OAC that is not rarely observed in real-life clinical practice.[104,113,115] In addition, AF in vast majority of cases has progressive course from paroxysmal AF via persistent AF to permanent arrhythmia[110,113] as an electrical and structural substrate for it is getting more advanced.[117] Furthermore, AF classification into paroxysmal, persistent, and permanent is somewhat mechanistic and does not always accurately reflect the temporal persistence of AF.[118] There is opportunity for bias when applying clinical AF classification, particularly between paroxysmal and persistent form, and when they are asymptomatic. For example, paroxysmal AF episodes are defined as self-limiting within 1 week, with a cardioversion allowed during that period; and episodes lasting more than 7 days are referred to as persistent and require pharmacologic or electrical cardioversion.[4]

Duration and arrhythmia burden are subject to high variability in paroxysmal AF; indeed, patients with one paroxysm a year are labeled as paroxysmal AF, as would a patient with paroxysms of AF 364 days/year, whereas patient with 2 weeks of persistent AF subsequently cardioverted can remain on sinus rhythm for a long period. The question as to how much "AF burden" is relevant to stroke risk is still controversial, especially with more sophisticated arrhythmia monitoring techniques that is discussed in Chapter 5 on subclinical AF.

Despite overall lower risk in paroxysmal AF compared with other AF types, many of them rate stroke or systemic embolism well above accepted threshold of 1%/year to gain positive net clinical benefit from OAC. Several metaanalyses evaluating stroke rates in patients with paroxysmal AF versus permanent AF were conducted.[119-121] In the most recent, 18 studies were included with a total of 239,528 patient-years of follow-up. The incidence of stroke or systemic embolism was 2.3% (95% CI 2.0%–2.7%) in patients with nonparoxysmal AF, whereas in those with paroxysmal AF it was 1.6% (95% CI 1.3%–2.0%) that corresponded 28% (20%–35%) risk reduction.[121] Of note the annual rate of thromboembolic events was decreased twofold with the increasing proportion of patients on OAC irrespectively of AF type: from 3.7% to 1.7% in nonparoxysmal AF, and from 2.5% to 1.2% in paroxysmal AF.[121]

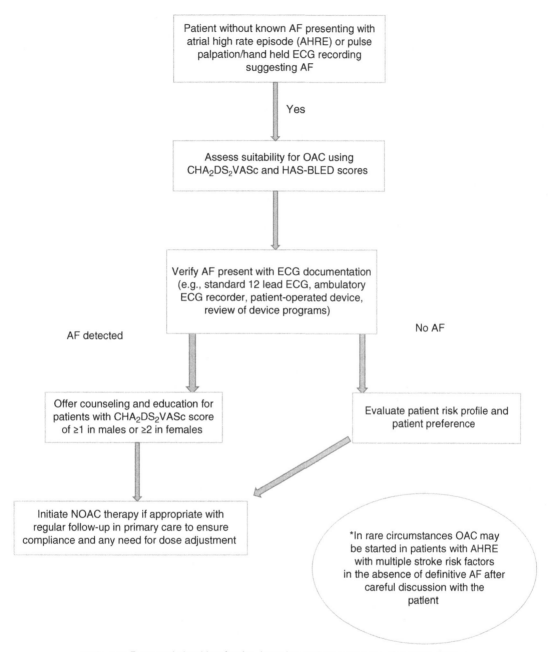

FIG. 4.2 Proposed algorithm for the detection and management of atrial fibrillation.

Fig. 4.2 provides an algorithm to aid in the detection and management of patients with possible AF. Net benefit analyses have consistently shown that patients who do not benefit from OAC are those at "low risk" with a CHA_2DS_2VASc score of 0 in males or 1 in females. Even in patients with a HAS-BLED score of 3, the net clinical benefit of stroke protection still outweighs bleeding risk. Hence, the default should be to offer stroke prevention unless the patient is at low risk, where OAC confers no advantage. Hence, the initial step should be to define low-risk patients (CHA_2DS_2VASc score of 0 in males or 1 in females) where no antithrombotic therapy is needed; the subsequent step is to offer stroke prevention (which is OAC) to those with stroke risk factors, irrespective of their absolute score point value.

Despite all stroke and bleeding risk scores having their benefits and limitations, complexity should be balanced against simplicity and practical use for everyday clinical practice in busy tertiary care settings. A pragmatic approach would be to use bleeding risk scores to focus the attention of clinicians and patients on distinguishing and reduction of correctable risk factors for bleeding (e.g., poorly controlled hypertension, labile INR, concurrent medication such as aspirin and nonsteroidal antiinflammatory medication, excessive alcohol consumption) as well as keep track of patients at risk of bleeding (important in the era of computerized electronic heart records and alert systems) for review and regular follow-up.

FUTURE DIRECTIONS TO IMPROVE RISK SCORES

There are many clinical risk factors for thromboembolism and bleeding that were not included into the current risk stratification schemes but had potential to improve their performance. For example, a history of both arterial (HR 1.39, 95% CI 1.08–1.79) and venous (HR 1.26, 95% CI 1.02–1.54) retinal vascular occlusions has been found to be associated with an increased risk of stroke/thromboembolism/TIA in patients with nonvalvular AF.[122] As cerebral circulation and retinal circulation are adjacent, it was suggested that retinal vascular occlusion could be considered as a previous thromboembolic event when evaluating stroke risk.[122]

Obesity is a clear risk factor for the development of new-onset AF and is a valid stroke risk factor in the general population, also having an independent predictive role for stroke development in patients with AF.[123] In the prospective Danish Diet, Cancer and Health study there was a 31% and 36% increase in risk of the composite endpoint of "ischemic stroke, thromboembolism, or death" in overweight and obese patients, respectively, even after adjustment for CHA_2DS_2-VASc score.[124] In anticoagulated patients, a TTR > 70% in patients with a BMI > 24 mitigated the risk of stroke and all-cause death in obese patients with AF.[125]

Ethnicity

Ethnic differences are important for stroke prediction. Specifically, Asians represent large population with overall higher burden of AF than in Western

countries.[126,127] Despite stroke risk factors being common for both populations, OAC is underused and decision-making does not correspond to individual risk, assessed via modern stratification schemes.[128]

Studies from Asia have suggested a higher RR of AF-related stroke than typically seen in the Western populations.[129] A population-based study conducted in Taiwan of nearly 13,000 non-anticoagulated AF subjects showed that male patients with only a single risk factor for stroke (i.e., CHA_2DS_2-VASc score of 1) had an annual risk of stroke 1.96%–3.50%. For female patients with one additional stroke-related risk factor (i.e., CHA_2DS_2-VASc score of 2), the annual stroke rate was 1.91%–3.34%.[129] Without optimal thromboprophylaxis up to 2.9 million Asians in 2050 are projected to suffer from AF-related stroke.[130] In addition, multiple studies have found that this ethnic population is more prone to developing intracerebral hemorrhage (ICH).[131,132] A large metaanalysis showed that Asian subjects have twice the incidence of ICH compared with those of Western countries (51.8 vs. 24.2/100,000 person-years).[133]

Why Asian patients are more prone to higher rates of bleeding on warfarin is not fully understood. Poorer TTRs have been proposed to be a possible factor contributing to these findings. The need to maintain TTR > 70% to achieve maximal benefits from anticoagulation with warfarin is well evidence based.[134] Data from major clinical trials of NOACs in AF show that the average TTRs were below 70% in the Asian cohorts, which may partly reflect the debatable practice within Asian countries to aim a lower INR range in the hope of reducing the risk of bleeding. Even in Asian patients with a prior ICH the use of warfarin may still be beneficial in those with a CHA_2DS_2-VASc ≥ 6.[135]

With the realization that risk stratification of stroke based on evidence from mainly Caucasian and Western population cannot be directly extrapolated to evaluate Asian patients a "modified" CHA_2DS_2-VASc score. The latter refers to one point assigned to patients aged 50–74 years given that the risk of stroke seems to rise from age 50 years in this population.[136]

The arrival of NOACs confers a potentially greater net clinical benefit than the Caucasian population in which they have been largely studied. A metaanalysis of data from the RE-LY, ROCKET-AF, ARISTOTLE, and ENGAGE AF-TIMI 48 trials compared NOACs with warfarin in Asian (>8000 patients) and non-Asian patients with regard to both efficacy and safety.[137] The results suggested that NOACs may be more effective and safer in Asians than in non-Asians compared with warfarin. Although NOACs significantly reduced the risk of stroke/systemic embolism both in Asian and non-Asian patients, the reduction was more prominent in Asian patients than in non-Asian patients (OR=0.65 for Asians vs. 0.85 for non-Asians; P interaction=0.045). NOACs reduced major bleeding more in Asian than in non-Asian patients (OR=0.57 for Asians vs. 0.89 for non-Asian patients; P interaction=0.004). ICH was significantly reduced in both cohorts with NOACs (OR=0.33 for Asians vs. 0.52 for non-Asian patients; p for interaction=0.059).

CONCLUSION

In essence, the aim of reducing risk in AF-related stroke patients is to find the balance of reducing stroke risk while minimizing bleeding risk. Net benefit analysis has consistently shown that the only patients not to benefit for OAC are low-risk patients, i.e., those with a CHA_2DS_2VASc of 0 in males or 1 in females.

Other risk scores have been studied but fail to provide superiority while maintaining practical use to assess stroke and bleeding risk of patients in busy tertiary care settings. Current guidelines recommend the use of the CHA_2DS_2VASc and HAS-BLED score in evaluating patients' stroke and bleeding risk on initiation of OAC. Both risk schemas have been validated in "real-world" studies and as such provide reassuring evidence for the effective yet efficient assessment of stroke and bleeding risk in patients with AF in need of OAC. At present attempts to provide greater predictability of stroke and bleeding risk using complex composite risk scores fail to provide superiority while resulting in less practical risk assessment. With the availability of NOACs, the use of OAC is likely to continue to rise and the use of such simple yet effective stroke risk scores should be implemented to ensure patients suitable are offered protection from AF-related stroke.

REFERENCES

1. Martinez C, Katholing A, Freedman SB. Adverse prognosis of incidentally detected ambulatory atrial fibrillation. A cohort study. *Thromb Haemost.* 2014;112:276–286.
2. Rivera-Caravaca JM, Roldan V, Esteve-Pastor MA, et al. Cessation of oral anticoagulation is an important risk factor for stroke and mortality in atrial fibrillation patients. *Thromb Haemost.* 2017;117(7):1448–1454.
3. Eikelboom JW, Weitz JI. 'Realworld' use of non-vitamin K antagonist oral anticoagulants (NOACs): lessons from the Dresden NOAC Registry. *Thromb Haemost.* 2015;113:1159–1161.
4. Kirchhof P, Benussi S, Kotecha D, et al. 2016 ESC guidelines for the management of atrial fibrillation developed in collaboration with EACTS. *Europace.* 2016;18:1609–1678.
5. Nielsen PB, Chao TF. The risks of risk scores for stroke risk assessment in atrial fibrillation. *Thromb Haemost.* 2015;113:1170–1173.
6. Banerjee A, Fauchier L, Bernard-Brunet A, Clementy N, Lip GY. Composite risk scores and composite endpoints in the risk prediction of outcomes in anticoagulated patients with atrial fibrillation. The Loire Valley Atrial Fibrillation Project. *Thromb Haemost.* 2014;111:549–556.
7. Gage BF, Waterman AD, Shannon W, Boechler M, Rich MW, Radford MJ. Validation of clinical classification schemes for predicting stroke: results from the National Registry of Atrial Fibrillation. *JAMA.* 2001;285:2864–2870.
8. Risk factors for stroke and efficacy of antithrombotic therapy in atrial fibrillation. Analysis of pooled data from five randomized controlled trials. *Arch Intern Med.* 1994;154:1449–1457.
9. Stroke Prevention in Atrial Fibrillation Investigators. Risk factors for thromboembolism during aspirin therapy in patients with atrial fibrillation: the stroke prevention in atrial fibrillation study. *J Stroke Cerebrovasc Dis.* 1995;5:147–157.
10. You JJ, Singer DE, Howard PA, et al. Antithrombotic therapy for atrial fibrillation: antithrombotic therapy and prevention of thrombosis, 9th ed: American College of Chest Physicians evidence-based clinical practice guidelines. *Chest.* 2012;141:e531S–e575S.
11. Fuster V, Ryden LE, Cannom DS, et al. ACC/AHA/ESC 2006 guidelines for the management of patients with atrial fibrillation: a report of the American College of Cardiology/American Heart Association Task Force on Practice Guidelines and the European Society of Cardiology Committee for Practice Guidelines (Writing Committee to Revise the 2001 guidelines for the management of patients with atrial fibrillation): developed in collaboration with the European Heart Rhythm Association and the Heart Rhythm Society. *Circulation.* 2006;114:e257–e354.
12. Lip GY, Skjoth F, Nielsen PB, Larsen TB. Non-valvular atrial fibrillation patients with none or one additional risk factor of the CHA2DS2-VASc score. A comprehensive net clinical benefit analysis for warfarin, aspirin, or no therapy. *Thromb Haemost.* 2015;114:826–834.
13. Camm AJ, Lip GY, De Caterina R, et al. 2012 focused update of the ESC Guidelines for the management of atrial fibrillation: an update of the 2010 ESC Guidelines for the management of atrial fibrillation. Developed with the special contribution of the European Heart Rhythm Association. *Eur Heart J.* 2012;33:2719–2747.
14. Cove CL, Albert CM, Andreotti F, Badimon L, Van Gelder IC, Hylek EM. Female sex as an independent risk factor for stroke in atrial fibrillation: possible mechanisms. *Thromb Haemost.* 2014;111:385–391.
15. Olesen JB, Torp-Pedersen C, Hansen ML, Lip GY. The value of the CHA2DS2-VASc score for refining stroke risk stratification in patients with atrial fibrillation with a CHADS2 score 0-1: a nationwide cohort study. *Thromb Haemost.* 2012;107:1172–1179.

16. Olesen JB, Torp-Pedersen C. Stroke risk in atrial fibrillation: do we anticoagulate CHADS2 or CHA2DS2-VASc >/=1, or higher? *Thromb Haemost.* 2015;113:1165–1169.

17. Aspberg S, Chang Y, Atterman A, Bottai M, Go AS, Singer DE. Comparison of the ATRIA, CHADS2, and CHA2DS2-VASc stroke risk scores in predicting ischaemic stroke in a large Swedish cohort of patients with atrial fibrillation. *Eur Heart J.* 2016;37(42):3203–3210.

18. Roldan V, Marin F, Manzano-Fernandez S, et al. Does chronic kidney disease improve the predictive value of the CHADS2 and CHA2DS2-VASc stroke stratification risk scores for atrial fibrillation? *Thromb Haemost.* 2013;109:956–960.

19. Lip GY, Nieuwlaat R, Pisters R, Lane DA, Crijns HJ. Refining clinical risk stratification for predicting stroke and thromboembolism in atrial fibrillation using a novel risk factor-based approach: the Euro Heart Survey on atrial fibrillation. *Chest.* 2010;137:263–272.

20. Fuster V, Ryden LE, Cannom DS, et al. ACC/AHA/ESC 2006 guidelines for the management of patients with atrial fibrillation–executive summary: a report of the American College of Cardiology/American Heart Association Task Force on Practice Guidelines and the European Society of Cardiology Committee for Practice Guidelines (Writing Committee to revise the 2001 guidelines for the management of patients with atrial fibrillation). *J Am Coll Cardiol.* 2006;48:854–906.

21. Kalra L, Lip GYH. Antithrombotic treatment in atrial fibrillation. *Heart.* 2007;93:39–44.

22. Lane DA, Lip GY. Use of the CHA(2)DS(2)-VASc and HAS-BLED scores to aid decision making for thromboprophylaxis in nonvalvular atrial fibrillation. *Circulation.* 2012;126:860–865.

23. Van Staa TP, Setakis E, Di Tanna GL, Lane DA, Lip GY. A comparison of risk stratification schemes for stroke in 79,884 atrial fibrillation patients in general practice. *J Thromb Haemost.* 2011;9:39–48.

24. Olesen JB, Lip GY, Hansen ML, et al. Validation of risk stratification schemes for predicting stroke and thromboembolism in patients with atrial fibrillation: nationwide cohort study. *BMJ.* 2011;342:d124.

25. Poli D, Lip GY, Antonucci E, Grifoni E, Lane D. Stroke risk stratification in a "real-world" elderly anticoagulated atrial fibrillation population. *J Cardiovasc Electrophysiol.* 2011;22:25–30.

26. Davis G, Johns EJ. Somatosensory regulation of renal function in the stroke-prone spontaneously hypertensive rat. *J Physiol.* 1994;481(Pt 3):753–759.

27. Mostofsky E, Wellenius GA, Noheria A, et al. Renal function predicts survival in patients with acute ischemic stroke. *Cerebrovasc Dis (Basel, Switzerland).* 2009;28:88–94.

28. Guo Y, Wang H, Zhao X, et al. Sequential changes in renal function and the risk of stroke and death in patients with atrial fibrillation. *Int J Cardiol.* 2013;168:4678–4684.

29. Piccini JP, Stevens SR, Chang Y, et al. Renal dysfunction as a predictor of stroke and systemic embolism in patients with nonvalvular atrial fibrillation: validation of the R(2)CHADS(2) index in the ROCKET AF (rivaroxaban once-daily, oral, direct factor Xa inhibition compared with vitamin K antagonism for prevention of stroke and embolism trial in atrial fibrillation) and ATRIA (anticoagulation and risk factors in atrial fibrillation) study cohorts. *Circulation.* 2013;127:224–232.

30. Friberg L, Benson L, Lip GYH. Balancing stroke and bleeding risks in patients with atrial fibrillation and renal failure: the Swedish atrial fibrillation cohort study. *Eur Heart J.* 2015;36:297–306.

31. Hippisley-Cox J, Coupland C, Brindle P. Derivation and validation of QStroke score for predicting risk of ischaemic stroke in primary care and comparison with other risk scores: a prospective open cohort study. *BMJ (Clin Res Ed).* 2013;346:f2573.

32. Singer DE, Chang Y, Borowsky LH, et al. A new risk scheme to predict ischemic stroke and other thromboembolism in atrial fibrillation: the ATRIA study stroke risk score. *J Am Heart Assoc.* 2013;2.

33. Go AS, Hylek EM, Borowsky LH, Phillips KA, Selby JV, Singer DE. Warfarin use among ambulatory patients with nonvalvular atrial fibrillation: the anticoagulation and risk factors in atrial fibrillation (ATRIA) study. *Ann Intern Med.* 1999;131:927–934.

34. Chao TF, Wang KL, Liu CJ, et al. Age threshold for increased stroke risk among patients with atrial fibrillation: a nationwide cohort study from Taiwan. *J Am Coll Cardiol.* 2015;66:1339–1347.

35. Lip GY, Nielsen PB, Skjoth F, Lane DA, Rasmussen LH, Larsen TB. The value of the European Society of Cardiology guidelines for refining stroke risk stratification in patients with atrial fibrillation categorized as low risk using the anticoagulation and risk factors in atrial fibrillation stroke score: a nationwide cohort study. *Chest.* 2014;146:1337–1346.

36. Nielsen PB, Larsen TB, Skjoth F, Overvad TF, Lip GY. Stroke and thromboembolic event rates in atrial fibrillation according to different guideline treatment thresholds: a nationwide cohort study. *Sci Rep.* 2016;6:27410.

37. Hijazi Z, Lindback J, Alexander JH, et al. The ABC (age, biomarkers, clinical history) stroke risk score: a biomarker-based risk score for predicting stroke in atrial fibrillation. *Eur Heart J.* 2016;37:1582–1590.

38. Garcia-Fernandez A, Roldan V, Rivera-Caravaca JM, et al. Does von Willebrand factor improve the predictive ability of current risk stratification scores in patients with atrial fibrillation? *Sci Rep.* 2017;7:41565.

39. Hijazi Z, Oldgren J, Siegbahn A, Wallentin L. Application of biomarkers for risk stratification in patients with atrial fibrillation. *Clin Chem.* 2017;63:152–164.

40. Hijazi Z, Oldgren J, Andersson U, et al. Cardiac biomarkers are associated with an increased risk of stroke and death in patients with atrial fibrillation: a randomized evaluation of long-term anticoagulation therapy (RE-LY) substudy. *Circulation.* 2012;125:1605–1616.

41. Roldan V, Marin F, Diaz J, et al. High sensitivity cardiac troponin T and interleukin-6 predict adverse cardiovascular events and mortality in anticoagulated patients with atrial fibrillation. *J Thromb Haemost.* 2012;10:1500–1507.
42. Hijazi Z, Siegbahn A, Andersson U, et al. Comparison of cardiac troponins I and T measured with high-sensitivity methods for evaluation of prognosis in atrial fibrillation: an ARISTOTLE substudy. *Clin Chem.* 2015;61:368–378.
43. Hijazi Z, Wallentin L, Siegbahn A, et al. N-terminal pro-B-type natriuretic peptide for risk assessment in patients with atrial fibrillation: insights from the ARISTOTLE Trial (apixaban for the prevention of stroke in subjects with atrial fibrillation). *J Am Coll Cardiol.* 2013;61:2274–2284.
44. Apostolakis S, Sullivan RM, Olshansky B, Lip GYH. Factors affecting quality of anticoagulation control among patients with atrial fibrillation on warfarin: the SAMe-TT(2)R(2) score. *Chest.* 2013;144:1555–1563.
45. Lip GY, Lane DA. Assessing bleeding risk in atrial fibrillation with the HAS-BLED and ORBIT scores: clinical application requires focus on the reversible bleeding risk factors. *Eur Heart J.* 2015;36:3265–3267.
46. Lip GY, Andreotti F, Fauchier L, et al. Bleeding risk assessment and management in atrial fibrillation patients. Executive summary of a position document from the European Heart Rhythm Association [EHRA], endorsed by the European Society of Cardiology [ESC] Working Group on Thrombosis. *Thromb Haemost.* 2011;106:997–1011.
47. Gage BF, Yan Y, Milligan PE, et al. Clinical classification schemes for predicting hemorrhage: results from the National Registry of Atrial Fibrillation (NRAF). *Am Heart J.* 2006;151:713–719.
48. Fang MC, Go AS, Chang Y, et al. A new risk scheme to predict warfarin-associated hemorrhage: the ATRIA (anticoagulation and risk factors in atrial fibrillation) study. *J Am Coll Cardiol.* 2011;58:395–401.
49. Pisters R, Lane DA, Nieuwlaat R, de Vos CB, Crijns HJGM, Lip GYH. A novel user-friendly score (HAS-BLED) to assess 1-year risk of major bleeding in patients with atrial fibrillation: the Euro Heart Survey. *Chest.* 2010;138:1093–1100.
50. Lip GYH, Frison L, Halperin JL, Lane DA. Comparative validation of a novel risk score for predicting bleeding risk in anticoagulated patients with atrial fibrillation: the HAS-BLED (hypertension, abnormal renal/liver function, stroke, bleeding history or predisposition, labile INR, elderly, drugs/alcohol concomitantly) score. *J Am Coll Cardiol.* 2011;57:173–180.
51. Kooiman J, van Hagen N, Iglesias Del Sol A, et al. The HAS-BLED score identifies patients with acute venous thromboembolism at high risk of major bleeding complications during the first six months of anticoagulant treatment. *PLoS One.* 2015;10:e0122520.
52. Omran H, Bauersachs R, Rubenacker S, Goss F, Hammerstingl C. The HAS-BLED score predicts bleedings during bridging of chronic oral anticoagulation. Results from the national multicentre BNK Online bRiDging REgistRy (BORDER). *Thromb Haemost.* 2012;108:65–73.
53. Smith JG, Wieloch M, Koul S, et al. Triple antithrombotic therapy following an acute coronary syndrome: prevalence, outcomes and prognostic utility of the HAS-BLED score. *EuroIntervention.* 2012;8:672–678.
54. Proietti M, Senoo K, Lane DA, Lip GYH. Major bleeding in patients with non-valvular atrial fibrillation: impact of time in therapeutic range on contemporary bleeding risk scores. *Sci Rep.* 2016;6:24376.
55. Pisters R, Lane DA, Nieuwlaat R, de Vos CB, Crijns HJ, Lip GY. A novel user-friendly score (HAS-BLED) to assess 1-year risk of major bleeding in patients with atrial fibrillation: the Euro Heart Survey. *Chest.* 2010;138:1093–1100.
56. Roldan V, Marin F, Manzano-Fernandez S, et al. The HAS-BLED score has better prediction accuracy for major bleeding than CHADS2 or CHA2DS2-VASc scores in anticoagulated patients with atrial fibrillation. *J Am Coll Cardiol.* 2013;62:2199–2204.
57. Senoo K, Proietti M, Lane DA, Lip GY. Evaluation of the HAS-BLED, ATRIA, and ORBIT bleeding risk scores in patients with atrial fibrillation taking warfarin. *Am J Med.* 2016;129:600–607.
58. Zhu W, He W, Guo L, Wang X, Hong K. The HAS-BLED score for predicting major bleeding risk in anticoagulated patients with atrial fibrillation: a systematic review and meta-analysis. *Clin Cardiol.* 2015;38:555–561.
59. Caldeira D, Costa J, Fernandes RM, Pinto FJ, Ferreira JJ. Performance of the HAS-BLED high bleeding-risk category, compared to ATRIA and HEMORR2HAGES in patients with atrial fibrillation: a systematic review and meta-analysis. *J Interv Card Electrophysiol.* 2014;40:277–284.
60. Gallego P, Roldan V, Marin F, et al. Cessation of oral anticoagulation in relation to mortality and the risk of thrombotic events in patients with atrial fibrillation. *Thromb Haemost.* 2013;110:1189–1198.
61. Fang MC, Go AS, Chang Y, et al. A new risk scheme to predict warfarin-associated hemorrhage: the ATRIA (anticoagulation and risk factors in atrial fibrillation) study. *J Am Coll Cardiol.* 2011;58:395–401.
62. O'Brien EC, Simon DN, Thomas LE, et al. The ORBIT bleeding score: a simple bedside score to assess bleeding risk in atrial fibrillation. *Eur Heart J.* 2015;36:3258–3264.
63. Hijazi Z, Oldgren J, Lindback J, et al. The novel biomarker-based ABC (age, biomarkers, clinical history)-bleeding risk score for patients with atrial fibrillation: a derivation and validation study. *Lancet.* 2016;387:2302–2311.
64. Kalantarian S, Ay H, Gollub RL, et al. Association between atrial fibrillation and silent cerebral infarctions: a systematic review and meta-analysis. *Ann Intern Med.* 2014;161:650–658.
65. Vermeer SE, Hollander M, van Dijk EJ, et al. Silent brain infarcts and white matter lesions increase stroke risk in the general population: the Rotterdam Scan Study. *Stroke.* 2003;34:1126–1129.
66. Udompanich S, Lip GY, Apostolakis S, Lane DA. Atrial fibrillation as a risk factor for cognitive impairment: a semi-systematic review. *QJM.* 2013;106:795–802.

67. Haeusler KG, Wilson D, Fiebach JB, Kirchhof P, Werring DJ. Brain MRI to personalise atrial fibrillation therapy: current evidence and perspectives. *Heart.* 2014;100:1408–1413.

68. Wang Z, van Veluw SJ, Wong A, et al. Risk factors and cognitive relevance of cortical cerebral microinfarcts in patients with ischemic stroke or transient ischemic attack. *Stroke.* 2016;47:2450–2455.

69. Gupta A, Giambrone AE, Gialdini G, et al. Silent brain infarction and risk of future stroke: a systematic review and meta-analysis. *Stroke.* 2016;47:719–725.

70. Cha MJ, Park HE, Lee MH, Cho Y, Choi EK, Oh S. Prevalence of and risk factors for silent ischemic stroke in patients with atrial fibrillation as determined by brain magnetic resonance imaging. *Am J Cardiol.* 2014;113:655–661.

71. Fanning JP, Wong AA, Fraser JF. The epidemiology of silent brain infarction: a systematic review of population-based cohorts. *BMC Med.* 2014;12:119.

72. Freedman B, Potpara TS, Lip GY. Stroke prevention in atrial fibrillation. *Lancet (London, England).* 2016;388:806–817.

73. Fisher M. MRI screening for chronic anticoagulation in atrial fibrillation. *Front Neurol.* 2013;4:137.

74. Horstmann S, Mohlenbruch M, Wegele C, et al. Prevalence of atrial fibrillation and association of previous antithrombotic treatment in patients with cerebral microbleeds. *Eur J Neurol.* 2015;22:1355–1362.

75. Poels MM, Vernooij MW, Ikram MA, et al. Prevalence and risk factors of cerebral microbleeds: an update of the Rotterdam scan study. *Stroke.* 2010;41:S103–S106.

76. Saito T, Kawamura Y, Tanabe Y, et al. Cerebral microbleeds and asymptomatic cerebral infarctions in patients with atrial fibrillation. *J Stroke Cerebrovasc Dis.* 2014;23:1616–1622.

77. Lim JS, Hong KS, Kim GM, et al. Cerebral microbleeds and early recurrent stroke after transient ischemic attack: results from the Korean Transient Ischemic Attack Expression Registry. *JAMA Neurol.* 2015;72:301–308.

78. Song TJ, Kim J, Lee HS, et al. The frequency of cerebral microbleeds increases with CHADS(2) scores in stroke patients with non-valvular atrial fibrillation. *Eur J Neurol.* 2013;20:502–508.

79. Paciaroni M, Agnelli G. Should oral anticoagulants be restarted after warfarin-associated cerebral haemorrhage in patients with atrial fibrillation? *Thromb Haemost.* 2014;111:14–18.

80. Wang DN, Hou XW, Yang BW, Lin Y, Shi JP, Wang N. Quantity of cerebral microbleeds, antiplatelet therapy, and intracerebral hemorrhage outcomes: a systematic review and meta-analysis. *J Stroke Cerebrovasc Dis.* 2015;24:2728–2737.

81. Olesen JB, Lip GY, Lindhardsen J, et al. Risks of thromboembolism and bleeding with thromboprophylaxis in patients with atrial fibrillation: a net clinical benefit analysis using a 'real world' nationwide cohort study. *Thromb Haemost.* 2011;106:739–749.

82. Murthy SB, Gupta A, Merkler AE, et al. Restarting anticoagulant therapy after intracranial hemorrhage. *Stroke.* 2017;48(6):1594–1600.

83. Gladstone DJ, Bui E, Fang J, et al. Potentially preventable strokes in high-risk patients with atrial fibrillation who are not adequately anticoagulated. *Stroke.* 2009;40:235–240.

84. Ogilvie IM, Newton N, Welner SA, Cowell W, Lip GY. Underuse of oral anticoagulants in atrial fibrillation: a systematic review. *Am J Med.* 2010;123:638–645.e4.

85. Lahaye S, Regpala S, Lacombe S, et al. Evaluation of patients' attitudes towards stroke prevention and bleeding risk in atrial fibrillation. *Thromb Haemost.* 2014;111:465–473.

86. Eckman MH, Singer DE, Rosand J, Greenberg SM. Moving the tipping point: the decision to anticoagulate patients with atrial fibrillation. *Circ Cardiovasc Qual Outcomes.* 2011;4:14–21.

87. Proietti M, Lip GY. Major outcomes in atrial fibrillation patients with one risk factor: impact of time in therapeutic range observations from the SPORTIF trials. *Am J Med.* 2016;129(10):1110–1116.

88. Martinez C, Katholing A, Wallenhorst C, Freedman SB. Therapy persistence in newly diagnosed non-valvular atrial fibrillation treated with warfarin or NOAC. A cohort study. *Thromb Haemost.* 2015;115:31–39.

89. van Walraven C, Hart RG, Connolly S, et al. Effect of age on stroke prevention therapy in patients with atrial fibrillation: the atrial fibrillation investigators. *Stroke.* 2009;40:1410–1416.

90. Lip GY. The role of aspirin for stroke prevention in atrial fibrillation. *Nat Rev Cardiol.* 2011;8:602–606.

91. Hart RG, Pearce LA, Aguilar MI. Meta-analysis: antithrombotic therapy to prevent stroke in patients who have nonvalvular atrial fibrillation. *Ann Intern Med.* 2007;146:857–867.

92. Mant J, Hobbs FD, Fletcher K, et al. Warfarin versus aspirin for stroke prevention in an elderly community population with atrial fibrillation (the Birmingham Atrial Fibrillation Treatment of the Aged Study, BAFTA): a randomised controlled trial. *Lancet (London, England).* 2007;370:493–503.

93. Gage BF, Birman-Deych E, Kerzner R, Radford MJ, Nilasena DS, Rich MW. Incidence of intracranial hemorrhage in patients with atrial fibrillation who are prone to fall. *Am J Med.* 2005;118:612–617.

94. Phelan EA, Mahoney JE, Voit JC, Stevens JA. Assessment and management of fall risk in primary care settings. *Med Clin.* 2015;99:281–293.

95. Deandrea S, Bravi F, Turati F, Lucenteforte E, La Vecchia C, Negri E. Risk factors for falls in older people in nursing homes and hospitals. A systematic review and meta-analysis. *Arch Gerontol Geriatr.* 2013;56:407–415.

96. Banerjee A, Clementy N, Haguenoer K, Fauchier L, Lip GY. Prior history of falls and risk of outcomes in atrial fibrillation: the Loire Valley Atrial Fibrillation Project. *Am J Med.* 2014;127:972–978.

97. Man-Son-Hing M, Nichol G, Lau A, Laupacis A. Choosing antithrombotic therapy for elderly patients with atrial fibrillation who are at risk for falls. *Arch Intern Med.* 1999;159:677–685.

98. Stöllberger C, Chnupa P, Abzieher C, et al. Mortality and rate of stroke or embolism in atrial fibrillation during long-term follow-up in the embolism in left atrial thrombi (ELAT) study. *Clin Cardiol.* 2004;27:40–46.

99. Cabin HS, Clubb KS, Hall C, Perlmutter RA, Feinstein AR. Risk for systemic embolization of atrial fibrillation without mitral stenosis. *Am J Cardiol.* 1990;65:1112–1116.

100. Hart RG, Pearce LA, Rothbart RM, McAnulty JH, Asinger RW, Halperin JL. Stroke with intermittent atrial fibrillation: incidence and predictors during aspirin therapy. Stroke Prevention in Atrial Fibrillation Investigators. *J Am Coll Cardiol.* 2000;35:183–187.

101. Hohnloser SH, Pajitnev D, Pogue J, et al. Incidence of stroke in paroxysmal versus sustained atrial fibrillation in patients taking oral anticoagulation or combined antiplatelet therapy: an ACTIVE W Substudy. *J Am Coll Cardiol.* 2007;50:2156–2161.

102. Friberg L, Hammar N, Rosenqvist M. Stroke in paroxysmal atrial fibrillation: report from the Stockholm cohort of atrial fibrillation. *Eur Heart J.* 2010;31:967–975.

103. Flaker G, Ezekowitz M, Yusuf S, et al. Efficacy and safety of dabigatran compared to warfarin in patients with paroxysmal, persistent, and permanent atrial fibrillation: results from the RE-LY (randomized evaluation of long-term anticoagulation therapy) study. *J Am Coll Cardiol.* 2012;59:854–855.

104. Disertori M, Franzosi MG, Barlera S, et al. Thromboembolic event rate in paroxysmal and persistent atrial fibrillation: data from the GISSI-AF trial. *BMC Cardiovasc Disord.* 2013;13:28.

105. van Latum JC, Koudstaal PJ, Venables GS, et al. Predictors of major vascular events in patients with a transient ischemic attack or minor ischemic stroke and with nonrheumatic atrial fibrillation. *Stroke.* 1995;26:801–806.

106. Vanassche T, Lauw MN, Eikelboom JW, et al. Risk of ischaemic stroke according to pattern of atrial fibrillation: analysis of 6563 aspirin-treated patients in ACTIVE-A and AVERROES. *Eur Heart J.* 2015;36:281–287a.

107. Steinberg BA, Hellkamp AS, Lokhnygina Y, et al. Higher risk of death and stroke in patients with persistent vs. paroxysmal atrial fibrillation: results from the ROCKET-AF trial. *Eur Heart J.* 2015;36:288–296.

108. Al-Khatib SM, Thomas L, Wallentin L, et al. Outcomes of apixaban vs. warfarin by type and duration of atrial fibrillation: results from the ARISTOTLE trial. *Eur Heart J.* 2013;34:2464–2471.

109. Link MS, Giugliano RP, Ruff CT, et al. Stroke and mortality risk in patients with various patterns of atrial fibrillation. *Circ Arrhythm Electrophysiol.* 2017;10.

110. Nieuwlaat R, Prins MH, Le Heuzey JY, et al. Prognosis, disease progression, and treatment of atrial fibrillation patients during 1 year: follow-up of the Euro Heart Survey on atrial fibrillation. *Eur Heart J.* 2008;29:1181–1189.

111. Palomaki A, Kiviniemi T, Mustonen P, et al. Mortality after stroke in patients with paroxysmal and chronic atrial fibrillation – the FibStroke study. *Int J Cardiol.* 2017;227:869–874.

112. Hohnloser SH, Shestakovska O, Eikelboom J, et al. The effects of apixaban on hospitalizations in patients with different types of atrial fibrillation: insights from the AVERROES trial. *Eur Heart J.* 2013;34:2752–2759.

113. Bosch RF, Kirch W, Theuer JD, et al. Atrial fibrillation management, outcomes and predictors of stable disease in daily practice: prospective non-interventional study. *Int J Cardiol.* 2013;167:750–756.

114. Lip GY, Frison L, Grind M, SPORTIF Investigators. Stroke event rates in anticoagulated patients with paroxysmal atrial fibrillation. *J Intern Med.* 2008;264:50–61.

115. Takabayashi K, Hamatani Y, Yamashita Y, et al. Incidence of stroke or systemic embolism in paroxysmal versus sustained atrial fibrillation: the Fushimi Atrial Fibrillation Registry. *Stroke.* 2015;46:3354–3361.

116. Dzeshka MS, Lip GY. Antithrombotic and anticoagulant therapy for atrial fibrillation. *Heart Fail Clin.* 2016;12:257–271.

117. Dzeshka MS, Lip GY, Snezhitskiy V, Shantsila E. Cardiac fibrosis in patients with atrial fibrillation: mechanisms and clinical implications. *J Am Coll Cardiol.* 2015;66:943–959.

118. Charitos EI, Purerfellner H, Glotzer TV, Ziegler PD. Clinical classifications of atrial fibrillation poorly reflect its temporal persistence: insights from 1,195 patients continuously monitored with implantable devices. *J Am Coll Cardiol.* 2014;63:2840–2848.

119. Lauw MN, Vanassche T, Masiero S, Eikelboom JW, Connolly SJ. Abstract 20413: pattern of atrial fibrillation and the risk of ischemic stroke – a systematic review and meta-analysis. *Circulation.* 2014;130:A20413.

120. Ganesan AN, Chew DP, Hartshorne T, et al. The impact of atrial fibrillation type on the risk of thromboembolism, mortality, and bleeding: a systematic review and meta-analysis. *Eur Heart J.* 2016;37:1591–1602.

121. Lilli A, Di Cori A, Zaca V. Thromboembolic risk and effect of oral anticoagulation according to atrial fibrillation patterns: a systematic review and meta-analysis. *Clin Cardiol.* 2017:641–647.

122. Christiansen CB, Lip GY, Lamberts M, Gislason G, Torp-Pedersen C, Olesen JB. Retinal vein and artery occlusions: a risk factor for stroke in atrial fibrillation. *J Thromb Haemost.* 2013;11:1485–1492.

123. Strazzullo P, D'Elia L, Cairella G, Garbagnati F, Cappuccio FP, Scalfi L. Excess body weight and incidence of stroke: meta-analysis of prospective studies with 2 million participants. *Stroke.* 2010;41:e418–e426.

124. Overvad TF, Rasmussen LH, Skjoth F, Overvad K, Lip GY, Larsen TB. Body mass index and adverse events in patients with incident atrial fibrillation. *Am J Med.* 2013;126:640.e9-17.

125. Proietti M, Lane DA, Lip GY. Relation of nonvalvular atrial fibrillation to body mass index (from the SPORTIF trials). *Am J Cardiol.* 2016;118:72–78.

126. Guo Y-T, Zhang Y, Shi X-M, et al. Assessing bleeding risk in 4824 Asian patients with atrial fibrillation: the Beijing PLA Hospital Atrial Fibrillation Project. *Sci Rep.* 2016;6:31755.

127. Guo Y, Wang H, Tian Y, Wang Y, Lip GY. Multiple risk factors and ischaemic stroke in the elderly Asian population with and without atrial fibrillation. An analysis of 425,600 Chinese individuals without prior stroke. *Thromb Haemost.* 2016;115:184–192.

128. Hamatani Y, Yamashita Y, Esato M, et al. Predictors for stroke and death in non-anticoagulated Asian patients with atrial fibrillation: the Fushimi AF registry. *PLoS One.* 2015;10:e0142394.

129. Chao T-F, Liu C-J, Wang K-L, et al. Should atrial fibrillation patients with 1 additional risk factor of the CHA2DS2-VASc score (beyond sex) receive oral anticoagulation? *J Am Coll Cardiol.* 2015;65:635–642.

130. Chiang CE, Wang KL, Lip GY. Stroke prevention in atrial fibrillation: an Asian perspective. *Thromb Haemost.* 2014;111:789–797.

131. Zhang LF, Yang J, Hong Z, et al. Proportion of different subtypes of stroke in China. *Stroke.* 2003;34:2091–2096.

132. Chau PH, Woo J, Goggins WB, et al. Trends in stroke incidence in Hong Kong differ by stroke subtype. *Cerebrovasc Dis (Basel, Switzerland).* 2011;31:138–146.

133. van Asch CJ, Luitse MJ, Rinkel GJ, van der Tweel I, Algra A, Klijn CJ. Incidence, case fatality, and functional outcome of intracerebral haemorrhage over time, according to age, sex, and ethnic origin: a systematic review and meta-analysis. *Lancet Neurol.* 2010;9:167–176.

134. Pastori D, Pignatelli P, Saliola M, et al. Inadequate anticoagulation by vitamin K antagonists is associated with major adverse cardiovascular events in patients with atrial fibrillation. *Int J Cardiol.* 2015;201:513–516.

135. Chao TF, Liu CJ, Liao JN, et al. Use of oral anticoagulants for stroke prevention in patients with atrial fibrillation who have a history of intracranial hemorrhage. *Circulation.* 2016;133:1540–1547.

136. Chao TF, Lip GY, Liu CJ, et al. Validation of a modified CHA2DS2-VASc score for stroke risk stratification in Asian patients with atrial fibrillation: a nationwide cohort study. *Stroke.* 2016;47:2462–2469.

137. Wang KL, Lip GY, Lin SJ, Chiang CE. Non-vitamin K antagonist oral anticoagulants for stroke prevention in Asian patients with nonvalvular atrial fibrillation: meta-analysis. *Stroke.* 2015;46:2555–2561.

CHAPTER 5

Subclinical Atrial Fibrillation: Definition, Prevalence, and Treatment Strategies

ABHINAV SHARMA, MD, FRCPC • RENATO D. LOPES, MD, MHS, PHD

INTRODUCTION

Atrial fibrillation (AF) is one of the most common arrhythmias worldwide. The presence of AF significantly increases the risk of strokes. Over 16% of strokes are attributable to a documented history of AF.[1] In addition, strokes related to AF, compared with non-AF-related strokes, are associated with an increased risk of mortality.[2]

Contemporary cardiovascular implantable devices including pacemakers and implantable cardioverter-defibrillators (ICDs) can continuously monitor atrial rhythm, and device-detected atrial high-rate arrhythmias are common among patients without a known history of AF.[3,4] Episodes that are asymptomatic, and have a short duration (minutes to hours), are referred to as subclinical AF.[5] Studies defining the consequences of subclinical AF have used cardiovascular implantable devices to detect AF.

Subclinical AF seems to differ from other forms of AF including permanent, persistent, and paroxysmal AF in which the diagnosis is made by various forms of surface electrocardiogram (ECG) monitoring. Subclinical AF is associated with an increased risk of stroke; however, the increase in risk seems to be lower than that with clinical AF.[4,6] Most studies that have demonstrated the efficacy of oral anticoagulation (OAC) therapy among patients with persistent or permanent AF have required documentation of AF by two or more ECGs.

Subclinical AF is common after stroke. Approximately 16.9 million incident strokes occur annually worldwide.[1] Overall, 1 in 4 strokes are cryptogenic or an embolic stroke of undetermined source, of which some are likely due to subclinical AF. Subclinical AF has been detected in 12%–16% of patients within 30 days of an ischemic stroke and in more than 30% of patients within 2 years after a stroke.[4–7] OAC can prevent approximately 60%–80% of strokes in patients with documented clinical AF.[8–11] However, the burden of subclinical AF that is required to increase the risk for stroke and the features that increase the risk for developing subclinical AF and stroke are unknown. Furthermore, there is uncertainty regarding the relative safety and efficacy of OAC to reduce stroke risk among people with subclinical AF. Given this therapeutic equipoise, the role of screening for subclinical AF also remains controversial.

In this chapter, we will review the definition of subclinical AF, the pathophysiology of this condition, the overall prevalence, stroke risk, OAC treatment options, health economics associated with screening, and future directions.

DEFINING SUBCLINICAL ATRIAL FIBRILLATION

There is significant variation in the nomenclature describing asymptomatic and undiagnosed atrial arrhythmia: device- or pacemaker-detected atrial tachycardia or AF; atrial high-rate episodes; silent AF; subclinical atrial tachyarrhythmias; undiagnosed AF, and subclinical AF. Overall, each carries certain connotations depending on the clinical context. Atrial high-rate episodes and device- or pacemaker-detected atrial tachycardia or AF are based on intracardiac electrograms (EGMs) versus surface electrocardiography. However, these device-based arrhythmias are dependent on the discriminatory capacity of implantable devices, which varies by the device, the manufacturer, and detection algorithms. Typically, atrial detection algorithms are defined by atrial rate counts below a certain cycle length, the rate and variability of ventricular depolarizations, and the exclusion of potential artifacts. The overall accuracy of these device-detected arrhythmias is high.[5]

Nonatrial-based devices often detect AF only after the ventricular response exceeds the preprogrammed ventricular arrhythmia detection rate. Episodes of AF with ventricular response rates below the threshold will not be captured.

AF may be detected noninvasively—traditionally through pulse palpation or surface ECG. Increasingly, novel devices such as smartphone photoplethysmography, oscillometry, or single-lead electrocardiographic recordings can record single or multiple events, can be patient-activated or continuous, and may lead to detection of AF. Unlike implanted devices, these methods typically detect permanent or persistent AF.

In summary, clinical AF can occur in the presence or absence of symptoms, is of long duration (hours to days), and traditionally has been captured by electrocardiography. In contrast, subclinical AF is asymptomatic, of short duration (seconds to minutes), and usually only detected with the use of long-term, continuous monitoring.

PREVALENCE OF SUBCLINICAL ATRIAL FIBRILLATION

The prevalence of subclinical AF has been primarily determined among patients who receive atrial-based implantable cardiac devices.[4,12–15] The Relationship Between Daily Atrial Tachyarrhythmia Burden From Implantable Device Diagnostics and Stroke Risk study (TRENDS) enrolled patients with a clinical indication for a pacemaker or ICD and at least one stroke risk factor.[12] Of the patients without a baseline history of AT/AF (n = 163), newly detected AT/AF was identified via the device in 45 patients (28%) over a mean follow-up of 1.1 ± 0.7 years.

The Asymptomatic Atrial Fibrillation and Stroke Evaluation in Pacemaker Patients and Atrial Fibrillation Reduction Atrial Pacing Trial (ASSERT) enrolled patients with a dual-chamber pacemaker for sinus node or atrioventricular node disease or with an ICD for any reason.[4] Overall, at least one AT was detected via an implanted device over 3 months among 10.1% of patients; an additional 24.5% of patients had AT identified within approximately 2.5 years of follow-up. Long-term continuous monitoring increases the chance of detecting not only AF that is present at the time of monitoring initiation but also AF that develops subsequently. Furthermore, long-term continuous monitoring seems to be far superior to intermittent rhythm monitoring (IRM) for the detection of AT/AF.

A study using computationally intensive simulations evaluated IRM in 647 patients with implantable cardiac monitoring device.[15] The sensitivity of intermittent monitoring of various frequencies and durations on the identification of AF recurrence was evaluated, and overall, prolonged duration intermittent monitoring was superior to shorter IRM ($P < .0001$). However,

even with aggressive intermittent monitoring strategies, AF recurrence was not detected in a great proportion of patients. Even at similar AF burdens, patients with high-density AF required higher frequency or prolonged duration of intermittent monitoring to achieve the same sensitivity as in low-density AF ($P < .0001$). Overall, it seems that patients with high-density, low-burden AF benefit the most from continuous for detection of AF recurrence.

Despite our knowledge of the prevalence of AF in these populations, our knowledge of the incidence of subclinical AF in patients at high risk of strokes is limited. There are several ongoing studies aiming to extend these findings. The Graz Study on the Risk of Atrial Fibrillation (GRAF)[16] is enrolling patients 18 years or older at high risk for stroke with no electrocardiographic evidence of AF. These patients are randomized to an implantable cardiac monitor with a Medtronic Reveal XT implantable loop recorder or no implantable device. Irrespective of the study arm to which they are randomized, patients in both study groups receive monthly and then quarterly in-person follow-up with electrocardiography for approximately 1 year.

The Prevalence of Subclinical Atrial Fibrillation Using an Implantable Cardiac Monitor in Patients With Cardiovascular Risk Factors study (ASSERT-II)[17] will enroll a single arm cohort to receive an implantable cardiac monitor for continuous monitoring over the study follow-up period to determine the incidence of subclinical AF. Patients will be 65 years or older, plus have a CHA_2DS_2-VASc score ≥ 2, obstructive sleep apnea (documented by polysomnography, ambulatory oximetry, positive Berlin Questionnaire, or requiring the use of CPAP/BiPAP), or BMI > 30. In addition, patients must have echocardiographic or biochemical evidence of increased risk of AF including left atrial enlargement on a clinical echocardiography at any time before enrollment (defined as LA volume ≥ 58 mL or LA diameter of ≥ 4.4 cm) or serum NT-ProBNP ≥ 290 pg/mL. These studies will help to further define the prevalence of subclinical AF in populations at higher risk for stoke.

The Incidence of AF in High-Risk Patients study (REVEAL-AF) enrolled patients 18 years or older and at high risk for stroke to receive a Medtronic REVEAL implantable cardiac monitor and will be followed up for 18 months (Table 5.1). Patients with a $CHADS_2$ score ≥ 3 (or $= 2$ with an additional AF risk factor) were included. Patients with AF detected on ≥ 24 h of screening external monitoring before ICM insertion were excluded. The primary endpoint for REVEAL-AF was AF detection rate at 18 months. In total, 385 patients

TABLE 5.1
Key Ongoing Studies of Implantable Cardiac Monitors to Detect Subclinical Atrial Fibrillation (AF)

Study	Population Enrolled	Comparison Group	Follow-up Duration	Primary Outcome of Interest
GRAF[16]	Patients aged ≥18 years with CHA$_2$DS$_2$-VASc score ≥4	Monthly and then quarterly in-person follow-up with ECG	12 months	Time to first diagnosis of AF
ASSERT-II[17]	Patients with cardiovascular risk factors including age ≥65 years and CHA$_2$DS$_2$-VASc score >2, obstructive sleep apnea, or BMI >30, as well as echocardiographic evidence of left atrial enlargement or elevated serum N-terminal pro-brain-type natriuretic peptide level ≥290 pg/mL	None	12 months	First AF of ≥5 min
REVEAL-AF[18]	Patients aged ≥18 years with CHADS$_2$ score ≥3 or 2 and at least one of the following: glomerular filtration rate 30–60 mL/min, sleep apnea, coronary artery disease, or chronic obstructive pulmonary disease	None	18 months	Time to first AF of ≥6 min

(median age 71.5 years) received an implantable cardiac monitor. The AF detection rate at 18 months was 29.3% with rates at 30 days, 6, 12, 24, and 30 months of 6.2%, 20.4%, 27.1%, 33.6%, and 40.0%, respectively. AF would have gone undetected in the majority of patients had monitoring been limited to 30 days. These results indicate the unrecognized burden of AF in patients with stroke risk factors.[18]

SUBCLINICAL ATRIAL FIBRILLATION AND STROKE RISK

Subclinical AF has been detected frequently among patients with cryptogenic stroke, who receive continuous[19] or triggered monitoring[20] compared with routine monitoring. In the Cryptogenic Stroke and Underlying AF (CRYSTAL-AF) trial, 441 patients with cryptogenic strokes were randomized to an insertable cardiac monitor versus conventional follow-up (control). Patients were 40 years of age or older with no baseline evidence of AF. The primary endpoint (time to first detection of AF lasting >30 s within 6 months) was detected in 8.9% of patients in the insertable cardiac monitor group (19 patients) versus 1.4% of patients in the control group (3 patients) [hazard ratio, 6.4; 95% confidence interval (CI), 1.9–21.7; $P < .001$][20] (Fig. 5.1).

However, given a lack of uniformity in study design, providing a quantitative value of stroke risk

that adequately represents findings across studies has proved challenging. Differences in the time window to detect subclinical AF, the specific definitions, and the study populations examined vary considerably by study. Stroke risk estimates are correspondingly heterogeneous, ranging from hazard ratios of 0.87 (95% CI, 0.58–1.31) to 9.40 (95% CI, 1.80–47.00) (Table 5.2).

The definition and duration of implantable-device detected subclinical AF varies in published studies has varied significantly from three consecutive premature atrial contractions across a 24-month period to longer than 3.8 h across a 24-h period (Table 5.2). In general, paroxysmal and permanent AF have been thought to have a comparable stroke risk, but recent evidence suggests that paroxysmal AF carries a lower absolute risk than persistent or permanent AF.[21]

The rates of stroke and systemic embolism were analyzed in 6563 aspirin-treated patients with AF from the ACTIVE-A/AVERROES databases.[21] Overall, yearly ischemic stroke rates were 2.1%, 3.0%, and 4.2% for paroxysmal, persistent, and permanent AF, respectively, with adjusted hazard ratio of 1.83 ($P < .001$) for permanent versus paroxysmal and 1.44 ($P = .02$) for persistent versus paroxysmal.[21] In comparison, the risk for stroke in patients with subclinical AF may be even lower. In the ASSERT study, the presence of subclinical tachyarrhythmia was associated with an annual stroke rate of 1.54%.[4]

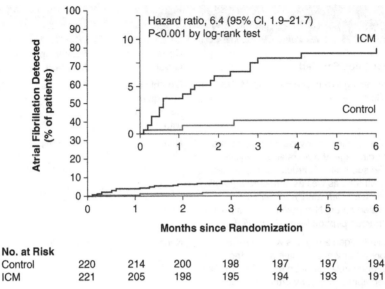

FIG. 5.1 Detection of atrial fibrillation using an insertable cardiac monitor after cryptogenic stroke. *ICM,* insertable cardiac monitor. (Adapted from Healey JS, Connolly SJ, Gold MR, et al. Subclinical atrial fibrillation and the risk of stroke. *N Engl J Med*. 2012;366(2):120–129. https://doi.org/10.1056/NEJMoa1105575.)

Most of the studies evaluating the risk of subclinical AF and stroke used prespecified cut points rather than empirically derived thresholds (Table 5.2). Although defining a threshold of subclinical AF is potentially useful, thresholds of AF duration and corresponding stroke risk vary by the presence of comorbidities.[14] A study assessed data from 568 patients with an implanted pacemaker and a history of AF was analyzed. Thromboembolic risk was quantified through $CHADS_2$ score and three AF groups were considered: patients with <5-min AF on 1 day (AF-free); patients with >5-min AF on 1 day but <24 h (AF-5 min); patients with AF episodes >24 h (AF-24 h). Three monitoring strategies were simulated including 24-h Holter, 1-week Holter, and 30-day Holter. Overall, 171 (30%) had $CHADS_2$ score = 0; 269 (47%) had $CHADS_2$ score = 1; 111 (20%) had $CHADS_2$ score = 2; and 17 (3%) had $CHADS_2$ score ≥ 3. During the follow-up period, 14 patients (2.5%) had an ischemic thromboembolic event. By combining AF presence/duration with $CHADS_2$ score, two subpopulations with markedly different risks of events were identified (0.8% vs. 5%, $P = .035$); the former corresponding to AF-free with $CHADS_2 ≤ 2$, or AF-5 min with $CHADS_2 ≤ 1$, or AF-24 h with $CHADS_2 = 0$. These results suggest that defining the risk of stroke with subclinical AF would vary significantly based on the presence or absence of cardiovascular comorbidities.

In addition to the intersection of comorbidities and subclinical AF stroke risk, emerging data indicate that a lower limit of AT/AF duration and stroke risk exists in certain populations.[22] A study of 5379 patients with pacemakers (N = 3141) or ICDs (N = 2238) at 225 US sites (median follow-up 22.9 months) adjudicated 37531 EGMs; 50% of patients had at least one episode of AT/AF. Short episodes of AT/AF were defined as episodes in which both the onset and offset of AT/AF were present within a single EGM recording. Short episodes of AT/AF were documented in 9% of pacemaker patients and 16% of ICD patients. Patients with clinical events were no more likely than those without to have short AT/AF (5.1% vs. 7.9% for pacemaker patients and 11.5% vs. 10.4% for ICD patients; $P = .21$ and .66, respectively).[22]

There is uncertainty regarding the temporal linkage between subclinical AF and subsequent stroke. One study indicates a temporal association between AF and stroke in a minority of cases.[23] Of 9850 patients with cardiac implantable electronic devices remotely monitored in the Veterans Administration Health Care System between 2002 and 2012, 187 patients were with acute ischemic stroke and continuous heart rhythm monitoring for 120 days before the stroke. Odds ratio for stroke was highest (17.4; 95% CI, 5.39–73.1) in the 5 days immediately after the occurrence of AF and

TABLE 5.2
Key Studies Evaluating the Duration and Burden of Subclinical Atrial Fibrillation

Study	Number of Patients	Study Design	Means of Detection	Adjudicated	Detection Criteria (bpm)	SCAF Burden	Detection Window	Primary Outcome	SCAF Event Rates	No SCAF Event Rate	HR (95% CI)[a]
Glotzer et al.[6]	312	Patients undergoing initial implantation of a dual-chamber pacemaker for sinus node dysfunction in sinus rhythm at the time of randomization	Dual-chamber pacemaker	No	>220	≥5 min	27 months	Stroke and mortality	NR	NR	2.79 (1.51–5.15)
Capucci et al.[26]	225	Patients with bradycardia and clear indication for dual-chamber pacing and a history of symptomatic atrial tachyarrhythmias	Dual-chamber pacemaker	No	Per physician detect	>1 day	22 months	Ischemic stroke, TIA, or peripheral arterial embolism	NR	NR	3.10 (1.10–10.5)
Glotzer et al.[3]	2486	Patients with a clear indication for an implantable device capable of long-term monitoring for arrhythmias and a $CHADS_2$ score >1b	CIED	No	>175	≥=5.5 h	30 days	Ischemic stroke, TIA, or systemic embolism	2.4	1.1	2.20 (0.96–5.05)
Shanmugam et al.[27]	560	Patients with heart failure and a cardiac resynchronization therapy device capable of long-term monitoring for arrhythmias via home monitoring and most home monitoring transmissions received during follow-up	Cardiac resynchronization therapy ± defibrillator	No	>180	>3.8h	24h	Stroke, TIA, and peripheral arterial embolism	NR	NR	9.40 (1.80–47.0)

Continued

TABLE 5.2
Key Studies Evaluating the Duration and Burden of Subclinical Atrial Fibrillation—cont'd

Study	Number of Patients	Study Design	Means of Detection	Adjudicated	Detection Criteria (bpm)	SCAF Burden	Detection Window	Primary Outcome	SCAF Event Rates	No SCAF Event Rate	HR (95% CI)[a]
Healey et al.[28]	2580	Patients with dual-chamber pacemakers capable of documenting AF	Dual-chamber pacemaker or defibrillator	Yes	>190	≥6 min	3 months	Ischemic stroke or systemic embolism	1.69	0.69	5.56 (1.28–4.85)
Boriani et al.[29]	10,016	Patients with an implantable device capable of measuring atrial tachyarrhythmia with available diagnostic data and without permanent AF	CIED	No	>175	5 min	24 h	Ischemic stroke	0.49	0.32	1.76 (1.02–3.02)
Swiryn et al.[22]	5379	Patients within 45 days of implantation of pacemaker or defibrillator that included an atrial lead	Pacemaker or defibrillator	Yes	>3 consecutive premature atrial contractions	Onset and offset within the same electrogram, or onset or offset not within the same electrogram	24 months	Stroke or TIA	NR	NR	0.87 (0.58–1.31) /1.51 (1.03–2.21)

AF, atrial fibrillation; *CHADS₂*, congestive heart failure, hypertension, age 75 years, diabetes mellitus, prior stroke or TIA, or thromboembolism; *CIED*, cardiovascular implantable electronic device; *HR*, hazard ratio; *NR*, not reported; *SCAF*, subclinical atrial fibrillation; *TIA*, transient ischemic attack.
[a]Cox proportional hazards models were adjusted for known thromboembolic risk factors.

decreased toward 1.0 as the period after the AF occurrence increased beyond 30 days.

However, several other studies suggest no temporal association exists between AF occurrence and subsequent stroke.[24,25] A substudy of the ASSERT identified that of 51 patients who experienced stroke or systemic embolism during follow-up, 26 (51%) had subclinical AF. In 18 patients (35%), subclinical AF was detected before stroke or systemic embolism. However, only four patients (8%) had subclinical AF detected within 30 days before stroke or systemic embolism, and only one of these four patients was experiencing subclinical AF at the time of the stroke (Fig. 5.2). In the 14 patients with SCAF detected >30 days before the stroke or systemic embolism event, the most recent episode occurred at a median interval of 339 days (25th–75th percentile, 211–619) earlier.[25] These contradictory findings may be related to differences in study designs or populations.

THE PATHOGENESIS OF SUBCLINICAL ATRIAL FIBRILLATION STROKE RISK

The pathogenesis of subclinical AF stroke risk is multifactorial, yet the major contributory factors remain unclear. AF and stroke have been associated in multiple epidemiologic and basic science studies indicating a true association between these conditions.[2,30] Overall, it is believed that potentially AF causes stroke, stroke causes AF, and AF is associated with other factors that cause stroke.[31] As described by Kamel and colleagues, the association of AF and stroke seems to satisfy many of the Bradford Hill criteria for association, namely, (1) strength of association, (2) consistency, (3) specificity, (4) temporality, (5) biologic gradient, (6) plausibility, (7) coherence, (8) accordance with experimental results, and (9) analogy. The strength of association, consistency, specificity of AF, and stroke relationship have been demonstrated in many studies and across multiple cohorts.[2,23,30,32]

Furthermore, the causal association is biologically plausible activity would result in the stasis of blood and should increase thromboembolic risk. However, there are some conflicting results.

Many studies have found a relationship between AF burden and stroke,[3,21] but this is not consistent across all studies.[33] In the RE-LY trial, after a mean follow-up of 2 years, the overall risk of stroke or systemic embolism in patients with paroxysmal, persistent, and permanent AF was similar (1.32%, 1.55%, and 1.49% per year, respectively).[33] The ASSERT study demonstrated

that a single brief episode of subclinical AF is associated with a twofold higher risk of stroke in older patients with vascular risk factors[4]; however, younger and healthy patients with clinically apparent AF do not face a significantly increased stroke risk.[34]

A study in Taiwan enrolled 509 males (CHA_2DS_2-VASc score = 0) and 320 females (CHA_2DS_2-VASc score = 1) with AF who were not receiving any antithrombotic therapy. These patients were selected from the National Health Insurance Research Database. To obtain controls, for each study patient, 10 age-matched and sex-matched subjects without AF and without any comorbidity from the CHA_2DS_2-VASc scheme were selected. During a follow-up of 57.4 months, 1.4% of patients experienced ischemic stroke. Overall, the event rate did not differ between groups with and without AF for male patients (1.6% vs. 1.6%; $P = .920$); however, AF was a significant risk factor for ischemic stroke among females with event rates of 4.4% and 0.7% for patients with and without AF ($P < .001$).[34]

These data highlight the conflicting information regarding the role of AF burden and risk of stroke. As the burden of subclinical AF, by definition, is substantially lower in patients with AF, it is unclear if the classic biologic hypothesis of increased atrial blood stasis and clot formation is the primary mechanism of the increased stroke risk.

Potentially, subclinical AF is a marker, rather than a cause of stroke.[24,25] In the ASSERT study, around 50% of patients had SCAF. Among these patients, 35% had SCAF detected before stroke systemic embolism, 8% within 30 days before stroke, and only one patient was experiencing SCAF at the time of the stroke. Finally, in 8 patients with both SCAF and an embolic event (16%), SCAF was detected only after the stroke or embolism, at a median interval of 101 days (25th to 75th percentile, 14–196 days) later.[25] These results further provide conflicting information on the causal role of subclinical AF and stroke risk.

The relationship between AF and stroke also does not satisfy the Bradford Hill criterion of specificity, namely if AF induces atrial blood stasis and subsequent thromboembolism, it should be specifically associated with embolic strokes.[31] There seems to be an especially strong association between AF and embolic strokes; however, 10% of patients with lacunar strokes have AF,[35] and among patients with AF, compared with those without, large-artery atherosclerosis is twice as common. The link between AF and noncardioembolic stroke indicates that stroke risk in AF cannot be entirely explained by AF directly causing stroke.

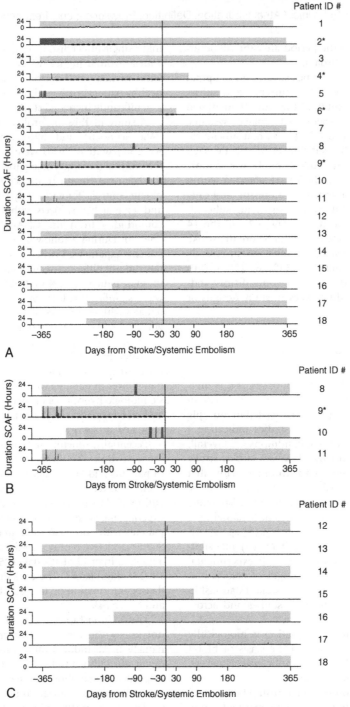

FIG. 5.2 Summary of subclinical atrial fibrillation occurring within 1 year of stroke or systemic embolism. **(A)** Each row represents data collected from each of 18 patients who had subclinical atrial fibrillation (SCAF) within 1 year before or after the event. Total hours of atrial episodes per day are denoted by the height of each *red vertical line*. *Gray shaded* areas correspond to the period of continuous monitoring with cardiac device. *Asterisks* and *black dashed lines* denote use and period of oral anticoagulation therapy. ID indicates identification. **(B)** Summary of SCAF events occurring within 30 days before stroke or systemic embolism. Each row represents data collected from each of four patients who had the last SCAF within 30 days before the event. **(C)** Summary of SCAF events occurring only after the stroke or systemic embolism. Each row represents data collected from each of seven patients who had SCAF within 1 year after the event. (Adapted from Brambatti M, Connolly SJ, Gold MR, et al. Temporal relationship between subclinical atrial fibrillation and embolic events. *Circulation*. 2014;129(21):2094–2099.)

STROKE RISK STRATIFICATION IN PATIENTS WITH SUBCLINICAL ATRIAL FIBRILLATION

The optimal strategy to identify patients with a substrate predisposing them to a higher risk for stroke continues to evolve. In the case of clinical AF, the $CHADS_2$ score (congestive heart failure; hypertension; age ≥75 years; diabetes mellitus; prior stroke, transient ischemic attack, or thromboembolism; range, 0–6, with higher scores indicating higher risk for stroke) and CHA_2DS_2-VASc score (congestive heart failure; hypertension; age ≥75 years; diabetes mellitus; prior stroke, transient ischemic attack, or thromboembolism; vascular disease; age 65–74 years; female sex; range, 0–9, with higher scores indicating higher risk for stroke) are the most commonly used risk prediction tools for the identification of stroke risk.[36] Whether this risk score extends into the patient population of subclinical AF remains to be evaluated. In the general public, factors that accurately predict stroke include left atrial size and structure, elevations of natriuretic peptide and troponin levels, and obstructive sleep apnea.[37,38] Significantly, the N-terminal fragment of pro–brain-type natriuretic peptide and high-sensitivity cardiac troponin play a prominent role in a biomarker-based risk score that performs better than the CHA_2DS_2-VASc score.[39–41] In addition, nontraditional risk factors, whether clinical factors or biomarkers, may also be prognostically important in linking AF and stroke. For example, previously underappreciated clinical factors include chronic obstructive pulmonary disease[42] and renal disease.[43] These risk factors have been used to enrich the populations of ongoing studies evaluating the burden of subclinical AF in various populations (Table 5.2). Whether these risk factors and associated scores play a role in patients with subclinical AF requires further study.

TREATMENT OF SUBCLINICAL ATRIAL FIBRILLATION

As OAC has been proven to reduce stroke risk in patients with clinical AF, such therapies may reduce stroke risk in patients with subclinical AF; however, the absolute risk for stroke associated with subclinical (vs. clinical) AF is lower, thereby potentially reducing the treatment effect and net clinical benefit of anticoagulation. In all trials that have assessed warfarin efficacy, most of these patients had persistent or permanent AF. Trials of non–vitamin K oral anticoagulation included patients with implantable device–detected AF when AF was not present at the time of enrollment, but patients with these devices were underrepresented, and the overall risk-benefit ratio was unknown.[8–11] Overall, no reliable evidence of OAC benefit was found in the subclinical AF population. In the current clinical practice, some patients with subclinical AF receive anticoagulation, whereas others do not,[44] suggesting clinical equipoise.

There are three ongoing studies that are assessing the feasibility of intermittent use of oral anticoagulant therapy based on the timing of AF episodes as detected by continuous monitoring with an implantable device: (1) Combined Use of BIOTRONIK Home Monitoring and Pre-defined Anticoagulation to Reduce Stroke Risk trial (IMPACT)[45]; (2) Rhythm Evaluation for Anticoagulation With Continuous Monitoring pilot study (REACT.COM)[46]; and (3) Tailored Anticoagulation for Non-Continuous Anticoagulation trial (TACTIC-AF).[47]

IMPACT evaluated the hypothesis that stroke risk may be highest around the time of AF episodes, and this risk could be mitigated with use of anticoagulation around the time of these episodes. Tailoring anticoagulant therapy accordingly would include stopping OAC therapy when AF episodes are not proximal. This strategy may potentially maintain the stroke reduction benefit of OAC therapy and minimize the bleeding risk. However, IMPACT was limited by a lack of adherence to a complex protocol.[45] Overall, 2718 patients with dual-chamber and biventricular defibrillators were randomized to start and stop anticoagulation based on remote rhythm monitoring versus usual office-based follow-up. The primary endpoint was the composite endpoint of stroke, systemic embolism, and major bleeding. The trial was stopped after 2 years median follow-up based on futility of finding a difference in primary endpoints between groups. Overall, 945 patients (34.8%) developed AT, 264 meeting study anticoagulation criteria. Primary events (2.4 vs. 2.3 per 100 patient-years) did not differ between groups (HR 1.06; 95% CI 0.75–1.51; $P = .732$) and major bleeding occurred at 1.6 versus 1.2 per 100 patient-years (HR 1.39; 95% CI 0.89–2.17; $P = .145$). Although AT burden was associated with thromboembolism, there was no temporal relationship between AT and stroke.[45]

TACTIC-AF is similarly designed to assess the feasibility of intermittent non–vitamin K antagonism use. Enrolled patients are assigned to intermittent OAC use based on implantable monitoring data or usual care.

Given the uncertainty of the risk/benefit ratio of OAC for stroke prevention in patients with device-detected subclinical AF, treatment patterns and guideline recommendations vary substantially. The 2016 European Society of Cardiology guidelines indicate uncertainty in whether subclinical AF requires the same therapeutic anticoagulation requirements as clinically overt AF, and recommend that patients with subclinical

AF should undergo further ECG monitoring to document AF before initiating anticoagulation therapy.[48] Conversely, the 2014 Canadian Cardiovascular Society Guidelines recommend OAC therapy for patients with subclinical AF who are ≥65 years of age, with a CHADS$_2$ score ≥1, and episodes that last more than 24 h, or for shorter episodes only if the patient is at high risk, such as having a history of recent cryptogenic stroke.[49] The question of whether this therapeutic approach is beneficial for patients with subclinical AF remained to be investigated in a large randomized trial.

There are two ongoing trials aiming to address the risk and benefit of non–vitamin K OAC therapy among patients free of AF but at high risk for stroke with a previously placed implantable device: (1) Apixaban for the Reduction of Thrombo-Embolism in Patients With Device-Detected Subclinical Atrial Fibrillation trial (ARTESiA)[50] and (2) Non–vitamin K Antagonist Oral Anticoagulants in Patients With Atrial High Rate Episodes trial (NOAH).[51]

In ARTESiA, approximately 4000 patients with at least one episode of device-detected subclinical AF (at least 6 min but less than 24 h) are randomized to apixaban versus low-dose aspirin. The primary efficacy outcome is stroke or systemic embolism and the key safety endpoint is major bleeding. In addition to having subclinical AF, eligible patients must have increased risk of stroke defined by the following: (1) previous stroke, or transient ischemic attack, or systemic embolism, or age 75 years or older; (2) age 65–74 years and two additional risk factors; or (3) age 55–64 years and three additional risk factors. The risk factors for stroke are female sex, hypertension, heart failure, diabetes, and vascular disease (coronary artery disease, peripheral artery disease, or aortic plaque).

In NOAH, a patient population (N=3400) similar to that in ARTESiA will be enrolled and randomized to edoxaban versus low-dose aspirin or placebo. The primary efficacy outcome will be stroke, systemic embolism, or cardiovascular death, whereas the principal safety endpoints are major bleeding or all-cause death.

Until evidence from these trials emerge to help guide treatment selection, there is a void in anticoagulation management strategies in these individuals. Patients with a CHA$_2$DS$_2$-VASc score of <2 are less likely to benefit from OAC regardless of the duration of subclinical AF. Those with a CHA$_2$DS$_2$-VASc score of ≥2 who experience longer episodes of AF (>24 h) may have similar stroke risk compared with those who have AF enrolled in historical anticoagulation trials clinical trials. These subclinical AF patients may warrant anticoagulation. For episodes shorter than 6 min

in patients with a CHA$_2$DS$_2$-VASc score of at least 2, the risk for stroke is likely very low, and not starting anticoagulation therapy would be a reasonable treatment option. Conversely, for episodes ranging from 6 min to 24 h in the setting of a CHA$_2$DS$_2$-VASc score of at least 2, there is little consensus on the risks to benefits ratio of starting OAC. Ongoing randomized trials will determine whether non–vitamin K oral anticoagulants can reduce the risk for stroke and systemic embolism in patients with AF lasting for several minutes but less than 24 h.

CONCLUSIONS
The burden of AF will grow as our population ages and the presence of comorbidities such as hypertension and obesity increases. The detection of subclinical AF remains an active area of research, and the optimal time when stroke risk increases remains to be determined. The optimal detection strategy is also under active evaluation as novel technologies, from handheld devices, to watches, to implantable monitors are now available and may facilitate the detection of subclinical AF. Ultimately, trials such as ARTESiA and NOAH will help to guide treatment strategies in patients with subclinical AF. Future directions of research will involve evaluating the detection of subclinical AF among patients with high-risk subgroups including heart failure and diabetes.

REFERENCES
1. Mozaffarian D, Benjamin EJ, Go AS, et al. Heart disease and stroke Statistics-2016 update: a report from the American heart association. *Circulation.* 2016;133(4):e38-e360. https://doi.org/10.1161/CIR.0000000000000350.
2. Wolf PA, Abbott RD, Kannel WB. Atrial fibrillation as an independent risk factor for stroke: the Framingham Study. *Stroke.* 1991;22(8):983-988. https://doi.org/10.1161/01.STR.22.8.983.
3. Glotzer TV, Daoud EG, Wyse DG, et al. The relationship between daily atrial tachyarrhythmia burden from implantable device diagnostics and stroke risk: the TRENDS study. *Circulation Arrhythmia Electrophysiol.* 2009;2(5):474-480. https://doi.org/10.1161/CIRCEP.109.849638.
4. Healey JS, Connolly SJ, Gold MR, et al. Subclinical atrial fibrillation and the risk of stroke. *N Engl J Med.* 2012;366(2):120-129. https://doi.org/10.1056/NEJMoa1105575.
5. Hess PL, Healey JS, Granger CB, et al. The role of cardiovascular implantable electronic devices in the detection and treatment of subclinical atrial fibrillation. *JAMA Cardiol.* 2017;2(3):324. https://doi.org/10.1001/jamacardio.2016.5167.

6. Glotzer TV, Hellkamp AS, Zimmerman J, et al. Atrial high rate episodes detected by pacemaker diagnostics predict death and stroke: report of the Atrial Diagnostics Ancillary Study of the MOde Selection Trial (MOST). *Circulation.* 2003;107(12):1614–1619. https://doi.org/10.1161/01.CIR.0000057981.70380.45.

7. Flint AC, Banki NM, Ren X, Rao VA, Go AS. Detection of paroxysmal atrial fibrillation by 30-day event monitoring in cryptogenic ischemic stroke: the stroke and monitoring for PAF in real time (SMART) registry. *Stroke.* 2012;43(10):2788–2790. https://doi.org/10.1161/STROKEAHA.112.665844.

8. Connolly SJ, Ezekowitz MD, Yusuf S, et al. Dabigatran versus warfarin in patients with atrial fibrillation. *N Engl J Med.* 2009;361(12):1139–1151. https://doi.org/10.1056/NEJMoa0905561.

9. Patel MR, Mahaffey KW, Garg J, et al. Rivaroxaban versus warfarin in nonvalvular atrial fibrillation. *N Engl J Med.* 2011;365(10):883–891. https://doi.org/10.1056/NEJMoa1009638.

10. Granger CB, Alexander JH, McMurray JJV, et al. Apixaban versus warfarin in patients with atrial fibrillation. *N Engl J Med.* 2011;365(11):981–992. https://doi.org/10.1056/NEJMoa1107039.

11. Giugliano RP, Ruff CT, Braunwald E, et al. Edoxaban versus warfarin in patients with atrial fibrillation. *N Engl J Med.* 2013;369(22):2093–2104. https://doi.org/10.1056/NEJMoa1310907.

12. Ziegler PD, Glotzer TV, Daoud EG, et al. Incidence of newly detected atrial arrhythmias via implantable devices in patients with a history of thromboembolic events. *Stroke.* 2010;41(2):256–260. https://doi.org/10.1161/STROKEAHA.109.571455.

13. Hindricks G, Pokushalov E, Urban L, et al. Performance of a new leadless implantable cardiac monitor in detecting and quantifying atrial fibrillation results of the XPECT trial. *Circulation Arrhythmia Electrophysiol.* 2010;3(2):141–147. https://doi.org/10.1161/CIRCEP.109.877852.

14. Botto GL, Padeletti L, Santini M, et al. Presence and duration of atrial fibrillation detected by continuous monitoring: crucial implications for the risk of thromboembolic events. *J Cardiovasc Electrophysiol.* 2008;20(3):241–248. https://doi.org/10.1001/archinte.167.3.246.

15. Charitos EI, Stierle U, Ziegler PD, et al. A comprehensive evaluation of rhythm monitoring strategies for the detection of atrial fibrillation recurrence: insights from 647 continuously monitored patients and implications for monitoring after therapeutic interventions. *Circulation.* 2012;126(7):806–814. https://doi.org/10.1161/CIRCULATIONAHA.112.098079.

16. NCT01461434. https://clinicaltrials.gov/ct2/show/NCT01461434.

17. NCT01694394. https://clinicaltrials.gov/ct2/show/NCT01694394.

18. http://www.abstractsonline.com/pp8/#!/4227/presentation/12996.

19. Sanna T, Diener H-C, Passman RS, et al. Cryptogenic stroke and underlying atrial fibrillation. *N Engl J Med.* 2014;370(26):2478–2486. https://doi.org/10.1056/NEJMoa1313600.

20. Gladstone DJ, Spring M, Dorian P, et al. Atrial fibrillation in patients with cryptogenic stroke. *N Engl J Med.* 2014;370(26):2467–2477. https://doi.org/10.1056/NEJMoa1311376.

21. Vanassche T, Lauw MN, Eikelboom JW, et al. Risk of ischaemic stroke according to pattern of atrial fibrillation: analysis of 6563 aspirin-treated patients in ACTIVE-A and AVERROES. *Eur Heart J.* 2015;36(5):281–287. https://doi.org/10.1093/eurheartj/ehu307.

22. Swiryn S, Orlov MV, Benditt DG, et al. Clinical implications of brief device-detected atrial tachyarrhythmias in a cardiac rhythm management device population: results from the registry of atrial tachycardia and atrial fibrillation episodes. *Circulation.* 2016;134(16):1130–1140. https://doi.org/10.1161/CIRCULATIONAHA.115.020252.

23. Turakhia MP, Ziegler PD, Schmitt SK, et al. Atrial fibrillation burden and short-term risk of stroke: case-crossover analysis of continuously recorded heart rhythm from cardiac electronic implanted devices. *Circulation Arrhythmia Electrophysiol.* 2015;8(5):1040–1047. https://doi.org/10.1161/CIRCEP.114.003057.

24. Daoud EG, Glotzer TV, Wyse DG, et al. Temporal relationship of atrial tachyarrhythmias, cerebrovascular events, and systemic emboli based on stored device data: a subgroup analysis of TRENDS. *Heart Rhythm.* 2011;8(9):1416–1423. https://doi.org/10.1016/j.hrthm.2011.04.022.

25. Brambatti M, Connolly SJ, Gold MR, et al. Temporal relationship between subclinical atrial fibrillation and embolic events. *Circulation.* 2014;129(21):2094–2099. https://doi.org/10.1161/CIRCULATIONAHA.113.007825.

26. Capucci A, Santini M, PADELETTI L, et al. Monitored atrial fibrillation duration predicts arterial embolic events in patients suffering from bradycardia and atrial fibrillation implanted with antitachycardia pacemakers. *J Am Coll Cardiol.* 2005;46(10):1913–1920. https://doi.org/10.1016/j.jacc.2005.07.044.

27. Shanmugam N, Boerdlein A, Proff J, et al. Detection of atrial high-rate events by continuous Home Monitoring: clinical significance in the heart failure-cardiac resynchronization therapy population. *Europace.* 2012;14(2):230–237. https://doi.org/10.1093/europace/eur293.

28. Healey JS, Merchant R, Simpson C, et al. Canadian cardiovascular society/canadian anesthesiologists' society/canadian heart rhythm society joint position statement on the perioperative management of patients with implanted pacemakers, defibrillators, and neurostimulating devices. *Can J Cardiol.* 2012;28(2):141–151. https://doi.org/10.1016/j.cjca.2011.08.121.

29. BORIANI G, Glotzer TV, Santini M, et al. Device-detected atrial fibrillation and risk for stroke: an analysis of >10,000 patients from the SOS AF project (Stroke prevention Strategies based on atrial fibrillation information from implanted devices). *Eur Heart J.* 2014;35(8):508–516. https://doi.org/10.1093/eurheartj/eht491.

30. Wolf PA, Dawber TR, Thomas HE, Kannel WB. Epidemiologic assessment of chronic atrial fibrillation and risk of stroke: the Framingham study. *Neurology.* 1978;28(10):973–977.
31. Kamel H, Okin PM, Elkind MSV, Iadecola C. Atrial fibrillation and mechanisms of stroke: time for a new model. *Stroke.* 2016;47(3):895–900. https://doi.org/10.1161/STROKEAHA.115.012004.
32. Hughes M, Lip GYH. Guideline development group, national clinical guideline for management of atrial fibrillation in primary and secondary care, national institute for health and clinical excellence. Stroke and thromboembolism in atrial fibrillation: a systematic review of stroke risk factors, risk stratification schema and cost effectiveness data. *Thromb Haemost.* 2008;99(2):295–304. https://doi.org/10.1160/TH07-08-0508.
33. Flaker G, Ezekowitz M, Yusuf S, et al. Efficacy and safety of dabigatran compared to warfarin in patients with paroxysmal, persistent, and permanent atrial fibrillation: results from the RE-LY (Randomized Evaluation of Long-Term Anticoagulation Therapy) study. *J Am Coll Cardiol.* 2012;59(9):854–855. https://doi.org/10.1016/j.jacc.2011.10.896.
34. Chao TF, Liu CJ, Chen SJ, et al. Atrial fibrillation and the risk of ischemic stroke: does it still matter in patients with a CHA2DS2-VASc score of 0 or 1? *Stroke.* 2012;43(10):2551–2555. https://doi.org/10.1161/STROKEAHA.112.667865.
35. Lodder J, Bamford JM, Sandercock PA, Jones LN, Warlow CP. Are hypertension or cardiac embolism likely causes of lacunar infarction? *Stroke.* 1990;21(3):375–381. https://doi.org/10.1161/01.STR.21.3.375.
36. Committee CTJMPFCW, Committee LSWMMFVCW, Member JSAMFFWC, et al. 2014 AHA/ACC/HRS guideline for the management of patients with atrial fibrillation: executive summary. *J Antimicrob Chemother.* 2014;64(21):2246–2280. https://doi.org/10.1016/j.jacc.2014.03.021.
37. Lip GYH, Nieuwlaat R, Pisters R, Lane DA, Crijns HJGM. Refining clinical risk stratification for predicting stroke and thromboembolism in atrial fibrillation using a novel risk factor-based approach: the Euro heart survey on atrial fibrillation. *Chest.* 2010;137(2):263–272. https://doi.org/10.1378/chest.09-1584.
38. Yaggi HK, Concato J, Kernan WN, Lichtman JH, Brass LM, Mohsenin V. Obstructive sleep apnea as a risk factor for stroke and death. *N Engl J Med.* 2005;353(19):2034–2041. https://doi.org/10.1056/NEJMoa043104.
39. Hijazi Z, Oldgren J, Andersson U, et al. Cardiac biomarkers are associated with an increased risk of stroke and death in patients with atrial fibrillation: a Randomized Evaluation of Long-term Anticoagulation Therapy (RE-LY) substudy. *Circulation.* 2012;125(13):1605–1616. https://doi.org/10.1161/CIRCULATIONAHA.111.038729.
40. Hijazi Z, Wallentin L, Siegbahn A, et al. High-sensitivity troponin T and risk stratification in patients with atrial fibrillation during treatment with apixaban or warfarin. *J Am Coll Cardiol.* 2014;63(1):52–61. https://doi.org/10.1016/j.jacc.2013.07.093.
41. Hijazi Z, Wallentin L, Siegbahn A, et al. N-terminal pro-B-type natriuretic peptide for risk assessment in patients with atrial fibrillation: insights from the ARISTOTLE Trial (Apixaban for the Prevention of Stroke in Subjects with Atrial Fibrillation). *J Am Coll Cardiol.* 2013;61(22):2274–2284. https://doi.org/10.1016/j.jacc.2012.11.082.
42. de Vos CB, Pisters R, Nieuwlaat R, et al. Progression from paroxysmal to persistent atrial fibrillation clinical correlates and prognosis. *J Am Coll Cardiol.* 2010;55(8):725–731. https://doi.org/10.1016/j.jacc.2009.11.040.
43. Piccini JP, Stevens SR, Chang Y, et al. Renal dysfunction as a predictor of stroke and systemic embolism in patients with nonvalvular atrial fibrillation clinical perspective. *Circulation.* 2013;127(2):224–232. https://doi.org/10.1161/CIRCULATIONAHA.112.107128.
44. Healey JS, Martin JL, Duncan A, et al. Pacemaker-detected atrial fibrillation in patients with pacemakers: prevalence, predictors, and current use of oral anticoagulation. *Can J Cardiol.* 2013;29(2):224–228. https://doi.org/10.1016/j.cjca.2012.08.019.
45. Martin DT, Bersohn MM, Waldo AL, et al. Randomized trial of atrial arrhythmia monitoring to guide anticoagulation in patients with implanted defibrillator and cardiac resynchronization devices. *Eur Heart J.* 2015;36(26):1660–1668. https://doi.org/10.1093/eurheartj/ehv115.
46. Passman R, Leong-Sit P, Andrei A-C, et al. Targeted anticoagulation for atrial fibrillation guided by continuous rhythm assessment with an insertable cardiac monitor: the rhythm evaluation for anticoagulation with continuous monitoring (REACT.COM) pilot study. *J Cardiovasc Electrophysiol.* 2016;27(3):264–270. https://doi.org/10.1111/jce.12864.
47. https://clinicaltrials.gov/ct2/show/NCT01650298.
48. Kirchhof P, Benussi S, Kotecha D, et al. 2016 ESC Guidelines for the management of atrial fibrillation developed in collaboration with EACTS. *Eur Heart J.* 2016;37(38):2893–2962. https://doi.org/10.1093/eurheartj/ehw210.
49. Macle L, Cairns J, Leblanc K, et al. 2016 Focused update of the Canadian cardiovascular society guidelines for the management of atrial fibrillation. *Can J Cardiol.* 2016;32(10):1170–1185. https://doi.org/10.1016/j.cjca.2016.07.591.
50. Lopes RD, Alings M, Connolly SJ, et al. Rationale and design of the apixaban for the reduction of thrombo-embolism in patients with device-detected sub-clinical atrial fibrillation (ARTESiA) trial. *Am Heart J.* 2017;189:137–145. https://doi.org/10.1016/j.ahj.2017.04.008.
51. Kirchhof P. *Non-vitamin K Antagonist Oral Anticoagulants in Patients with Atrial High Rate Episodes (NOAH).* NCT02618577. ClinicalTrials. gov (4 July 2016); 2016.

CHAPTER 6

The New Anticoagulation Clinic

ANNE E. ROSE, PHARMD

INTRODUCTION

In the United States, millions of patients are anticoagulated with warfarin, and there are approximately 3000 established anticoagulation clinics to assist with the management of this medication.[1] Compared with usual care, anticoagulation clinics are associated with better control of anticoagulation, decreased thrombotic and bleeding events, and decreased hospitalizations and emergency room visits.[2] Despite the known benefits of specialized anticoagulation care, many patients do not have access to anticoagulation clinics because of patient or provider preference, access through insurance coverage, or lack thereof, or regional location.

The challenges with warfarin management are well known. The narrow therapeutic window, variable dosing, multitude of drug interactions, dietary restrictions, and risk for bleeding complications have created the need for specialized clinics to assist with the management of warfarin to both enhance efficacy through increased time in therapeutic range (TTR) and decrease adverse events associated with anticoagulants.[3–5]

Whether by a specialized anticoagulation clinic or by a primary care provider, anticoagulation therapy should be closely monitored, as it can be associated with increased bleeding complications, especially if not well controlled.[5] Warfarin-related adverse drug events (ADEs) continue to be the most common reason for emergency hospitalization. A review of ADEs in an elderly population identified hematologic agents as the drug class with the highest percentage of hospitalizations compared with all other drug categories in the study. Warfarin was the medication associated with the most hospitalizations (33%) compared with all other medications in the study. Other common medications associated with hospitalizations included insulins (13.9%), antiplatelets (13.3%), and oral hypoglycemic agents (10.7%). Emergency department visits and hospitalizations related to hematologic agents were most commonly due to intracranial hemorrhage (ICH), gastrointestinal bleeding, and hemoptysis.[6]

For decades, warfarin was the only oral anticoagulant available. Today, the use of direct oral anticoagulant (DOAC) therapy continues to increase, with DOACs now accounting for 62% of all new prescriptions for anticoagulants since 2013.[7] The increase in use has been attributed to nationally recognized guidelines and guidance papers recommending DOACs over warfarin for treatment of venous thromboembolism (VTE) and atrial fibrillation (AF), the availability of a reversal agent, and overall physician awareness and comfort level with this new drug class.[8–12]

With the development of the DOACs, some of the previous challenges seen with anticoagulant therapy have been resolved, as they provide standardized dosing, require minimal monitoring, have fewer drug interactions, and are associated with a decreased risk of bleeding complications when compared with warfarin. However, the DOACs are not without their own challenges. Because of the short half-lives of these agents, a missed dose could leave the patient underanticoagulated; therefore, patient compliance is a big factor to consider when selecting a DOAC. Additionally, there are specific conditions where data for DOAC use are limited, for example, obesity, low body weight, hemodialysis, cancer, and hypercoagulable disease states and where warfarin is still the preferred anticoagulant (i.e., mechanical heart valves).[13–17]

In the era of a new anticoagulant drug class and the changing healthcare environment where there is a push to keep comprehensive care in the patient's medical home, anticoagulation clinics are challenged with the need to adapt to remain relevant in the anticoagulation management space. The aim of this chapter is to expand on how specialized anticoagulation clinics can and have been evolving during this transition and will explore areas to consider for further expansion.

FUNCTION OF ANTICOAGULATION CLINICS

Vitamin K antagonists (VKAs), i.e., warfarin, are associated with adverse events mostly because of the narrow therapeutic range. The narrow therapeutic range often equates to frequent dose adjustments and laboratory monitoring to find the maintenance dose that is most appropriate for the patient. The degree of anticoagulation can be affected by many factors including compliance, dietary intake of vitamin K, alcohol consumption, interacting medications, activity level, and illness. These patient-specific factors should be taken into consideration when developing a warfarin dosing plan.[3–5] This level of management can be burdensome to a primary care provider who is expected to stay on a specified time schedule for patient appointments or the provider's nurse who is triaging multiple clinic calls per day in addition to assisting with patient care needs. To combat this, specialized anticoagulation clinics were created to assist with the complex management of VKAs.[2,18,19]

Anticoagulation clinics typically employ pharmacists, nurses, or a combination of both to assist with the management of warfarin via a delegation protocol or collaborative practice agreement. The variability in staffing the clinic is determined by both personnel and financial resources available within a healthcare system. Although there have been some reported differences in the quality of care between pharmacist-managed and nurse-managed anticoagulation clinics, both models of care have demonstrated improved outcomes when compared with traditional physician management.[2,18–23] This is discussed further in the chapter.

There is no standardized model for how an anticoagulation clinic is designed, as this is driven by the resources of the health system. An example of a common model of care is telephonic management. This is when the international normalized ratio (INR) is performed by a venipuncture laboratory sample and the patient is contacted by his/her anticoagulation provider via telephone to complete the warfarin management. Other models of care are outlined in Table 6.1.[2,21,22,24–31]

There are studies that have compared anticoagulation clinic models of care to determine the best strategy for warfarin management. When in-clinic, face-to-face appointments are compared with telephone management, the face-to-face visits trend toward improved TTR, decreased adverse events, and decreased hospitalizations.[2,24] However, there are also studies that show similar clinical outcomes between these two models.[25,26]

Patient self-testing (PST) is a model that continues to grow in popularity among anticoagulation clinic models of care. In PST the patient uses a point-of-care INR meter in a home setting and communicates the INR result through either an electronic portal or telephone to their anticoagulation provider to complete the management plan. PST has been compared with anticoagulation clinics for management and INR testing. These studies have shown an improvement in TTR and clinical outcomes with PST.[30,32,33] The Home INR Study (THINRS) was a prospective, randomized, multicenter study comparing PST with face-to-face INR management. PST was associated with a higher TTR but no advantage over clinical outcomes including time to first stroke, major bleeding, or death compared with patients managed in a clinic setting.[27] For patients who do not have access to transportation, who have work responsibilities

---

TABLE 6.1
Examples of Models of Care Within Anticoagulation Clinics[16,20,21,23–30]

Anticoagulation Clinic Model of Care	Process for INR Management
Clinic management	Patient is seen by appointment in the clinic for INR management. The INR is typically performed by point-of-care (POC) method during appointment or by venipuncture draw before appointment.
Telephonic management	Patient is contacted by telephone for INR management. The INR is performed by venipuncture draw in a laboratory setting before phone call.
Telehealth management	Patient is contacted through the electronic medical record (i.e., personal healthcare portal or interface) or via video chat for INR management. INR is performed by venipuncture or home INR meter before contact.
Patient self-testing	Patient is contacted by telephone or through telehealth option. INR is performed by the patient with a home INR meter before contact.
Patient self-management	Patient is provided with a warfarin dose adjustment scale. INR is performed by home INR meter. Clinic may become involved for high INR readings (i.e., INR > 5), if initiated by patient, or at set times throughout the year.

INR, international normalized ratio.

during clinic hours, or whose living situation may not be near the clinic, the frequent monitoring of the INR can be challenging to incorporate into their daily lives. Self-testing may be an appropriate alternative for some of these patients.[34]

Patient self-management (PSM), which includes a self-tested INR and warfarin dose adjustments per the patient, has not been vastly utilized in the United States. Some limitations to PSM include finding a reliable patient who is not only willing and able to test the INR but also able to follow a warfarin dose adjustment scale. It also requires training and identifying a physician or anticoagulation clinic who would be willing to oversee the patient. Although there are limited data on PSM, the data that are available suggest similar management outcomes with PSM compared with anticoagulation clinics.[32,33,35,36]

Although the best model for how to manage warfarin therapy has yet to be established in the literature, it is widely agreed on that for those assisting with warfarin management it should be done following a standardized approach. Warfarin management should incorporate consistent INR testing and follow-up, utilization of a dosing nomogram, patient education, and clear communication, and ideally the clinician should be trained in these aspects of warfarin management.[5]

ROLE OF THE ANTICOAGULATION CLINICIAN

There is little difference in the role of the anticoagulation clinician if the patient is being seen face-to-face in clinic, managed over the phone, or through other care models. Before developing a management plan, it is the responsibility of the anticoagulation clinician to conduct a thorough evaluation of the patient. The evaluation of the patient for each resulted INR should include the following[3-5]:

- Verification of indication and target INR range
- Assessment of factors that could affect INR and/or warfarin dose:
  - Comorbidities
  - Compliance
  - Changes to medication list
  - Significant drug interactions
  - Dietary changes
  - Social behaviors (i.e., alcohol intake)
  - Signs and symptoms of illness (i.e., vomiting, diarrhea, fevers)
  - Signs and symptoms of bleeding
  - Signs and symptoms of clotting

- Signs and symptoms of stroke
- Need for periprocedural planning (as applicable)

Once the assessment is completed, the clinician can develop a warfarin dose plan and determine the time to next INR check. Another significant part of the role of the anticoagulation clinician is to ensure adequate follow-up and to stress compliance. This is often performed through patient education.

The clinician plays an important role in patient education. Patients are more likely to use their medication safely when they have an understanding of why they are taking it, the reason for repeated monitoring, the potential for drug interactions, and how to respond to ADEs or side effects.[37]

With the known complexities of warfarin regarding dose adjustments, frequency of monitoring, dietary restrictions, and the other factors that can affect the INR, it is understandable that patients may struggle with therapy. This is why education when a patient initially starts warfarin and continuous education throughout his/her length of therapy is very important. It can help minimize the risk for errors. Studies have shown that warfarin education provided by pharmacists increased patients' understanding of warfarin therapy and led to improvements in compliance, INR control, and decreased adverse events. This results in decreased emergency department visits, hospitalizations, and cost to the health system.[38,39]

QUALITY OF CARE

The overall goal of an anticoagulation clinic is to improve on the outcomes of anticoagulation care. This is commonly measured by the following:

- Decreased adverse events from warfarin (i.e., bleeding and thrombotic events)
- Decreased hospitalizations and/or emergency room visits
- Improved time within therapeutic INR range (TTR)
- Reduction in critical INR values
- Improved patient satisfaction
- Improved provider satisfaction

There is no clear advantage in clinical outcomes between the models of care provided by the anticoagulation clinic, i.e., telephonic versus in-clinic visit; however, there are studies that consistently support when warfarin is managed by pharmacists, compared with other healthcare providers; there are positive effects on clinical outcomes. This includes significant decreases in warfarin-related hospitalizations, improvement in patient compliance and understanding of warfarin, improvement in TTR, and positive impacts on both patient and physician satisfaction.[2,18-23,38]

EVOLVING ROLE OF THE ANTICOAGULATION CLINIC

With the availability and increased utilization of the DOACs, it has become a natural progression to begin incorporating management programs for these anticoagulants into the anticoagulation clinic setting. Anticoagulation providers have the specialized skills and knowledge to assist with drug selection and initial dosing based on indication for use and patient-specific factors, screen for drug interactions, provide education, and ensure affordability through insurance coverage or patient assistance programs. Although DOACs do not require monitoring of anticoagulant effect to achieve a target range, they do still require periodic monitoring of serum creatinine (Scr) and creatinine clearance (CrCl) for possible dose adjustments, and hemoglobin (Hgb) and platelets (PLTs) for early identification of bleeding complications.[40] Additionally, the DOACs are not truly a "one dose fits all" drug class, and as real-world data would suggest, challenges do exist with the initial prescribing of these medications. Studies show prescribing of incorrect dosing based on indication, renal function, hepatic function, drug interactions, and race.[41-47] One study showed that less than half of patients received appropriate baseline laboratory monitoring (i.e., complete blood count [CBC], Scr, liver function test [LFT]) before starting on DOAC therapy.[40] Initiation of an incorrect dose can increase the risk of bleeding or thrombosis, if a patient is either overdosed or underdosed.

This was described in a retrospective registry review done by Trujillo-Santos et al. This group reviewed an international, multisite registry of 1635 patients who were managed with DOACs for acute VTE and 1725 patients who received long-term DOAC therapy. They found that 18% (n=287) of rivaroxaban-treated and 50% of apixaban-treated (n=22) patients did not receive the initial higher lead in dose when used for treatment of VTE. For maintenance dosing, 14% (n=217) of rivaroxaban-treated, 36% (n=29) of apixaban-treated, and 46% (n=15) of dabigatran-treated patients did not received the recommended dose for VTE treatment. Common reasons for incorrect dosing were advanced age (>70 years), the presence of active cancer, low body weight (<60 kg), and renal insufficiency (CrCl < 30 mL/min). Patients on lower than recommended doses did have a trend toward higher incidence of recurrent VTE with no difference in bleeding. Of all the adverse events noted in this study, 75% of them occurred within the first 3 months of therapy.[48]

Race can also be a factor in prescribing unapproved dosing strategies. This happens more commonly in the Asian population where underdosing occurs. Data show that Asians have a higher rate of ICH with warfarin; because of this physicians often target a lower INR goal or prescribe lower dosing of oral anticoagulation to decrease this risk.[46,47] However, this practice may not be appropriate for the DOACs. Data show that the risk for ICH from DOACs is the same when lower doses are used versus standard dosing. This places the patient at risk for increased ischemic outcomes with no benefit in bleeding outcomes.[46,49,50]

Similar to warfarin, it seems that the first few months of DOAC therapy may also be a significant time to ensure the most appropriate management starting with drug selection, dosing, and baseline monitoring. Because there are no head-to-head trials comparing these agents to one another, it may be challenging for providers to determine which therapy is best for their patient. An important part of DOAC management programs is to assist with the selection of therapy based on both drug-specific and patient-specific factors. When selecting a DOAC, there are many patient-specific factors to consider when determining the most appropriate drug and dosing regimen. Patient-specific factors to consider include the following[40,51]:

- Age
- Weight
- Renal function
- Hepatic function
- Indication for use
- Drug interactions
- Bleeding history
- Affordability
- Compliance history

Because of the perceived ease of use of DOACs, it may be challenging to find support for the anticoagulation clinic to absorb the management of these patients. Providers may feel less likely to consult these specialized services and instead maintain the management in the medical home. A study by Howard et al. retrospectively reviewed patients initiated on DOAC therapy by a family practice, internal medicine, or geriatrics provider to identify prescribing and monitoring practices in real-world practice sites. This study found that nearly 15% (24/167) of patients were initiated on an incorrect dose. Of the 24 patients on an incorrect dose, 7 (29%) were on a higher than recommended dose and 15 (62.5%) were on a lower than recommended dose. Risk factors of patients who were initiated on an incorrect dose included females (20.6% vs. 10.2%; $P < .05$) and age greater than 75 years (23.5%; $P < .05$). The most common reason for prescribing an

TABLE 6.2
Patients With Laboratory Monitoring Before Initiation of DOAC Therapy—(Adapted)[52]

Laboratory Test	Number of Patients With Monitoring
Hemoglobin	119/167 (71.3%)
Creatinine	129/167 (77.2%)
Alanine aminotransferase	80 (47.9%)
Total bilirubin	60 (35.9%)

DOAC, direct oral anticoagulant.
Adapted from Howard M, Lipshutz A, Roess B, et al. Identification of risk factors for inappropriate and suboptimal initiation of direct oral anticoagulants. *J Thromb Thrombolysis.* 2017;43:149–156.

TABLE 6.3
Examples of DOAC Management Services Provided—(Adapted)[53]

Service provided	Activities included
Patient selection	Appropriate indication Review of contraindications Compliance assessment
Patient education	Appropriate storage Reason for use Adverse effects Adherence Missed doses Risk for falls Drug interactions Dosing
Patient monitoring	Adherence monitoring Adverse event Periprocedural planning Laboratory testing (Scr, liver function, complete blood count)

DOAC, direct oral anticoagulant; *Scr,* serum creatinine.
Adapted from Shore S, Ho M, Lambert-Kerzner A, et al. Site-level variation in and practices associated with dabigatran adherence. *JAMA.* 2015;313(14):1443–1450.

inappropriate dose was renal function. This study also evaluated if appropriate laboratory monitoring was complete before initiating DOAC therapy, with the results outlined in Table 6.2. The authors concluded that it would be beneficial to incorporate a DOAC management program into an anticoagulation clinic setting to ensure proper dosing and monitoring of DOACs.[52]

DOAC management programs are a relatively new concept for both clinicians and anticoagulation clinics. There is no established standard of care associated with how often to contact patients, how often to monitor laboratory data, what laboratory data should be monitored, and the role of the anticoagulation clinic. There have been some examples of DOAC management programs provided in the literature with positive findings in improving prescribing practices and adherence.[53,54]

The Veterans Health Administration (VHA) was one of the first health systems to publish on their experience with DOAC management programs. At the time of publication, the VHA did not have a standardized process for how each site was participating in and managing DOAC therapy. The goal was to evaluate site variation and determine best practices by monitoring patient adherence associated with the level of service the site was providing. Sites were included in the data analysis if at least one of the services listed in Table 6.3 was provided and if the site had at least 20 patients with an active prescription for dabigatran. Of a possible 67 sites, a total of 41 sites met criteria for inclusion.[53]

Overall, they found that 40/41 (98%) of sites were assisting with patient selection activities, 30/41 (73%) were completing patient education, and 28/41 (68.3%)

were offering a patient monitoring program for dabigatran. Patient adherence ranged widely across all 67 practice sites with an overall mean of 72% (42%–93%). Higher adherence rates were seen at sites offering at least one of the services listed in Table 6.3: patient selection (75% vs. 69%), patient education (76% vs. 66%), and patient monitoring (77% vs. 65%). It was also noted that the longer the patient was followed, the higher the adherence rate.[53]

The DOAC management program of a large academic health system was described in a recent publication that also included data on improved prescribing and adherence. In this pharmacist-led program, patients are contacted by phone to review current DOAC regimens. During the initial encounter, the pharmacist confirms correct dosing and duration based on the indication, evaluates pertinent laboratory data (i.e., Scr), and provides patient education. If needed, pharmacists make recommendations for changes to therapy and/or order any additional laboratory testing. Follow-up with the patient occurred 2 weeks after the initial contact, then again in 3–6 months, and continued every 3–6 months while the patient remained on DOAC therapy. For data evaluation, patients followed by the pharmacist's

TABLE 6.4					
DOAC Monitoring for the First 12 Months of Therapy—(UW Health Example)					
	Anticoagulation Clinic Visit (In Person)	Patient Assessment (Via Phone or EMR Portal)	Hgb/PLTs	Cr (w/CrCl)	ALT
Baseline	✓		✓	✓	✓
1 week		✓			
1 month		✓			
3 months		✓	✓	✓	
6 months		✓	✓	✓	
12 months		✓	✓	✓	✓

CrCl, creatinine clearance; DOAC, direct oral anticoagulant; EMR, electronic medical record; Hgb, hemoglobin; PLTs, platelets.

management (n = 129 patients) were matched to those managed with usual care (n = 129 patients). The following results were described:

- Patients in the pharmacist group were more likely to have the correct DOAC and dose prescribed based on the indication compared with the usual care group (93% vs. 79.1%; P = .009).
- A higher percentage of medication adherence was seen in the pharmacist-managed group (91.8%) versus usual care (79.3%) P = .0014.

When it came to prescribing a DOAC, the most common reason for prescribing an incorrect dose was the inappropriate use of a lower-dose option. This was followed by incorrect dosing per indication, incorrect dosing frequency, and incorrect dose based on renal dose adjustments. Study investigators concluded that pharmacists have more drug knowledge, time to educate, and time to counsel and can promote compliance, assist with finding programs to afford medications, and provide time for continued follow-up compared with their physician counterparts.[54]

When developing a DOAC management program, it is important to consider available staff resources, care models, and the expected number of patients that would be included in the program. Design and implementation of the DOAC management program should fit with the anticoagulation clinic's abilities to provide consistent care. For example, an anticoagulation clinic may be able to absorb the health system's DOAC patients if the majority of the management was completed through telephone or telehealth care models. Tables 6.4–6.6 provide an example of a DOAC management program designed by the University of Wisconsin that incorporates an initial face-to-face visit, where in-depth patient education is provided, and scheduled telephone/telehealth follow-up, for clinical and laboratory assessment.

EXPANDING THE ROLE OF THE ANTICOAGULATION CLINIC

In addition to expanding into the realm of DOAC management, anticoagulation clinics and health systems have also begun to explore other areas where offering additional specialized care can positively affect patients. One area is by expanding anticoagulation programs to include periprocedural planning for all anticoagulated patients within a health system. Other areas include expanding roles to include total wellness options for patients during anticoagulation clinic visits, shifting toward becoming complex medication management clinics, or focusing on population health and disease-specific initiatives.[40,55-62] These ideas will be reviewed in more detail in this section of the chapter.

PERIPROCEDURAL PLANNING

Approximately 10%–15% of anticoagulated patients will have a surgical or other invasive procedure that requires a temporary interruption in therapy each year. New recommendations for initiating a short-acting anticoagulant (i.e., low molecular weight heparin [LMWH]) during the interruption of a long-acting anticoagulant (i.e., warfarin), commonly referred to as bridging, show that this practice is associated with an increased risk for bleeding without reducing the risk of thrombotic events.[63] It is now recommended to bridge patients requiring temporary interruptions only if they are considered at high risk for thromboembolic events.[63-65] With these new recommendations for

TABLE 6.5
DOAC Monitoring After at Least 12 Months of Therapy—(UW Health Example)

Patient Characteristic	Schedule	Patient Assessment (Via Phone or EMR Portal)	Hgb/PLTs[a]	Cr (w/ CrCl)[a]	ALT[a]
CrCl: 15–29 mL/min	Q 3 months	✓		✓	
	Annually		✓		✓
CrCl: 30–60 mL/min or age ≥ 75 years	Q 6 months	✓		✓	
	Annually		✓		✓
CrCl: >60 mL/min	Annually	✓	✓	✓	✓

[a]Laboratory results that fall outside of normal limits should be repeated at least every 3–6 months.
CrCl, creatinine clearance; DOAC, direct oral anticoagulant; EMR, electronic medical record; Hgb, hemoglobin; PLTs, platelets.

TABLE 6.6
DOAC Monitoring Patient Assessment Questions—(UW Health Example)

Question	Response
1. Able to afford medication	Yes or No
2. Missed doses	Yes or No
3. Recent medication, over-the-counter, or supplement changes	Yes or No
4. Unusual bruising, bleeding, or serious fall or injury	Yes or No
5. New or unexplained trouble breathing, pain or swelling in the legs, sudden confusion or weakness along one side of the body, or difficulty speaking	Yes or No
6. Upcoming procedures or surgery	Yes or No

DOAC, direct oral anticoagulant.

when to initiate bridging and with newer oral anticoagulants to consider, periprocedural management can be challenging for clinicians who are unfamiliar with current recommendations and drug therapies. A recent survey showed just how complex development of a bridge plan for temporary anticoagulation interruption can be in the clinic setting. The survey showed there are often a many clinicians involved in the process including primary care physicians, surgeons, advanced practice providers, pharmacists, and anticoagulation clinics. Because of the complexities of periprocedural anticoagulation management, the authors promoted the use of standardized care pathways or protocols to simplify the process and decrease the risk for adverse outcomes.[55]

One such study demonstrated the benefits of having a standardized management plan for patients requiring temporary interruption of anticoagulation. In this study, LMWH was used as the short-acting anticoagulant for bridging purposes. The anticoagulation clinic was utilized to provide the patient or his/her caregiver education on the periprocedural anticoagulant plan, injection techniques for LMWH, and signs and symptoms of bleeding complications and thromboembolic events. The anticoagulation clinic was also involved in the postprocedural setting and helped to coordinate when to resume anticoagulation postprocedure. Through the use of a standardized process and utilizing anticoagulation specialists, this study showed low risks of both thromboembolic and major bleeding complications.[56]

TOTAL WELLNESS OPTIONS
In current practice within an anticoagulation clinic, not all interventions are related to anticoagulation therapy. The anticoagulation specialist often assists with coordinating other aspects of the patient's medical care. To have a better understanding of how often this occurs, a retrospective, single-center cohort sought to describe these non-anticoagulation-related interventions and reviewed all patients with at least one intervention outside of the usual anticoagulation care. The study included 252 patients with a total of 2222 interventions identified and classified into six major categories. The results are outlined in Table 6.7. This study noted that medication reconciliation and assisting with the continuity of care were the two categories with the highest interventions.[57] As described by this study, the anticoagulation specialists have a significant role in assisting with the overall care of the patient, and

TABLE 6.7
Non-anticoagulation-Related Activities Documented by an Anticoagulation Clinic—(Adapted)[57]

Non-anticoagulation-Related Intervention Categories (With Examples)	Number of Interventions (%)
Continuity of care • Obtain medical records • Facilitate refills • Education on follow-up care • Schedule appointments with other care providers • Facilitate obtaining a PCP • Communication of medical information to other care providers	252 (11.3)
Health assessment and triage • Counsel on symptom management • Referral to PCP or ED for treatment of acute event	206 (9.3)
Acquire necessary diagnostics • Order or consult a physician to order laboratories, radiology tests, etc.	16 (0.7)
Reconcile medications • Identify medication discrepancies	1591 (71.6)
Modify therapy • Recommend medication/dose change based on drug interactions, contraindications, adverse drug reactions, cost, lack of efficacy, duplication, no indication, inappropriate dose, etc.	27 (1.2)
Drug information and counseling	130 (5.9)

ED, emergency department; PCP, primary care provider.
Adapted from Hicho MD, Rybarczyk A, Boros M. Interventions unrelated to anticoagulation in a pharmacist-managed anticoagulation clinic. Am J Health Syst Pharm. 2016;73(suppl 3):S80–S87.

activities outside of usual anticoagulation care should be tracked.

Another total wellness idea a health system implemented was to offer influenza vaccines to both patients and accompanying caregivers during their anticoagulation clinic visits. Patients were screened when they checked in for their visit for interest in receiving the vaccine. If agreeable, the pharmacist administered the influenza vaccine during the visit for warfarin management. Within this health system, the anticoagulation clinic vaccinated about one-third or approximately 540 patients during the influenza season. It was seen as a successful program, and there are plans to continue at the current site and expand to additional anticoagulation clinic sites within their system.[58]

COMPLEX MEDICATION MANAGEMENT
Anticoagulants are not the only complex drug class that requires close monitoring. Amiodarone is another cardiac medication that is frequently prescribed but not consistently monitored for adverse effects. Amiodarone has been associated with liver, thyroid, and pulmonary

toxicity. It is recommended to monitor for these toxicities during therapy to identify any toxicities early in an effort to reverse or minimize the effect.[66] Studies have shown low rates of compliance with monitoring amiodarone, 23%–50%.[59] When pharmacists are involved in an amiodarone monitoring program, compared with usual care, significant improvements with monitoring liver and thyroid function were seen, as well as baseline chest X-rays.[60]

Mineralocorticoid receptor antagonists (i.e., spironolactone) are also a class of medications that should be monitored closely because of their association with increased hospital admissions and death from hyperkalemia.[67] However, one study showed only 7.2% of patients receiving mineralocorticoid receptor antagonists receive appropriate monitoring of potassium and Scr.[61]

Finally, another direction toward shifting to complex medication management clinics is to incorporate the monitoring the use of antiplatelet agents. The use of dual and triple antiplatelet therapy is associated with a significant increased risk for bleeding. Although indicated for patients with a need for

TABLE 6.8
Length of Antithrombotic Therapy in Atrial Fibrillation and Cardiac Disease—(Adapted)[11]

	ACUTE CORONARY SYNDROME		ELECTIVE PCI	
	Low Bleed Risk	**High Bleed Risk**	**Low Bleed Risk**	**High Bleed Risk**
Triple therapy (oral anticoagulant, aspirin, clopidogrel)	Complete 6 months	Complete 1 month	Complete 1 month	Complete 1 month
Dual therapy (oral anticoagulant and antiplatelet)	Complete additional 6 months	Complete additional 11 months	Complete additional 11 months	Complete additional 5 months
Monotherapy (oral anticoagulant)	Maintenance after 1 year of antiplatelet therapy	Maintenance after 1 year of antiplatelet therapy	Maintenance after 1 year of antiplatelet therapy	Maintenance after 1 year of antiplatelet therapy

Reference 11 Kirchhof P, *Euro Heart J.* 2016.

long-term anticoagulants and cardiac disease, the length of dual and triple antiplatelet therapy should be monitored closely.[11] The goal should be to balance the risk for bleeding while also ensuring an adequate length of antiplatelet therapy. The recent European Society of Cardiology's management of AF guideline provides recommendations for how to risk stratify patients based on cardiac indication and bleeding risks. This is described in Table 6.8. The length of therapy for both dual and triple antiplatelet therapy differs between both cardiac indications and bleeding risk. This may be a source of confusion for providers, especially patients who are not being closely followed by a cardiologist. Anticoagulation clinics could assist with ensuring patients are closely monitored for bleeding events and assist with adjusting antiplatelet therapy at the correct time to ensure patients are not continued on dual or triple therapy longer than necessary.

POPULATION HEALTH

Studies have shown a benefit in patient adherence to treatment, patient understanding of disease state and medications, disease state outcomes, and cost benefits when pharmacists are involved in chronic disease management clinics. Within these clinics, the pharmacist's roles include medication management, symptom monitoring, adverse event monitoring, and patient education. Chronic disease states where benefit has been seen include asthma, hyperlipidemia, hypertension, heart failure, and smoking cessation.[68–70] Although many population health clinics are focused on the primary care setting, anticoagulation clinics can adapt and

expand into areas that are better suited to their areas of expertise. One area to consider is partnering with other specialty areas to provide seamless transitions from inpatient to outpatient management and provide comprehensive patient care in a single ambulatory location. An example of this practice is with pulmonary embolism management clinics.

DISEASE STATE CLINICS: PULMONARY EMBOLISM MANAGEMENT

With the increase in popularity of multidisciplinary disease state management teams, for example, pulmonary embolism response teams (PERTs) in the inpatient setting, this concept of continuing a multidisciplinary approach has also moved into the ambulatory setting. The example of a PERT clinic is a relatively new concept. A PERT clinic functions to care for patients newly diagnosed with PE after hospital discharge and have been designed to include care from a variety of specialties such as hematology, vascular medicine, pulmonology, and cardiology. As the needs of the patient are identified, they may be managed by an individual specialty; however, the multidisciplinary team will discuss all patients seen in clinic to discuss and create a treatment plan.[62]

While including anticoagulation clinics have not been widely incorporated into PERT clinics, as described in the literature, it is an area for possible involvement. The anticoagulation specialist can assist with the selection of anticoagulation therapy, evaluate the patient's individual risk of VTE recurrence, and use this to determine the length of therapy and to monitor patients closely to better manage complications and

symptoms. The anticoagulation specialist will often follow up the patient more frequently than the medical
specialist and can assist with identifying any complications or symptoms quickly and can refer to the multidisciplinary team to evaluate.[62]

CONCLUSION

As the landscape of anticoagulation management continues to change with new therapeutic options so must
the traditional approach to patient management. Anticoagulation clinics are still an important and relevant
part of this management. Patients who are managed by
specialized clinicians through a standardized approach
have consistently demonstrated better outcomes with
less thromboembolic and major bleeding events,
improvement in patient adherence to medication regimens, and overall disease state understanding, and they
experience a decrease in emergency room visits and
hospitalizations.

However, as new therapeutic options continue to
emerge and grow in popularity, traditional anticoagulation clinics must also adapt to incorporate these
new therapies into their management programs. Some
ideas have been to develop management programs to
fit the DOACs, whereas others have been more expan-
sive to include monitoring other complex medications.
Additionally, complete disease state management from
inpatient to the ambulatory setting has also been proposed as an idea to evolve the role of the anticoagulation clinic.

Ultimately, the evolution of the anticoagulation
clinic should match the needs of the health system and
patients within that health system to maximize both
the clinical and financial outcomes that can be appreciated through specialized care.

REFERENCES

1. Barnes GD, Lucas E, Alexander GC, Goldberger ZD. National trends in ambulatory oral anticoagulant use. *Am J Med.* 2015;128:1300–1305.
2. Chiquette E, Amato M, Bussey H. Comparison of an anticoagulation clinic with usual medical care. *Arch Intern Med.* 1998;158:1641–1647.
3. Ageno W, Gallus AS, Wittkowsky A, Crowther M, Hylek EM, Palareti G. Oral anticoagulant therapy: antithrombotic therapy and prevention of thrombosis, 9th ed: American College of Chest Physicians evidence-based clinical practice guidelines. *Chest.* 2012;141:e44s–e88s.
4. Holbrook AM, Pereira JA, Labiris R, et al. Systematic overview of warfarin and its drug and food interactions. *Arch Intern Med.* 2005;165:1095–1106.
5. Holbrook A, Schulman S, Witt DM, et al. Evidence-based management of anticoagulant therapy: antithrombotic therapy and prevention of thrombosis, 9th ed: American College of Chest Physicians evidence-based clinical practice guidelines. *Chest.* 2012;141:e152s–e184s.
6. Budnitz DS, Lovegrove MC, Shehab N, Richards CL. Emergency hospitalizations for adverse drug events in older Americans. *N Engl J Med.* 2011;365:2002–2012.
7. Desai NR, Krumme AA, Schneeweiss S. Patterns of initiation of oral anticoagulants in patients with atrial fibrillation: quality and cost implications. *Am J Med.* 2014;127:1075–1082.
8. January CT, Wann LS, Alpert JS, et al. 2014 AHA/ACC/HRS guideline for the management of patients with atrial fibrillation: a report of the American College of Cardiology/American Heart Association Task Force on Practice Guidelines and the Heart Rhythm Society. *Circulation.* 2014;130(23):e199–e267.
9. Kearon C, Akl EA, Ornelas J, et al. Antithrombotic therapy for VTE disease: CHEST guideline and expert panel report. *Chest.* 2016;149(2):315–352.
10. Streiff MB, Agnelli G, Connors JM, et al. Guidance for the treatment of deep vein thrombosis and pulmonary embolism. *J Thromb Thrombolysis.* 2016;41:32–67.
11. Kirchhof P, Benussi S, Kotecha D, et al. 2016 ESC guidelines for the management of atrial fibrillation developed in collaboration with EACTS. *Eur Heart J.* 2016;37(38):2893–2962.
12. Badreldin H, Nichols H, Rimsans J, Carter D. Evaluation of anticoagulation selection for acute venous thromboembolism. *J Thromb Thrombolysis.* 2017;43(1):74–78.
13. Li A, Lopes RD, Garcia DA. Use of direct oral anticoagulants in special populations. *Hematol Oncol Clin North Am.* 2016;30(5):1053–1071.
14. Martin K, Beyer-Westendorf J, Davidson BL, Huisman MV, Sandset PM, Moll S. Use of the direct oral anticoagulants in obese patients: guidance from the SSC of the ISTH. *J Thromb Haemost.* 2016;14:1308–1313.
15. Sardar P, Chatterjee S, Herzog E, et al. New oral anticoagulants in patients with cancer: current state of evidence. *Am J Ther.* 2015;22:460–468.
16. Schaefer JK, McBane RD, Black DF, Williams LN, Moder KG, Wysokinski WE. Failure of dabigatran and rivaroxaban to prevent thromboembolism in antiphospholipid syndrome: a case series of three patients. *Thromb Haemost.* 2014;112(5):947–950.
17. Eikelboom JW, Connolly SJ, Brueckmann M, et al. Dabigatran versus warfarin in patients with mechanical heart valves. *N Engl J Med.* 2013;369:1206–1214.
18. Nichol M, Knight T, Dow T, et al. Quality of anticoagulation monitoring in nonvalvular atrial fibrillation patients: comparison of anticoagulation clinic versus usual care. *Ann Pharmacother.* 2008;42:62–70.
19. Hall D, Buchanan J, Helms B, et al. Health care expenditures and therapeutic outcomes of a pharmacist-managed anticoagulation service versus usual medical care. *Pharmacotherapy.* 2011;31:686–694.

20. Lee YP, Schommer JC. Effect of a pharmacist-managed anticoagulation clinic on warfarin-related hospital readmissions. *Am J Health Syst Pharm*. 1996;53:1580–1583.

21. Garwood C, Dumo P, Baringhaus S, Laban K. Quality of anticoagulation care in patients discharged from a pharmacist-managed anticoagulation clinic after stabilization of warfarin therapy. *Pharmacotherapy*. 2008;28:20–26.

22. Rudd K, Dier J. Comparison of two different models of anticoagulation management services with usual medical care. *Pharmacotherapy*. 2010;30:330–338.

23. Rose AE, Robinson EN, Premo JA, Hauschild LJ, Trapskin PJ, McBride AM. Improving warfarin management within the medical home: a health-system approach. *Am J Med*. 2016;130(3):365.e7–e12.

24. Stoudenmire LG, DeRemer CE, Elewa H. Telephone versus office-based management of warfarin: impact on international normalized ratios and outcomes. *Int J Hematol*. 2014;100:119–124.

25. Wittkowsky A, Nutescu EA, Blackburn J, et al. Outcomes of oral anticoagulant therapy managed by telephone vs in-office visits in an anticoagulation clinic settings. *Chest*. 2006;130(5):1385–1389.

26. Goldberg Y, Meytes D, Shabtai E, et al. Monitoring oral anticoagulant therapy by telephone communication. *Blood Coagul Fibrinolysis*. 2005;16:227–230.

27. Matchar DB, Jacobson A, Dolor R, et al. Effect of home testing of international normalized ratio on clinical events. *N Engl J Med*. 2010;363(17):1608–1620.

28. Gadisseur AP, Breukink-Engbers WG, van der Meer FJ, et al. Comparison of the quality of oral anticoagulant therapy through patient self-management and management by specialized anticoagulation clinics in The Netherlands. *Arch Intern Med*. 2003;163(21):2639–2646.

29. Garcia-Alamino JM, Ward AM, Alonso-Coello P, et al. Self-monitoring and self-management of oral anticoagulation. *Cochrane Database Syst Rev*. 2010;(4):CD003839.

30. Bloomfield HE, Krause A, Greer N, et al. Meta-analysis: effect of patient self-testing and self-management of long-term anticoagulation on major clinical outcomes. *Ann Intern Med*. 2011;154(7):472–482.

31. Barcellona D, Fenu L, Marongiu F. Point-of-care testing INR: an overview. *Clin Chem Lab Med*. 2017;55(6):800–805.

32. Watzke HH, Forberg E, Svolba G, Jimenez-Boj E, Krinninger B. A prospective controlled trial comparing weekly self-testing and self-dosing with standard management of patients on stable oral anticoagulation. *Thromb Haemost*. 2000;83:661–665.

33. Heneghan CJ, Garcia-Alamino JM, Spencer EA, et al. Self-monitoring and self-management of oral anticoagulation. *Cochrane Database Syst Rev*. 2016;(7):CD003839.

34. Jacobson AK. The North American experience with patient self-testing of the INR. *Semin Vasc Med*. 2003;3(3):295–302.

35. Cosmi B, Palareti G, Carpanedo M, et al. Assessment of patient capability to self-adjust oral anticoagulant dose: a multicenter study on home use of portable prothrombin time monitor (COAGUCHECK). *Haematologica*. 2000;85:826–831.

36. Nagler M, Bachmann LM, Schmid P, Raddatz-Muller P, Wuillemin WA. Patient self-management of oral anticoagulation with vitamin K antagonist in everyday practice: efficacy and safety in a nationwide long-term prospective cohort study. *PLoS One*. 2014;9(4):e95761.

37. Russell TM. Warfarin and beyond: an update on oral anticoagulation therapy. *US Pharm*. 2011;36(2):26–43.

38. Krittathanmakul S, Silapachote P, Pongwecharak J, Wongsatit U. Effects of pharmacist counseling on outpatients receiving warfarin at Songklanagarind Hospital. *Songkla Med J*. 2006;24(2):93–99.

39. Willey ML, Chagan L, Sisca TS, et al. A pharmacist-managed anticoagulation clinic: six-year assessment of patient outcomes. *Am J Health Syst Pharm*. 2003;60: 1033–1037.

40. Barnes GD, Nallamothu BK, Sales AE, Froehlich JB. Re-imaging anticoagulation clinics in the era of direct oral anticoagulants. *Circ Cardiovasc Qual Outcomes*. 2016;9: 182–185.

41. Rieser KN, Rosenberg EI, Vogel-Anderson K. Evaluation of the appropriateness of direct oral anticoagulant selection and monitoring in the outpatient setting. *J Pharm Technol*. 2017;33(3):108–113.

42. Tran E, Duckett A, Fisher S, et al. Appropriateness of direct oral anticoagulant dosing for venous thromboembolism treatment. *J Thromb Thrombolysis*. 2017; 43(4):505–513.

43. Rose AJ, Reisman JI, Allen AL, Miller DR. Potentially inappropriate prescribing of direct-acting oral anticoagulants in the Veterans Health Administration. *Am J Pharm Benefits*. 2016;8(4):e75–e80.

44. Simon J, Hawes E, Deyo Z, Bryant-Shilliday B. Evaluation of prescribing and patient use of target specific oral anticoagulants in outpatient setting. *J Clin Pharm Ther*. 2015;40(5):525–530.

45. Tellor KB, Patel S, Armbruster AL, Daly MW. Evaluation of the appropriateness of dosing, indication and safety of rivaroxaban in a community hospital. *J Clin Pharm Ther*. 2015;40(4):447–451.

46. Chen CH, Chen MC, Gibbs H, et al. Antithrombotic treatment for stroke prevention in atrial fibrillation: the Asian agenda. *Int J Cardiol*. 2015;191:244–253.

47. Chan YH, Yen KC, See LC, et al. Cardiovascular, bleeding, and mortality risks of dabigatran in Asians with nonvalvular atrial fibrillation. *Stroke*. 2016;47:441–449.

48. Trujillo-Santos J, Di Micco P, Dentall F, et al. Real-life treatment of venous thromboembolism with direct oral anticoagulants: the influence of recommended dosing and regimens. *Thromb Haemost*. 2017;117:382–389.

49. Wang KL, Giugliano RP, Goto S, et al. Standard dose versus low dose non-vitamin K antagonist oral anticoagulants in Asian patients with atrial fibrillation: a meta-analysis of contemporary randomized controlled trials. *Heart Rhythm*. 2016;13(12):2340–2347.

50. Hori M, Matsumoto M, Tanahashi N, et al. Rivaroxaban vs. warfarin in Japanese patients with atrial fibrillation: the J-ROCKET AF study. *Circ J*. 2012;76:2104–2111.

51. Gladstone DJ, Geerts WH, Douketis J, Ivers N, Healey JS, Leblanc K. How to monitor patients receiving direct oral anticoagulants for stroke prevention in atrial fibrillation: a practice tool endorsed by Thrombosis Canada, the Canadian Stroke Consortium, the Canadian Cardiovascular Pharmacists Network, and the Canadian Cardiovascular Society. *Ann Intern Med.* 2015;163(5):382–385.

52. Howard M, Lipshutz A, Roess B, et al. Identification of risk factors for inappropriate and suboptimal initiation of direct oral anticoagulants. *J Thromb Thrombolysis.* 2017;43:149–156.

53. Shore S, Ho M, Lambert-Kerzner A, et al. Site-level variation in and practices associated with dabigatran adherence. *JAMA.* 2015;313(14):1443–1450.

54. Ashjian E, Kurtz B, Renner E, Yeshe R, Barnes G. Evaluation of a pharmacist-led outpatient direct oral anticoagulant service. *Am J Health Syst Pharm.* 2017;74:483–489.

55. Flaker GC, Theriot P, Binder LG, et al. Management of periprocedural anticoagulation: a survey of contemporary practice. *J Am Coll Cardiol.* 2016;68(2):217–226.

56. Douketis JD, Johnson JA, Turpie AG. Low-molecular weight heparin as bridging anticoagulation during interruption of warfarin. *Arch Intern Med.* 2004;164:1319–1326.

57. Hicho MD, Rybarczyk A, Boros M. Interventions unrelated to anticoagulation in a pharmacist-managed anticoagulation clinic. *Am J Health Syst Pharm.* 2016;73(suppl 3):S80–S87.

58. Thompson CA. Anticoagulation clinics offer seasonal influenza vaccination. *Am J Health Syst Pharm.* 2016;73(19):1480–1482.

59. Raebel MA, Lyons EE, Chester EA, et al. Improving laboratory monitoring at initiation of drug therapy in ambulatory care. *Arch Intern Med.* 2005;165(20):2395–2401.

60. Spence MM, Polzin JK, Weisberger CL, Martin JP, Rho JP, Willick GH. Evaluation of a pharmacist-managed amiodarone monitoring program. *J Manag Care Pharm.* 2011;17:513–522.

61. Cooper LB, Hammill BG, Peterson ED, et al. Consistency of laboratory monitoring during initiation of mineralocorticoid receptor antagonist therapy in patients with heart failure. *JAMA.* 2015;314:1973–1975.

62. Dudzinski DM, Piazza G. Multidisciplinary pulmonary embolism response teams. *Circulation.* 2016;133:98–103.

63. Douketis JD, Spyropoulos AC, Kaatz S, et al. Perioperative bridging anticoagulation in patients with atrial fibrillation. *N Engl J Med.* 2015;373(9):828–833.

64. Steinberg BA, Peterson ED, Kim S, et al. Use and outcomes associated with bridging during anticoagulation interruptions in patients with atrial fibrillation: findings from the Outcomes Registry for Better Informed Treatment of Atrial Fibrillation (ORBIT-AF). *Circulation.* 2015;131(5):488–494.

65. Clark NP, Witt DM, Davies LE, et al. Bleeding, recurrent venous thromboembolism and mortality risks during warfarin interruption for invasive procedures. *JAMA Intern Med.* 2015;175(7):1163–1168.

66. Siddoway LA. Amiodarone: guidelines for use and monitoring. *Am Fam Physician.* 2003;68(11):2189–2196.

67. Juurlink DN, Mamdani MM, Lee DS, et al. Rates of hyperkalemia after publication of the randomized aldactone evaluation study. *N Engl J Med.* 2004;351:543–551.

68. Joseph T, Hale GM, Eltaki SM, et al. Integration strategies of pharmacists in primary care-based accountable care organizations: a report from the accountable care organization research network, services, and education. *J Manag Care Spec Pharm.* 2017;23(5):541–548.

69. Parajuli DR, Franzon J, McKinnon RA, Shakib S, Clark RA. Role of the pharmacist for improving self-care and outcomes in heart failure. *Curr Heart Fail Rep.* 2017;14(2):78–86.

70. Chisholm-Burns MA, Kim Lee J, Spivey CA, et al. U.S. pharmacists' effect as team members on patient care: systematic review and meta-analyses. *Med Care.* 2010;48:923–933.

CHAPTER 7

Management of Bleeding Associated With Anticoagulation

GENO J. MERLI, MD, MACP, FSVM, FHM • LYNDA THOMSON, PHARMD

BACKGROUND

Nonvalvular atrial fibrillation (NVAF) is the most common sustained cardiac arrhythmia that predisposes patients to an increased risk of embolic stroke and has a higher mortality than sinus rhythm.[1,2] As the population ages, the incidence of NVAF in the United States is expected to more than double between 2010 and 2030[2] and is reported to have approximately doubled in the last decade across Europe.[3]

In subjects with NVAF, the incidence of stroke is increased nearly fivefold over that observed in subjects without NVAF.[4] In persons aged 80–89 years, NVAF was found to be the only cardiovascular condition with an independent effect on the incidence of stroke.[4] This complication of NVAF is a major financial burden on healthcare systems globally and will only grow if not prevented by anticoagulation.[5,6]

The vitamin K antagonist (VKA) warfarin has been shown to be clinically effective in the prevention of stroke in NVAF. The direct oral anticoagulants (DOACs) have emerged to fulfill an unmet need for anticoagulation in NVAF.[7] These agents have demonstrated a favorable risk-benefit profile compared with the VKA and their use is increasing worldwide. With the increased use of anticoagulation in NVAF will come need to be prepared to manage major bleeding in this patient population.

INCIDENCE MAJOR BLEEDING

Before we proceed with the approach to the management of bleeding associated with anticoagulation in patients with NVAF, an understanding of the incidence of major bleeding in the patient population associated with warfarin and DOACs is important.[8]

Apixaban

In the Apixaban for Reduction in Stroke and Other Thromboembolic Events in Atrial Fibrillation (ARISTOTLE) study, 18,201 patients with atrial fibrillation

(AF) and at least one additional risk factor for stroke were randomized to apixaban or warfarin and followed for a median 1.8 years.[9] The rate of major bleeding was 2.13%/year in the apixaban group versus 3.09%/year in the warfarin group (hazards ratio [HR] 0.69; 95% CI 0.60–0.80; $P < .001$). The rate of intracranial bleeding was reduced with apixaban (0.33%/year) versus warfarin (0.80%/year; HR 0.42; 95% CI 0.30–0.58; $P < .001$). In contrast, the rate of gastrointestinal bleeding (GIB) did not differ between apixaban (0.76%/year) and warfarin (0.86%/year; HR 0.89; 95% CI 0.70–1.15; $P = .37$) (Table 7.1).[8]

In a separate analysis, Hylek et al. evaluated clinical outcomes associated with major bleeding in the ARISTOTLE patient cohort.[15] Baseline factors that were independently associated with major hemorrhage were older age, prior hemorrhage, prior stroke or transient ischemic attack(TIA), diabetes, lower creatinine clearance (<85 mL/min/1.73 m²), decreased hematocrit level (<45%), aspirin therapy, and use of nonsteroidal antiinflammatory drugs.[15] Adverse events associated with major extracranial hemorrhage occurred less frequently in the apixaban versus warfarin group, including fewer hospitalizations (apixaban, 1.05 vs. warfarin, 1.41; HR 0.75; 95% CI 0.61–0.92; $P = .0052$) and fewer transfusions (apixaban, 0.89 vs. warfarin, 1.25; HR 0.71; 95% CI 0.57–0.89; $P = .0025$). In addition, death following major hemorrhage occurred half as often in the apixaban (36 events) versus warfarin (71 events) group (HR 0.50; 95% CI 0.33–0.74; $P < .001$).

Rivaroxaban

In the Rivaroxaban Once Daily Oral Direct Factor Xa Inhibition Compared With Vitamin K Antagonism for Prevention of Stroke and Embolism Trial in Atrial Fibrillation (ROCKET AF), 14,264 patients with NVAF who were at moderate-to-high risk for stroke were randomized to rivaroxaban or warfarin and followed up for median 1.94 years.[16] The rates of any major bleeding event were similar between the rivaroxaban group

TABLE 7.1

Primary Safety Outcomes Data From Phase 3 Studies of DOACs Versus Warfarin by Type of Bleeding[8]

Primary Safety Outcome (Percentage of Patients with an Adverse Event)[a]	RE-LY[10,b]			ROCKET AF[11,12]		ARISTOTLE[13]		ENGAGE-AF TIMI 48[14]		
	Dabigatran 150 mg (n=6076)	Dabigatran 110 mg (n=6015)	Warfarin (n=6022)	Rivaroxaban (n=7111)	Warfarin (n=7125)	Apixaban (n=9088)	Warfarin (n=9052)	Edoxaban 60 mg (n=7012)	Edoxaban 30 mg (n=7002)	Warfarin (n=7012)
Major bleeding	3.11%/year	2.71%/year	3.36%/year	3.6%/year	3.4%/year	2.13%/year	3.09%/year	2.75%/year	1.61%/year	3.43%/year
Hazard ratio (95% CI)	0.93 (0.81–1.07)	0.80 (0.69–0.93)	–	1.04 (0.90–1.20)	–	0.69 (0.60–0.80)	–	0.80 (0.71–0.91)	0.47 (0.41–0.55)	–
P-value	0.31	0.003		0.58		<0.001		<0.001	<0.001	
Intracranial bleeding	0.30%/year	0.23%/year	0.74%/year	0.5%/year	0.7%/year	0.33%/year	0.80%/year	0.39%/year	0.26%/year	0.85%/year
Hazard ratio (95% CI)	0.40 (0.27–0.60)	0.31 (0.20–0.47)	–	0.67 (0.47–0.93)	–	0.42 (0.30–0.58)	–	0.47 (0.34–0.63)	0.30 (0.21–0.43)	–
P-value	<0.001	<0.001		0.02		<0.001		<0.001	<0.001	
Gastrointestinal bleeding	1.51%/year	1.12%/year	1.02%/year	2.00%/year	1.24%/year	0.76%/year	0.86%/year	1.51%/year	0.82%/year	1.23%/year
Hazard ratio (95% CI)	1.50 (1.19–1.89)	1.10 (0.86–1.41)	–	1.61 (1.30–1.99)	–	0.89 (0.70–1.15)	–	1.23 (1.02–1.50)	0.67 (0.53–0.83)	–
P-value	<0.001	0.43		<0.0001		0.37		0.03	<0.001	

ARISTOTLE, Apixaban for Reduction in STroke and Other ThromboemboLic Events in Atrial Fibrillation; *CI*, confidence interval; *DOAC*, direct oral anticoagulant; *ENGAGE-AF TIMI 48*, Effective aNti-coaGulation with factor Xa next GEneration in Atrial Fibrillation–Thrombolysis in Myocardial Infarction study 48; *RE–LY*, Randomized Evaluation of long-term anticoagulation therapY; *ROCKET AF*, Rivaroxaban Once daily oral direct factor Xa inhibition Compared with vitamin K antagonism for prevention of stroke and Embolism Trial in Atrial Fibrillation.

[a]Data are presented as reported in each publication. Proportion of patients with an adverse event is described as an event rate (percentage/year)[10,13,14] or event rate number/100 patient-years.[11,12]

[b]Rates of the primary safety outcomes from the RE–LY trial are reported as relative risk, not as hazard ratios.

(3.6%) and the warfarin group (3.4%) (HR 1.04; 95% CI, 0.90–1.20; $P=.58$).[16] Rates of ICH were reduced in the rivaroxaban group (HR 0.67; 95% CI, 0.47–0.93; $P=.02$) compared with warfarin. Events of GIB were identified in 3.2% of patients treated with rivaroxaban versus 2.2% of warfarin-treated patients ($P<.001$) (Table 7.1).[8]

In a subgroup analysis by Hankey et al., the efficacy and safety of rivaroxaban versus warfarin was consistent among subgroups of patients who did or did not experience a previous stroke or TIA (interaction $P=.23$ and $P=.08$, respectively), thus supporting its use as an alternative to warfarin for prevention of initial and recurrent stroke in patients with AF.[17] Additional safety results were reported in a multivariate analysis of the ROCKET AF cohort, which demonstrated that age, sex, diastolic blood pressure, prior GIB, prior aspirin use, and anemia were independently associated with increased risk of major bleeding.[18] History of GIB was the only independent predictor of major bleeding that was associated with treatment type ($P=.002$). Patients treated with rivaroxaban versus warfarin had a higher risk of major bleeding if they had a history of GIB (HR 2.33; 95% CI 1.39–3.88).

Edoxaban

In the Effective Anticoagulation With Factor Xa Next Generation in Atrial Fibrillation—Thrombolysis in Myocardial Infarction 48 (ENGAGE-AF TIMI 48) trial, 21,105 patients with moderate-to-high-risk AF were randomized to warfarin, high-dose (HD) edoxaban (60 mg) or low-dose (LD) edoxaban (30 mg), and followed up for a median 2.8 years.[19] Patients in either edoxaban group were eligible to receive half the dose if they met prespecified clinical factors at randomization or during the course of the study. The annualized rate of major bleeding in patients who initiated with HD edoxaban was 2.75% (HR 0.80; 95% CI, 0.71–0.91; $P<.001$) and 1.61% in patients who initiated with LD edoxaban (0.47; 0.41–0.55; $P<.001$) versus 3.43% in the warfarin group. Rates of ICH were reduced with HD edoxaban (0.39%; HR 0.47; 95% CI 0.34–0.63) and LD edoxaban (0.26%; 0.30; 0.21–0.43) versus warfarin (0.85%; both doses $P<.001$). GIB occurred more frequently with HD edoxaban (1.51%; HR 1.23; 95% CI 1.02–1.50; $P=.03$) and less frequently with LD edoxaban (0.82%; 0.67; 0.53–0.83; $P<.001$) versus warfarin (1.23%) (Table 7.1).[8]

In a subgroup analysis of the ENGAGE-AF TIMI cohort, both doses of edoxaban were associated with reductions in various subtypes of ICH, including parenchymal, subarachnoid, and subdural or epidural bleeds.[20] Both edoxaban doses also reduced the composite outcome of death, nonfatal stroke, or ICH (HR 0.88; $P=.003$ for HD edoxaban, and HR, 0.90; $P=.021$ for LD edoxaban) compared with warfarin. In a separate subgroup analysis, Ruff et al. reported that reducing edoxaban dose based on clinical factors decreased the risk of bleeding compared with warfarin.[21] Edoxaban dose reductions, which correlated with lower anti-FXa activity, provided even greater reductions in major bleeding risk. Risk of ICH was reduced in the LD edoxaban group, but not in the HD group. The risk of GIB was not affected by reducing the dose of edoxaban.

Dabigatran

In the Randomized Evaluation of Long-Term Anticoagulation Therapy (RE-LY) study, 18,113 patients who had NVAF and risk of stroke were randomized to dabigatran 110 or 150 mg twice daily or warfarin and followed up for a median 2.0 years.[10] In the primary publication of the RE-LY study, rates of major bleeding were 3.11%/year in the dabigatran 150 mg group (HR 0.93; 95% CI 0.81–1.07; $P=.31$) and 2.71%/year in the dabigatran 110 mg group (HR 0.80; 95% CI 0.69–0.93; $P=.003$) versus 3.36%/year in the warfarin group.[10] Dabigatran 150 and 110 mg significantly reduced the relative risk (RR) of intracranial bleeding (both doses $P<.001$) and only dabigatran 150 mg increased the RR of GIB ($P<.001$) versus warfarin (Table 7.1).[8] After the completion of the study, additional primary efficacy and safety outcome events were identified and the rates of major bleeding were revised to 3.32% in the dabigatran 150 mg group (HR 0.93; 95% CI 0.81–1.07; $P=.32$) and 2.87% in the dabigatran 110 mg group (HR 0.80; 95% CI 0.70–0.93; $P=.003$) versus 3.57% in the warfarin group.[11] Inclusion of the newly identified events did not change the study conclusions. The recommended dosage of dabigatran to reduce the risk of stroke and systemic embolism in patients with NVAF and creatinine clearance > 30 mL/min is 150 mg, twice daily.

In a subgroup analysis of the RE-LY cohort, the incidence of ICH during anticoagulation therapy was evaluated by site (intracerebral, subdural, or subarachnoid), risk factors, and outcomes.[12] The clinical spectrum of ICH was similar among patients treated with dabigatran and warfarin. Independent predictors of all ICHs were randomization to warfarin, aspirin use during follow-up, age, previous stroke/TIA, and white race. Mortality associated with all sites of ICH was not increased with dabigatran 150 mg (13/37; 35%) or dabigatran 110 mg (11/27; 41%) versus warfarin (32/90; 36%), and the RR of intracerebral hemorrhage was significantly reduced with dabigatran 150 mg (RR 0.23; 95% CI 0.12–0.45; P<.001) and dabigatran 110 mg (RR 0.30; 95% CI 0.16–0.54; P<.001) versus warfarin.[12] The RR of subdural hemorrhages was only reduced with dabigatran 110 compared with warfarin (P<.001).

In summarizing all the above studies, major bleeding risk was reduced with apixaban, edoxaban (60 and 30 mg), and dabigatran 110 mg versus warfarin, and rivaroxaban and dabigatran 150 mg had a similar bleeding risk versus warfarin. GIB risk was similar between apixaban and warfarin, and increased with rivaroxaban and dabigatran 150 mg versus warfarin. The risk of GIB with edoxaban was greater with edoxaban 60 mg and lower with edoxaban 30 mg. Intracranial bleeding risk was reduced with all DOACs that were compared with warfarin. The post hoc and subgroup analyses of all the above trials have provided greater detail with regard to the major bleeding risk.

PATHWAY FOR MANAGING THE BLEEDING PATIENT
Step 1: Bleeding Definitions and Initial Assessment
Bleeding definitions
Major bleeding. Major bleeding is defined as fatal bleeding or symptomatic bleeding in a critical area or organ, such as intracranial, intraspinal, intraocular, retroperitoneal, intraarticular or pericardial, or intramuscular with compartment syndrome.[13] Another criterion of major bleeding is a drop of ≥2 g/dL in hemoglobin level or administration of ≥2 units of packed red blood cells.[13] Bleeding events causing a hemoglobin drop of ≥2 g/dL or requiring transfusion of RBCs have been associated with a significantly increased mortality risk.[14] Patients with cardiovascular disease, defined as history of angina, myocardial infarction, heart failure, or peripheral artery disease, have an increased risk of mortality associated with a hemoglobin drop during their hospitalization.[14,22]

Clinically relevant nonmajor bleeding. Clinically relevant nonmajor bleeding is defined as a bleeding event that is clinically overt and that satisfies none of the above major bleeding criteria and leads to (1) hospital admission for bleeding or (2) physician-guided medical or surgical treatment for bleeding or (3) a change in antithrombotic therapy.

Initial assessment. This patient population frequently presents to the emergency department as an acute event, is a transfer from an outside hospital, or

is a hospitalized patient with bleeding. The first step in managing bleeding in the NVAF patient on a VKA or DOAC is stopping the anticoagulant and identifying the location of bleeding followed by defining whether it is major and clinically relevant nonmajor. During the initial evaluation, a focused history and physical examination, with documentation of vital signs and laboratory testing, should be obtained aimed at determining timing of the last dose of VKA or DOAC, whether there was an intentional or unintentional overdose, as well as the onset and severity of bleeding. Hemodynamic stability should be assessed immediately and evaluated frequently with the patient being closely monitored in a critical care setting. Comorbidities must be documented because they could contribute to further bleeding and would require additional approaches to management (e.g., renal failure, liver disease, thrombocytopenia, chemotherapy, medication that enhance anticoagulant effect of VKAs or DOACs, antiplatelet therapy). Whether all patients with suspected acute upper GIB require nasogastric tube placement is controversial, in part because studies have failed to demonstrate a benefit with regard to clinical outcomes.

Step 2: Fluid Resuscitation
In patients with localized major bleeding such as an expanding traumatic hematoma or large laceration, measures such as pressure and packing should be used. For those with major bleeding and hemodynamic instability, aggressive volume resuscitation with intravenous isotonic crystalloids such as 0.9% NaCl or Ringer's lactate with the goal of achieving hemodynamic stability.[23,24] The literature does not appear to show a benefit of colloids over crystalloids.[25] Hypothermia and acidosis should be corrected as they may worsen the coagulopathy and perpetuate the bleeding. Urgent consultation with the appropriate service for site of bleeding is critical (e.g., Neurologic Surgery, Vascular Surgery, Interventional Radiology, Gastroenterology). Supportive measures should include blood product transfusion as appropriate. Randomized trial data by Villanueva et al. and Clinical Practice Guidelines from the American Association of Blood Bankers recommend a restrictive transfusion threshold maintaining a hemoglobin level of >7 g/dL versus a liberal strategy of >9 g/dL in hospitalized adult patients who are hemodynamically stable and including critically ill patients since this approach improves survival and reduces the risk of recurrent bleeding in patients presenting with severe acute upper GIB.[26,27] For patients with underlying coronary artery disease, a more liberal transfusion approach targeting a hemoglobin

level of ≥9 g/dL with appropriate monitoring for fluid overload is recommended.[28] Platelets should be transfused to maintain a platelet count ≥ 50,000 and cryoprecipitated to maintain a fibrinogen > 100 mg/dL.[29,30] For patients requiring ≥3 units of packed red cells within 1 h of significant trauma, activation of a massive transfusion protocol should be considered.[31] Ionized calcium levels should be monitored and supplemented as indicated. Some centers transfusion protocols use goal-directed with thromboelastography or rotational thromboelastometry for management.[32] Early administration of tranexamic acid for trauma patients within the first 3 h of presentation is associated with decreased bleeding and overall mortality and should be considered with appropriate consultation from Hematology or Trauma Surgery.[33] We recommend further resuscitation using a goal-directed strategy guided by the results of laboratory testing.

Step 3: Laboratory Testing

Sequentially in the process of managing the bleeding patient, laboratory testing should include complete blood count, serum creatinine, prothrombin time (PT/INR), and an activated partial thromboplastin time (aPTT). Other testing should be obtained depending on existing patient comorbidities. In patients on a VKA, the PT/INR will be the guide to degree of anticoagulation and planning the intervention to rescue the patient from the major bleeding event. In the case of DOAC major bleeding, laboratory measurement is more complex because the best assays are not widely available. The PT and aPTT in DOAC bleeding have important limitation in their interpretation of degree of anticoagulation.

The best tests for measuring the concentration of dabigatran include the dilute thrombin time, ecarin clotting time, and ecarin chromogenic assay (Table 7.2).[34] These tests correlate closely with dabigatran levels measured by the reference standard method, liquid chromatography-tandem mass spectrometry.[34] Unfortunately, these assays are not widely available, particularly on an emergent basis. In their absence, the thrombin time (TT) and aPTT may be used for qualitative assessment (Table 7.2). The TT is very sensitive to dabigatran, even at very low drug concentrations. A normal TT excludes clinically important dabigatran levels, but a prolonged TT does not discriminate between clinically important and insignificant drug concentrations. A prolonged aPTT suggests the presence of dabigatran but does not discriminate on the anticoagulant effect. A normal aPTT does not exclude the presence of dabigatran levels, especially when a relatively insensitive aPTT reagent is used.[35,36] The preferred test for rivaroxaban, apixaban, and edoxaban is a chromogenic anti-Xa assay (Table 7.2). When the assay is calibrated with the drug of interest, the results correlate closely with drug. This testing is not widely available.

Step 4: Managing Vitamin K Antagonist or Direct Oral Anticoagulant Major Bleeding (Table 7.3)
Vitamin K antagonist (warfarin)
Three options exist for rescue from VKA-based anticoagulation, which include administration of vitamin K, prothrombin complex concentrates (PCCs), and fresh frozen plasma (FFP).

Vitamin K is a rescue agent for VKA because it restores intrinsic hepatic carboxylation of vitamin K–dependent factors (II, VII, IX, X) by overcoming VKA in a dose-dependent manner.[37] It can be given orally, subcutaneously, or intravenously. Slow intravenous administration (15–30 min in 50 mL normal saline)

TABLE 7.2
Laboratory Testing Direct Oral Anticoagulants

Strength of Labs	Apixaban	Rivaroxaban	Edoxaban	Dabigatran
Strong	Chromogenic Anti-Xa	Chromogenic Anti-Xa	Chromogenic Anti-Xa	ECT
				TT or dTT
				aPTT
		PT*	PT*	
Weak				PT/INR

aPTT, activated partial thromboplastin time; *dTT*, dilute thrombin time; *ECT*, ecarin clotting time; *PT**, reagent neoplastin has the most linear correlation; *PT/INR*, prothrombin time/international normalized ratio; *TT*, thrombin time.

TABLE 7.3
Rescue or Reversal Agents

Rescue or Reversal Agent	Vitamin K Antagonist Warfarin	Factor IIa Inhibitor Dabigatran	Factor Xa Inhibitor Apixaban, Edoxaban, Rivaroxaban
Vitamin K	Vitamin K, 10 mg in 50 mL normal saline, IV over 15–30 min with concomitant use PCC or fresh frozen plasma (see below)	Not indicated	Not indicated
4-Factor PCC	First-line treatment INR 2–4: 25 U/kg INR 4–6: 35 U/kg INR>6: 50 U/kg may repeat Q12 h as indicated	Second-line treatment If idarucizumab not available, 50 U/kg, IV, may repeat as indicated	First-line treatment 50 U/kg, IV, may repeat as indicated
Fresh frozen plasma	If 4-factor PCC not available 10–15 mL/kg	Not indicated	Not indicated
Activated PCC	Not indicated	Second-line treatment 50 units/kg, IV	Not indicated
Idarucizumab	Not indicated	First-line treatment 2.5 g, IV over 5–10 min followed by second 2.5 g vial	Not indicated
Andexanet[a] Not approved by FDA	Not indicated	Not indicated	First-line treatment

[a]Use of apixaban or rivaroxaban>7 h: bolus 400 mg, IV and then infusion 480 mg over 2 h or use of enoxaparin, edoxaban, rivaroxaban 7 h or less: bolus 800 mg, IV and then infusion 960 mg over 2 h.

effects a more predictable and rapid reduction in the international normalized ratio (INR) (approximately 4–6 h) compared with oral (approximately 18–24 h). Subcutaneous dosing is not recommended because of unreliable absorption and the need for urgent intervention. Anaphylactic reactions reported in the past with IV administration are not encountered with current preparations.[37] Administration of vitamin K does not result in an immediate correction of coagulopathy and must be accompanied by a rescue strategy with PCC. FFP is used if massive volume replenishment is required or only if 4F-PCC is unavailable.

PCCs contain purified vitamin K–dependent factors obtained from pooled human plasma and are free of viral contaminants. Nonactivated 3-factor PCCs contain factors II, IX, and X with negligible factor VII and proteins C and S, whereas nonactivated 4-factor PCCs contain factors II, VII, IX, X, and proteins C and S. The amount of each factor varies with a listing on every vial. Only 4F-PCC is FDA approved for rapid VKA rescue. They do not require ABO compatibility and can be stored at room temperature as a lyophilized powder, which allows rapid reconstitution for infusion. They

are dosed based on INR and body weight as follows: INR 2–4 at 25 IU/kg, INR 4–6 at 35 IU/kg, and INR>6 at 50 IU/Kg; max dose 5000 IU capped at 100 kg body weight for VKA rescue. Per unit volume, 4F-PCCs contain approximately 25 times (25 IU/mL) the concentration of vitamin K–dependent factors as compared with FFP (1 IU/mL). In addition, the small volume of PCC can be administered rapidly reducing any issues related to volume overload.[38] The other aspect of concern for clinicians is the concern for thromboembolic events caused by the infusion of nonactivated and activated 3- or 4-factor PCC. This stems from anecdotal reports of thrombotic events associated with the extended use of 3F/4F-PCCs in patients with hemophilia. Recent randomized clinical trials comparing 4F-PCC with plasma for VKA rescue showed similar thromboembolic incidence in both groups.[39]

At the present time, the conversion from FFP to PCCs for rescue in VKA major bleeding is appropriate because FFP requires ABO blood type matching and a 30-min thawing time and has allergic reactions and the risk of transfusion acute lung injury, which could affect lifesaving treatment. These complications are not observed with PCC, making them the preferred choice for rescue in VKA major bleeding.

Factor Xa inhibitors (rivaroxaban, apixaban, edoxaban)

Currently andexanet alfa (andexanet), a reversal agent, has been studied in patients with major bleeding or requiring urgent surgery but has not yet been approved by the FDA. As we await confirmation, supplementation with 3- or 4-factor PCC or activated PCC has been studied as a potential nonspecific rescue strategy for the direct factor Xa inhibitors, primarily based on data from in vitro studies, animal models, ex vivo human samples spiked with factor Xa inhibitors, and in healthy volunteer subjects receiving factor Xa inhibitors. None of these agents has demonstrated efficacy or safety in factor Xa inhibitor–treated patients with bleeding or requirement for urgent surgery.[40,41] 4-Factor-PCC is the most extensively studied nonspecific rescue strategy for factor Xa inhibitors and is the only agent studied in vivo in humans. Three randomized studies evaluated the effect of 4-factor-PCC or comparator (placebo or 3-factor-PCC) in human volunteer subjects administered an oral direct factor Xa inhibitor.[42–44] All three trials evaluated the effect of 4-factor-PCC on coagulation laboratory parameters (coagulation tests and thrombin generation), and one study evaluated bleeding following punch biopsy. There was correction of anticoagulant-induced laboratory abnormalities, but results were not consistent across all parameters and all studies. Bleeding duration following punch biopsy was reduced with the highest dose of 4-factor-PCC evaluated (50 IU/kg). Based on these limited data, 4-factor-PCC (50 IU/kg maximum dose as per product monograph) is a reasonable option for emergency rescue for major bleeding or patients requiring urgent surgery in anticoagulated patients with oral direct factor Xa inhibitors. The use of activated PCC has been used in hemophilia patients, but there are no randomized data regarding use in FXa inhibitor major bleeding.

Andexanet alfa (andexanet): reversal agent factor Xa inhibitors

Two recent publications have demonstrated the effectiveness of andexanet in reversing the anticoagulant effect of rivaroxaban and apixaban. This agent is currently under evaluation by the FDA. It is a recombinant protein with a similar structure to endogenous factor Xa, which binds factor Xa inhibitors, but is not enzymatically active.[45] A bolus and 2-h infusion of andexanet rapidly reversed the anticoagulant effects of rivaroxaban and apixaban in older healthy volunteers.[46]

Andexanet is being evaluated in FXa inhibitor–treated patients with major bleeding who had taken rivaroxaban or apixaban within 18 h. In a preliminary analysis of 67 patients, andexanet reduced antifactor Xa activity and active drug levels by over 90%, and clinical hemostasis was adjudicated as good/excellent in 79% of patients.[47] Because of the short half-life of andexanet, some anticoagulant effects of DOACs return within 1–3 h of stopping the infusion, which is a concern regarding the optimal duration of infusion and/or need for repeat administration.[46,47] In healthy volunteers, andexanet increased biomarkers of thrombin generation with no clinical thrombosis. Thrombotic risk following andexanet treatment was reported in 18% of patients within 30 days of the infusion with 92% of the patients not restarting anticoagulant therapy. It is unclear whether this rate of thrombosis is higher than would be expected in bleeding patients at increased baseline thrombotic risk in whom anticoagulation was discontinued.

Management factor IIa inhibitors (dabigatran)

Idarucizumab is FDA approved for reversing the anticoagulant effect of dabigatran in patients with major bleeding. If idarucizumab is not available, then the use of activated charcoal at 50 g can be used when the drug has been taken 2–4 h before presentation of major bleeding.[48] In addition dabigatran is mostly nonprotein bound in the plasma, and hemodialysis can be used to remove 60% of the drug, especially in patients with renal impairment.[48,49] If the preceding interventions cannot be used, then PCC rescue therapy should be used. Unfortunately, studies using PCC have demonstrated inconsistent results. Eerenberg et al. demonstrated that PCC immediately and completely reverses the anticoagulant effect of rivaroxaban in healthy subjects but had no effect on the anticoagulant action of dabigatran.[42] Other smaller case series did not demonstrate improvement in coagulation studies using PCC.[50–53] From these data, it is recommended that 3- or 4-factor PCC not be used for rescue treatment in dabigatran major bleeding. Recently, Shulman et al. reported on 14 patients treated for dabigatran-associated major bleeding with activated PCC (APCC).[54] All patients had good to moderate reversal of bleeding as described by the treating physician and there were no posttreatment thrombotic events. The study was terminated early because of the availability of idarucizumab. Two ex-vivo studies demonstrated effectiveness in reversing prolonged thrombin generation in healthy individuals treated with dabigatran using APCC.[55,56] In two separate case reports, one with dabigatran-associated pericardial tamponade and the second an emergency surgery on dabigatran, APCC was effective in reversing major bleeding.[57,58] In the scenario where idarucizumab is not available, the use of APCC should be considered and the development of postinfusion thromboembolic complications be followed.

Idarucizumab (praxabind): reversal agent factor IIa inhibitor

In the study by Pollack C et al., dabigatran-treated patients with anticoagulation emergencies ongoing either severe or life-threatening hemorrhage or emergency procedures on therapy were given 5 g of idarucizumab as a fixed-dose IV infusion of two 2.5 g aliquots.[59] The study's primary endpoint of maximum reversal of the anticoagulant effect of dabigatran within 4 h was 100% as measured by dilute thrombin time or ecarin clotting time. Among patients with bleeding, cessation was achieved within a median time of 3.5–4.5 h, depending on the location of the bleed. In patients undergoing procedures or surgery, the attending surgeon judged hemostasis to be normal in 92% of patients during their procedure. In the full cohort analysis, thrombotic events occurred in 24 of the 503 patients 4.8% (14 with life-threatening bleeding [Group A] and 10 undergoing surgery or invasive procedure [Group B]) within 30 days after treatment and in 34 of 503 patients 6.8% (19 Group A and 15 Group B) within 90 days.[60]

Anti-idarucizumab antibodies were detected in 5.6% (28/501) of patients who could be assessed.[60] Of those 28 patients, 19 tested positive for preexisting antibodies that were cross-reactive with idarucizumab before its administration and 9 had antibodies that developed during treatment.[60] The antibody titers were generally low, and the preexisting antibodies had no detectable effect on idarucizumab activity.

Other factors may contribute to the thrombotic risk when anticoagulation with DOACs is discontinued for major bleeding such as the following: increased coagulation activation in setting of bleeding, urgent surgery, NVAF with high CHA2DS2-VASc scores, history of recurrent thromboembolic event, active cancer, and continued immobility. Idarucizumab has not been studied outside the above emergency reversal scenarios.

Step 5: Restarting Anticoagulation Following Major Bleeding

After a patient has had a major bleeding event on a VKA or DOAC, the indication for anticoagulation should be reassessed to determine if and when anticoagulation therapy should be resumed. In the studies using idarucizumab or andexanet, postdiscontinuation and reversal therapy demonstrated a risk for thrombotic events including stroke, venous thromboembolism (VTE), and myocardial infarction as noted in reversal section. During the 90-day follow-up in the idarucizumab study, antithrombotic therapy including treatment with prophylactic or therapeutic doses of an anticoagulant or with an antiplatelet drug was restarted in 72.8% of the patients in group A and in 90.1% in group B, at a mean of 13.2 and 3.5 days, respectively, after the administration of idarucizumab.[60] In the andexanet study, only 27% of patients resumed anticoagulation within 30 days.[47] Let us review the data on the safety of anticoagulation resumption in patients following a major bleeding event or after a major surgical procedure.

Gastrointestinal bleeding

GIB is a relatively common hemorrhagic complication of chronic oral anticoagulant therapy (OAC). Anticoagulant therapy is frequently discontinued in a substantial proportion of patients despite evidence of benefit with resuming the OAC. In a systematic review of observational studies, patients with OAC-associated GIB who resumed anticoagulation had a lower risk of thromboembolism (9.9% vs. 16.4%; HR, 0.68, 95%: 0.52–0.88) and death (24.6% vs. 39.2%; HR, 0.76, 95% CI 0.66–0.88) compared with those who did not restart, with a nonsignificant increase in the risk of recurrent bleeding (10.1% vs. 5.5%, HR, 1.20, 95% CI: 0.97–1.48).[61] The timing of restarting anticoagulation has not been systematically studied and is highly variable, although a prospective study in which anticoagulation was restarted at the time of discharge in patients with a median length of stay of 5 days demonstrated fewer thromboembolic events at 90 days with no increase in bleeding events, and in AF patients restarting warfarin >7 days after a bleed was associated with improved survival and decreased thromboembolism without an increased risk of recurrent GIB.[62,63] Deciding to resume warfarin or DOAC therapy becomes more challenging in cases where the bleeding source cannot be identified. Each of the above studies demonstrated that the resumption of anticoagulation between 7 and 90 days following a major GIB showed a reduction in thromboembolic events and mortality without increasing recurrent GIB. Based on the above studies, resumption of anticoagulation with warfarin or a DOAC requires a full assessment of rebleeding versus the thromboembolic risk for each individual patient. Although there are no clinical trials on the safety of using alternate DOACs in patients with major bleeding, extrapolating to the bleeding incidence from the NVAF trials could serve as a reasonable approach to selecting a DOAC with lower bleeding risk than warfarin. On the other hand, the selection of another DOAC in the face of a DOAC-associated major bleed lacks clinical evidence, but it would be reasonable to select a DOAC that has lower major bleeding. A clinically reasonable recommendation would be to assess the CHA2DS$_2$-VASc and HAS-BLED scores and delay resumption of full dose anticoagulation until the patient hemoglobin status remains stable. The lower extremity external pneumatic compression for VTE prophylaxis should be applied to all patients during this risk period. If the patient has a mechanical heart valve and AF, starting an unfractionated heparin infusion and dose adjusting to therapeutic anticoagulation would be a clinically reasonable option for management.

Intracranial hemorrhage

Intracranial hemorrhage (ICH) is the most catastrophic complication of anticoagulant therapy with a reported 30-day mortality rate of approximately 50%.[64] Approximately 20% of spontaneous ICHs are related to anticoagulation therapy. Resumption of anticoagulation in this patient population requires an individualized approach. Factors associated with a higher risk of recurrent bleeding include the mechanism of ICH either spontaneous or traumatic, lobar location of the initial bleed (suggesting amyloid angiopathy), the presence and number of microbleeds on MRI, size of the bleed, and need for ongoing anticoagulation.[65]

Limited data exist on the reinitiation of OAC after an ICH. Depending on bleed characteristics, risk factor modification, and the indication for anticoagulation, restarting OAC after a nonlobar ICH may be considered.[65] In observational studies of patients with warfarin-associated ICH, resumption of anticoagulation appears to confer a 70% lower risk of thrombosis and 50%–70% lower risk of death without a significant increased risk of recurrent bleeding compared with discontinuation.[66-71] Optimization of modifiable cardiovascular risk factors such as hypertension is important before OAC resumption. Lobar ICH secondary to amyloid angiopathy either spontaneous or related to warfarin use and spontaneous subdural hematomas are associated with a high risk of rebleeding. Restarting anticoagulation in these settings should be approached with caution in consultation with either neurology or neurologic surgery. DOACs are associated with a lower risk of ICH than warfarin, but the safety of switching a patient with an ICH to a DOAC has not been evaluated.[9,65]

The timing of anticoagulation resumption following an ICH has not been systematically studied and varies widely in observational studies (72 h to 30 weeks) reflecting a lack of consensus. In patients without mechanical heart valves, guidelines recommend avoiding anticoagulation for at least 4 weeks, and if indicated, aspirin monotherapy may be restarted in the days after an ICH.[65] In a large retrospective study that demonstrated benefits associated with OAC resumption, the median time to restart OAC was approximately 4 weeks after the bleeding event.[66] I agree with the recommendations of resuming anticoagulation 4 weeks following an ICH as per the AHA/ASA guidelines.[65]

Restarting anticoagulation after a surgery/procedure. If anticoagulation was discontinued and rescued or reversed for an urgent or emergent surgery/procedure without a preceding bleeding event and adequate postprocedural hemostasis has been achieved, anticoagulation should be resumed based on the postprocedure bleeding risk. For procedures that carry a low bleeding risk, anticoagulation can be restarted within 24 h. If the postprocedural bleeding risk is high, therapeutic dose anticoagulation should be delayed for 48–72 h.[72] It should be kept in mind that patients will require VTE prophylaxis following major procedures. The use of prophylactic anticoagulants is not adequate to prevent stroke but serve to reduce the risk of developing postoperative VTE. A recent study demonstrated that bridge therapy with low molecular weight heparin or unfractionated heparin in a low-risk CHADS$_2$ score population had increased the risk of major bleeding.[73] There are limited data regarding the efficacy and safety of using intravenous unfractionated heparin in the subset of patients with a high or very high thrombotic and bleeding risk following surgery, who will be restarting warfarin therapy. In these patients, the ability to titrate parenteral anticoagulation may be the most reasonable clinical option for bridging to warfarin. If a DOAC is used postprocedurally, bridging anticoagulation should not be used. It must be remembered that the NVAF DOAC dose is higher than the DOAC VTE prophylaxis dose in hip and knee replacement surgery. A reasonable approach in this patient population would be to use the orthopedic DOAC dose for 2 weeks and then convert to the full DOAC dose. For surgeries/procedures performed to control bleeding, restarting anticoagulation after the procedure may carry a higher bleeding risk. This depends on the characteristics of the bleed and the surgical management. If the source of bleeding was identified and completely corrected with adequate hemostasis, restarting anticoagulation in a similar fashion as discussed above may be reasonable. Individualized strategies with close clinical monitoring apply for patients in whom surgical/procedural management was not successful at controlling bleeding as described herein for bleeding complications managed without procedural intervention.

CONCLUSION (FIG. 7.1)

Because of the relatively short half-lives of the DOACs, management of minor to moderate anticoagulant-associated bleeding may only require discontinuation of therapy and supportive management. In situations involving major bleeding, including noncompressible hemorrhages, use of a reversal agent is necessary because of the need for rapid achievement of hemostasis. The FDA approval of a specific reversal agent, idarucizumab, for dabigatran-associated bleeding has been beneficial in expanding our armamentarium for management and has a rapid onset of action. Currently, there is a pending FDA approval for andexanet as a reversal agent for the orally administered direct factor

Xa inhibitors. In the interim, the use of PCCs has demonstrated fairly rapid achievement of hemostasis and can be employed for major bleeding. Another reversal agent, ciraparantag, is currently under investigation for reversing direct thrombin inhibitors, factor Xa inhibitors, low molecular weight heparins, and heparin.

The management of major bleeding for patients with NVAF on a VKA or DOAC is changing rapidly with better rescue therapies and reversal agents as reviewed in this paper. The challenge we face is establishing a structured organized approach for the treatment of this patient population. A team pathway approach to operationalizing the assessment and management of major bleeding in patients with NVAF on OACs could be as follows:

1. Bleeding alert team activated
2. Define major bleeding as hemodynamic instability, bleeding at a critical site, a drop of $\geq 2\,\text{g/dL}$ in hemoglobin level and transfusion of >2 units RBCs
3. History and physical examination, laboratory testing, imaging
4. Fluid resuscitation
5. Rescue or reversal therapy for VKA and DOACs
6. Posttreatment resumption of anticoagulation based on etiology for bleeding (GI, ICH, postsurgery)

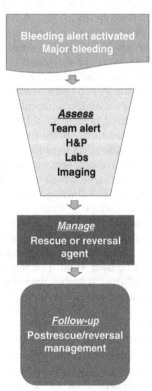

FIG. 7.1 Approach to Major Bleeding in patients taking Vitamin K Antagonist or Direct Thrombin Inhibitors

REFERENCES

1. Camm A, Lip GY, De Caterina R, et al. 2012 focused update of the ESC Guidelines for the management of atrial fibrillation: an update of the 2010 ESC Guidelines for the management of atrial fibrillation. Developed with the special contribution of the European Heart Rhythm Association. *Eur Heart J.* 2012;33(21):2719–2747.
2. Colilla S, Crow A, Petkun W, et al. Estimates of current and future incidence and prevalence of atrial fibrillation in the U.S. adult population. *Am J Cardiol.* 2013;112:1142–1147.
3. Zoni-Berisso M, Lercari F, Carazza T, et al. Epidemiology of atrial fibrillation: European perspective. *J Clin Epidemiol.* 2014;6:213–220.
4. Wolf P, Abbott R, Kannel W. Atrial fibrillation as an independent risk factor for stroke: the Framingham study. *Stroke.* 1991;22:983–988.
5. Luengo-Fernandez R, Gray A, Rothwell P. Population-based study of determinants of initial secondary care costs of acute stroke in the United Kingdom. *Stroke.* 2006;37:2579–2587.
6. Demaerschalk B, Hwang H, Leung G. US cost burden of ischemic stroke: a systematic literature review. *Am J Manag Care.* 2010;16:525–533.
7. Ruff C, Giugliano R, Braunwald E, et al. Comparison of the efficacy and safety of new oral anticoagulants with warfarin in patients with atrial fibrillation: a meta-analysis of randomized trials. *Lancet.* 2014;383:955–962.

8. Eikelboom J, Merli G. Bleeding with direct oral anti-coagulants vs warfarin: clinical experience. *Am J Med.* 2016;129:S33–S40.

9. Granger CB, Alexander JH, McMurray JJ, et al. Apixaban versus warfarin in patients with atrial fibrillation. *N Engl J Med.* 2011;365:981–992.

10. Connolly SJ, Ezekowitz MD, Yusuf S, et al. Dabigatran versus warfarin in patients with atrial fibrillation. *N Engl J Med.* 2009;361:1139–1151.

11. Eikelboom JW, Wallentin L, Connolly SJ, et al. Risk of bleeding with 2 doses of dabigatran compared with war-farin in older and younger patients with atrial fibrilla-tion: an analysis of the randomized evaluation of long-term anticoagulant therapy (RE-LY) trial. *Circulation.* 2011;123:2363–2372.

12. Hart RG, Diener HC, Yang S, et al. Intracranial hemor-rhage in atrial fibrillation patients during anticoagula-tion with warfarin or dabigatran: the RE-LY trial. *Stroke.* 2012;43:1511–1517.

13. Smilowitz NR, Oberweis BS, Nukala S, et al. Association between anemia, bleeding, and 31 transfusion with long-term mortality following noncardiac surgery. *Am J Med.* 2016;129. 315–332 23 e2. 33.

14. Fakhry SM, Fata P. How low is too low? Cardiac risks with anemia. *Crit Care.* 2004;8(suppl 2):S11–S514.

15. Hylek EM, Held C, Alexander JH, et al. Major bleeding in patients with atrial fibrillation receiving apixaban or warfarin: the ARISTOTLE Trial (apixaban for reduction in stroke and other thromboembolic events in atrial fibrilla-tion): predictors, characteristics, and clinical outcomes. *J Am Coll Cardiol.* 2014;63:2141–2147.

16. Patel MR, Mahaffey KW, Garg J, et al. Rivaroxaban versus warfarin in nonvalvular atrial fibrillation. *N Engl J Med.* 2011;365:883–891.

17. Hankey G, Stevens S, Piccini J, et al. Intracranial hem-orrhage among patients with atrial fibrillation anti-coagulated with warfarin or rivaroxaban: the rivar-oxaban once daily, oral, direct factor Xa inhibition compared with vitamin K antagonist for prevention of stroke and embolism trial in atrial fibrillation. *Stroke.* 2014;45:1304–1312.

18. Goodman SG, Wojdyla DM, Piccini JP, et al. Factors as-sociated with major bleeding events: insights from the ROCKET AF trial (rivaroxaban once-daily oral direct factor Xa inhibition compared with vitamin K antagonism for prevention of stroke and embolism trial in atrial fibrilla-tion). *J Am Coll Cardiol.* 2014;63:891–900.

19. Giugliano RP, Ruff CT, Braunwald E, et al. Edoxaban ver-sus warfarin in patients with atrial fibrillation. *N Engl J Med.* 2013;369:2093–2104.

20. Giugliano RP, Ruff CT, Rost NS, et al. Cerebrovascular events in 21,105 patients with atrial fibrillation rand-omized to edoxaban versus warfarin: effective antico-agulation with factor Xa next generation in atrial fibril-lation-thrombolysis in myocardial infarction 48. *Stroke.* 2014;45:2372–2378.

21. Ruff CT, Giugliano RP, Braunwald E, et al. Association between edoxaban dose, concentration, anti-factor Xa activity, and outcomes: an analysis of data from the ran-domised, double-blind ENGAGE AF-TIMI 48 trial. *Lancet.* 2015;385:2288–2295.

22. Damluji AA, Macon C, Fox A, et al. The association between in-hospital hemoglobin changes, 36 cardiovascular events, and mortality in acute decompensated heart failure: results from the 37 ESCAPE trial. *Int J Cardiol.* 2016;222:531–537.

23. Baradarian R, Ramdhaney S, Chapalamadugu R, et al. Early intensive resuscitation of patients with upper gastro-intestinal bleeding decreases mortality. *Am J Gastroenterol.* 2004;99:619–622.

24. Spoerke N, Michalek J, Schreiber M, et al. Crystalloid re-suscitation improves survival in trauma patients receiving low ratios of fresh frozen plasma to packed red blood cells. *J Trauma.* 2011;71(2 suppl 3):S380–S383.

25. Perel P, Roberts I, Ker K. Colloids versus crystalloids for fluid resuscitation in critically ill patients. *Cochrane Data-base Syst Rev.* 2013;(2):CD000567.

26. Villanueva C, Colomo A, Bosch A, et al. Transfusion strat-egies for acute upper gastrointestinal bleeding. *N Engl J Med.* 2013;368:11–21.

27. Carson JL, Guyatt G, Heddle NM, et al. Clinical practice guidelines from the AABB: red blood cell transfusion thresholds and storage. *JAMA.* 2016;316:2025–2035.

28. Retter A, Wyncoll D, Pearse R, et al. Guidelines on the management of anaemia and red cell transfusion in adult critically ill patients. *Br J Haematol.* 2013;160:445–464.

29. Contreras M. Final statement from the consensus conference on platelet transfusion. *Transfusion.* 1998;1738(8):796–797.

30. Razzaghi A, Barkun AN. Platelet transfusion threshold in patients with upper gastrointestinal bleeding: a systematic review. *J Clin Gastroenterol.* 2012;46:482–486.

31. Dzik WH, Blajchman MA, Fergusson D, et al. Clinical review: Canadian National Advisory 20 Committee on blood and blood products–massive transfusion consen-sus conference 2011: 21 report of the panel. *Crit Care.* 2011;15:242.

32. Holcomb JB, Tilley BC, Baraniuk S, et al. Transfusion of plas-ma, platelets, and red blood cells in a 23 1:1:1 vs a 1:1:2 ratio and mortality in patients with severe trauma: the PROPPR randomized 24 clinical trial. *JAMA.* 2015;313:471–482.

33. Roberts I, Bautista R, Caballero J, et al. Effects of tranexam-ic acid on death, vascular occlusive 29 events, and blood transfusion in trauma patients with significant haemor-rhage (CRASH-2): a randomised, placebo-controlled trial. *Lancet.* 2010;376:23–32.

34. Cuker A. Laboratory measurement of the non-vitamin K antagonist oral anticoagulants: selecting 41 the optimal assay based on drug, assay availability, and clinical indica-tion. *J Thromb Thrombolysis.* 2016;41:241–247.

35. Samuelson BT, Cuker A, Siegal DM, et al. Laboratory assessment of the anticoagulant activity of 44 direct oral anticoagulants: a systematic review. *Chest.* 2017; 151:127–138.

36. Cuker A, Siegal DM, Crowther MA, et al. Laboratory measurement of the anticoagulant activity of the non-vitamin K oral anticoagulants. *J Am Coll Cardiol*. 2014; 64:1128–1139.

37. Britt RB, Brown JN. Characterizing the severe reactions of parenteral vitamin K1. *Clin Appl Thromb Hemost*. 2016. https://doi.org/10.1177/1076029616674825.

38. Sarode R, Milling Jr TJ, Refaai MA, et al. Efficacy and safety of a 4-factor prothrombin complex concentrate in patients on vitamin K antagonists presenting with major bleeding: a randomized, plasma-controlled, phase IIIb study. *Circulation*. 2013;128:1234–1243.

39. Milling Jr TJ, Refaai MA, Sarode R, et al. Safety of a four-factor prothrombin complex concentrate versus plasma for vitamin K antagonist reversal: an integrated analysis of two phase IIIb clinical trials. *Acad Emerg Med*. 2016;23:466–475.

40. Crowther M, Crowther MA. Antidotes for novel oral anticoagulants: current status and future potential. *Arterioscler Thromb Vasc Biol*. 2015;35:1736–1745.

41. Siegal DM. Managing target-specific oral anticoagulant associated bleeding including an update on pharmacological reversal agents. *J Thromb Thrombolysis*. 2015; 39:395–402.

42. Eerenberg ES, Kamphuisen PW, Sijpkens MK, et al. Reversal of rivaroxaban and dabigatran by prothrombin complex concentrate: a randomized, placebo-controlled, crossover study in healthy subjects. *Circulation*. 2011;124(14):1573–1579.

43. Levi M, Moore KT, Castillejos CF, et al. Comparison of three-factor and four-factor prothrombin complex concentrates regarding reversal of the anticoagulant effects of rivaroxaban in healthy volunteers. *J Thromb Haemost*. 2014;12:1428–1436.

44. Zahir H, Brown KS, Vandell AG, et al. Edoxaban effects on bleeding following punch biopsy and reversal by a 4-factor prothrombin complex concentrate. *Circulation*. 2015;131:82–90.

45. Lu G, DeGuzman FR, Hollenbach SJ, et al. A specific antidote for reversal of anticoagulation by direct and indirect inhibitors of coagulation factor Xa. *Nat Med*. 2013;19:446–451.

46. Siegal DM, Curnutte JT, Connolly SJ, et al. Andexanet alfa for the reversal of factor Xa inhibitor activity. *N Engl J Med*. 2015;373:2413–2424.

47. Connolly SJ, Milling Jr TJ, Eikelboom JW, et al. Andexanet alfa for acute major bleeding associated with factor Xa inhibitors. *N Engl J Med*. 2016;375:1131–1141.

48. van Ryn J, Stangier J, Haertter S, et al. Dabigatran etexilate–a novel, reversible, oral direct thrombin inhibitor: interpretation of coagulation assays and reversal of anticoagulant activity. *Thromb Haemost*. 2010;103(6):1116–1127.

49. Stangier J, Rathgen K, Stahle H, et al. Influence of renal impairment on the pharmacokinetics and pharmacodynamics of oral dabigatran etexilate: an open-label, parallel-group, single-centre study. *Clin Pharmacokinet*. 2010;49:259–268.

50. Marlu R, Hodaj E, Paris A, et al. Effect of non-specific reversal agents on anticoagulant activity of dabigatran and rivaroxaban: a randomised crossover ex vivo study in healthy volunteers. *Thromb Haemost*. 2012;108:217–224.

51. Zhou W, Schwarting S, Illanes S, et al. Hemostatic therapy in experimental intracerebral hemorrhage associated with the direct thrombin inhibitor dabigatran. *Stroke*. 2011;42:3594–3599.

52. Pragst I, Zeitler SH, Doerr B, et al. Reversal of dabigatran anticoagulation by prothrombin complex concentrate (Beriplex P/N) in a rabbit model. *J Thromb Haemost*. 2012;10:1841–1848.

53. Hoffman M, Volovyk Z, Monroe DM. Reversal of dabigatran effects in models of thrombin generation and hemostasis by factor VIIa and prothrombin complex concentrate. *Anesthesiology*. 2015;122:353–362.

54. Schulman S, Ritchie B, Goy JK, et al. Activated prothrombin complex concentrate for dabigatran-associated bleeding. *Br J Haematol*. 2014;164:308–310.

55. Majeed A, Shulman S. Bleeding and antidotes new oral anticoagulants. *Best Pract Res Clin Haematol*. 2013;26:191–202.

56. Lindahl TL, Wallstedt M, Gustafsson KM, et al. More efficient reversal of dabigatran inhibition of coagulation by activated prothrombin complex concentrate or recombinant factor VIIa than by four-factor prothrombin complex concentrate. *Thromb Res*. 2015;135:544–547.

57. Wong H, Keeling D. Activated prothrombin complex concentrate for the prevention of dabigatran-associated bleeding. *Br J Haematol*. 2014;166:152–153.

58. Dager A. Roberts, reversing dabigatran with FEIBA in a patient with a transseptal perforation during cardiac ablation. *Crit Care Med*. 2011;39(suppl):243.

59. Pollack Jr CV, Reilly PA, Eikelboom J, et al. Idarucizumab for dabigatran reversal. *N Engl J Med*. 2015;373:511–520.

60. Pollack Jr CV. *Idarucizumab for Dabigatran Reversal: Updated Results of the RE-VERSE AD Study 20 American Heart Association Scientific Sessions 2016 New Orleans, Louisiana*; 2016.

61. Chai-Adisaksopha C, Hillis C, Monreal M, et al. Thromboembolic events, recurrent bleeding and mortality after resuming anticoagulant following gastrointestinal bleeding. A meta-analysis. *Thromb Haemost*. 2015;114:819–825.

62. Sengupta N, Feuerstein JD, Patwardhan VR, et al. The risks of thromboembolism vs. recurrent gastrointestinal bleeding after interruption of systemic anticoagulation in hospitalized inpatients with gastrointestinal bleeding: a prospective study. *Am J Gastroenterol*. 2015;110:328–335.

63. Qureshi W, Mittal C, Patsias I, et al. Restarting anticoagulation and outcomes after major gastrointestinal bleeding in atrial fibrillation. *Am J Cardiol*. 2014;113:662–668.

64. Cervera A, Amaro S, Chamorro A. Oral anticoagulant-associated intracerebral hemorrhage. *J Neurol*. 2012;259:212–224.

65. Hemphill 3rd JC, Greenberg SM, Anderson CS, et al. Guidelines for the management of spontaneous intracerebral hemorrhage: a guideline for healthcare professionals from the American Heart Association/American Stroke Association. *Stroke*. 2015;46:2032–2060.

66. Kuramatsu JB, Gerner ST, Schellinger PD, et al. Anticoagulant reversal, blood pressure levels, and anticoagulant resumption in patients with anticoagulation-related intracerebral hemorrhage. *JAMA.* 2015;313:824–836.

67. Milling Jr TJ, Spyropoulos AC. Re-initiation of dabigatran and direct factor Xa antagonists after a major bleed. *Am J Med.* 2016;129:S54–S63.

68. Witt DM, Delate T, Hylek EM, et al. Effect of warfarin on intracranial hemorrhage incidence and fatal outcomes. *Thromb Res.* 2013;132:770–775.

69. Yung D, Kapral MK, Asllani E, et al. Reinitiation of anticoagulation after warfarin-associated intracranial hemorrhage and mortality risk: the best practice for reinitiating anticoagulation therapy after intracranial bleeding (BRAIN) study. *Can J Cardiol.* 2012;28:33–39.

70. Nielsen PB, Larsen TB, Skjoth F, et al. Restarting anticoagulant treatment after intracranial hemorrhage in patients with atrial fibrillation and the impact on recurrent stroke, mortality, and bleeding: a nationwide cohort study. *Circulation.* 2015;132:517–525.

71. Hawryluk GW, Austin JW, Furlan JC, et al. Management of anticoagulation following central nervous system hemorrhage in patients with high thromboembolic risk. *J Thromb Haemost.* 2010;8:1500–1508.

72. Doherty JU, Gluckman TJ, Hucker WJ, et al. 2017 ACC expert consensus decision pathway for periprocedural management of anticoagulation in patients with nonvalvular atrial fibrillation: a report of the American College of Cardiology Clinical Expert Consensus Document Task Force. *J Am Coll Cardiol.* 2017;69(7):871–898.

73. Douketis JD, Spyropoulos AC, Kaatz S, et al. Perioperative bridging anticoagulation in patients with atrial fibrillation. *N Engl J Med.* 2015;373:823–833.

FURTHER READING

1. Patel MR, Hellkamp AS, Fox KA, ROCKET AF Executive Committee and Investigators. Point-of-care warfarin monitoring in the ROCKET AF trial. *N Engl J Med.* 2016;374:785–788.

Periprocedural Management of Anticoagulation in Patients With Atrial Fibrillation

RICHARD WEACHTER, MD • GREG FLAKER, MD

BACKGROUND

Annually 10%–15% of patients who receive oral anti-coagulant (AC) therapy will have treatment interruption for an invasive procedure or surgery.[1,2] Patients with atrial fibrillation account for the greatest percentage for whom periprocedural decisions regarding anticoagulation will be made.[3] The decision to either continue or interrupt anticoagulation must take into account two primary factors—the risk of periprocedural thromboembolic event (TE) with interruption of anticoagulation and the risk of periprocedural bleeding, especially for those with highest risk for TE for whom parenteral bridging anticoagulation may be prescribed.

For patients undergoing an invasive procedure or surgery at low risk for bleeding, no interruption of oral anticoagulation might be considered. For patients undergoing an invasive procedure or surgery at high risk for bleeding but low risk for a TE, interruption of anticoagulation without parenteral anticoagulation might be considered. For patients undergoing an invasive procedure or surgery at moderate to high TE and bleeding risk, a variety of strategies have been developed incorporating parenteral bridging anticoagulation, typically with unfractionated heparin (UFH) or low molecular weight heparin (LMWH), during interruption of oral anticoagulation. A number of periprocedural antithrombotic strategies have been proposed[4] (Fig. 8.1).

Additionally, the prescribed oral AC will have an impact on decisions made. Warfarin, requiring several days for its AC effect to dissipate when discontinued preprocedurally, and to be reestablished when resumed postprocedurally, may necessitate for some patients parenteral bridging anticoagulation. The new direct oral anticoagulants (DOACs), having shorter half-lives than warfarin, take far less time for their AC effect to dissipate preprocedurally and to be reestablished

postprocedurally, thereby potentially avoiding the need for parenteral bridging anticoagulation.

GENERAL PRINCIPLES FOR PERIPROCEDURAL MANAGEMENT OF ANTICOAGULATION

The initial assessments and subsequent decisions to be made periprocedurally to achieve the lowest possible periprocedural TE and bleeding risk should include the following:

1. estimation of TE risk during anticoagulation interruption
2. estimation of procedural bleeding risk
3. determination of the need for oral AC discontinuation
4. determination of the need for parenteral bridging anticoagulation
5. determining when to resume anticoagulation postprocedure

IDENTIFICATION OF THE PATIENT AT HIGH RISK FOR A THROMBOEMBOLIC EVENT DURING ANTICOAGULATION INTERRUPTION

The most effective manner to identify patients at high risk for a TE with interruption of anticoagulation therapy is not known.[1,5] The $CHADS_2$ score (congestive heart failure, hypertension, age, diabetes, stroke) was used in the BRIDGE (Bridging Anticoagulation in Patients Who Require Temporary Interruption of Warfarin Therapy for an Elective Procedure or Surgery) trial to identify patients who required interruption of anticoagulation therapy before an invasive procedure or surgery.[6] The rationale for using the $CHADS_2$ score to identify patients at risk for TE in the periprocedural period had been extrapolated from the past experience

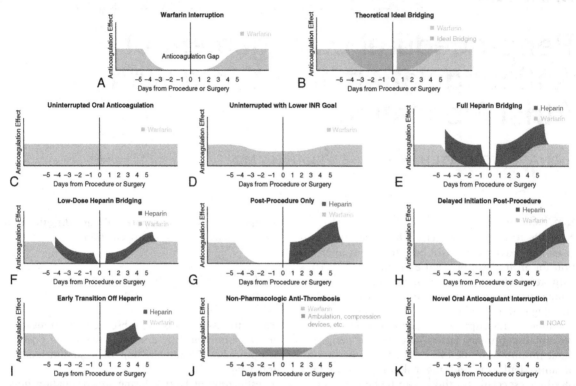

FIG. 8.1 Periprocedural antithrombotic strategies. *NOAC*, novel oral anticoagulant. (From Rechenmacher SJ, Fang JC. Bridging anticoagulation primum non nocere. *J Am Coll Cardiol.* 2015;66:1392–1403.)

with mechanical heart valves. Major embolism (leading to death, stroke, or peripheral ischemia requiring surgery) occurs in 4% of patients with mechanical heart valves annually without anticoagulation and in 1% annually with warfarin.[7,8] Based in part on these late 1990s data, it was recommended that preoperative and/or postoperative heparin prophylaxis be considered to prevent thromboembolism when the international normalized ratio (INR) fell below 2.0.[9] The 2001 CHEST guidelines commented that "until clinical trials that specifically target the perioperative management of patients with valvular heart disease requiring warfarin anticoagulation prior to surgical procedure are performed, treatment of such patients will remain controversial."[10] Because the yearly risk of stroke in atrial fibrillation patients with a $CHADS_2$ score ≥ 4 was reported to be 8%,[11] most clinicians thought the risk of TE to be sufficiently high to warrant parenteral bridging anticoagulation when oral anticoagulation therapy was interrupted in these patients.

However, in a recent survey on the practice of periprocedural management of anticoagulation in the

United States, the use of the CHA_2DS_2-VASc score (congestive heart failure, hypertension, age, diabetes, stroke, vascular disease, female) was preferred over the $CHADS_2$ score by a 4:1 margin[12] (Fig. 8.2).

Neither the $CHADS_2$ nor CHA_2DS_2-VASc scores have been validated to be predictive of TE with interruption of anticoagulation, but because CHA_2DS_2-VASc has replaced $CHADS_2$ as a scoring system to determine when to use oral anticoagulation,[13] its use in this regard seems logical.

IDENTIFICATION OF THE PATIENT AT LOW RISK FOR THROMBOEMBOLIC EVENT DURING ANTICOAGULATION INTERRUPTION

A prospective, observational cohort study assessed the safety of brief (≤5 days) periprocedural interruption of warfarin for patients undergoing a minor outpatient intervention (colonoscopy, oral or dental surgery, ophthalmologic surgery, prostate or breast biopsy, epidural injection, and dermatologic procedure). The

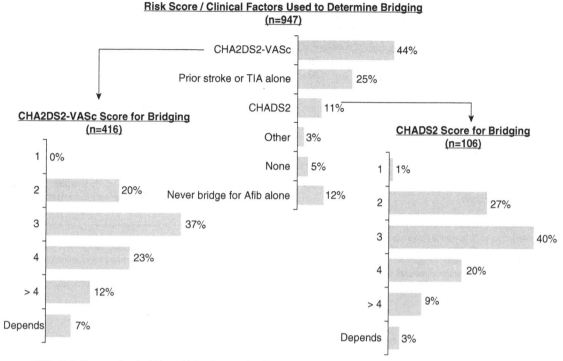

FIG. 8.2 Nonmechanical Heart Valve Patient for Surgery: Risk Score/Clinical Factors Used and Bridging Threshold. *Afib*, atrial fibrillation; *TIA*, transient ischemic attack. (From Flaker G, Theriot P, Binder L, et al. A survey of the management of periprocedural anticoagulation in contemporary practice. *J Am Coll Cardiol.* 2016;68:217–226.)

most common indication for anticoagulation was atrial fibrillation (54%) followed by deep vein thrombosis/pulmonary embolus (PE) (14%), prosthetic heart valve (13%), and stroke (9%). Only 0.7% of patients, none receiving periprocedural parenteral bridging anticoagulation, experienced a postprocedure thromboembolism, whereas 2.3% had a significant bleeding episode, of which 61% received periprocedural heparin bridging.[3]

Analysis of RE-LY (Randomized Evaluation of Long-term Anticoagulation Therapy), ROCKET-AF (Rivaroxaban Once daily, oral, direct, factor Xa inhibition Compared with vitamin K antagonism for prevention of stroke and Embolism Trial in Atrial Fibrillation), and ARISTOTLE (Apixaban for Reduction in Stroke and Other Thromboembolic Events in Atrial Fibrillation) data has further assessed the relationship between anticoagulation and outcomes among atrial fibrillation patients treated with long-term anticoagulation who underwent temporary interruption of AC therapy.

RE-LY (comparing dabigatran with warfarin) reported periprocedural bleeding and TE risk 7 days before and 30 days after an invasive procedure or surgery. Over 2 years, 25% of RE-LY patients (mean CHADS₂ score 2.1) underwent an invasive procedure or surgery. Most commonly performed procedures included pacemaker/defibrillator implantation, dental procedure, cataract removal, colonoscopy, and joint replacement. Periprocedural bridging anticoagulation was used in 20% of RE-LY patients. Periprocedural TE risk was low: 0.5% for stroke or systemic embolism and 1.3% for the composite endpoint of cardiovascular death, stroke, systemic embolism, and PE. The need for urgent surgery was associated with a more than four-fold increased incidence of ischemic stroke or systemic embolism.[14]

ROCKET-AF (comparing rivaroxaban with warfarin) reported TE risk from initial temporary interruption of AC therapy to 30 days after resumption of study drug. 33% of ROCKET-AF patients (mean CHADS₂ score 3.4) had temporary interruption of anticoagulation. Most commonly performed procedures included colonoscopy/gastrointestinal endoscopy, dental work, abdominal/thoracic/orthopedic surgery, dermatologic/tissue biopsy,

TABLE 8.1

Thromboembolic Risk (Stroke/Systemic Embolus) During Temporary Interruption of Anticoagulation: Analysis of RE-LY, ROCKET-AF, and ARISTOTLE

	At-Risk Period	CHADS$_2$ (Mean)	Bridging Anticoagulation (%)	TE Risk (%)
RE-LY (comparing dabigatran with warfarin)	7 days preprocedure→30 days postprocedure	2.1	20	0.5% (0.69% warfarin treated, 0.46% dabigatran treated)
ROCKET-AF (comparing rivaroxaban with warfarin)	from TI→30 days after resumption of study drug	3.4	9	0.36% (0.41% warfarin treated, 0.30% rivaroxaban treated)
ARISTOTLE (comparing apixaban with warfarin)	30 days postprocedure	2.1	12	0.46% (0.57% warfarin treated, 0.35% apixaban treated)

TE, thromboembolic; TI, temporary interruption.

Adapted from Healey JS, Eikelboom J, Douketis J, et al. Periprocedural bleeding and thromboembolic events with dabigatran compared with warfarin. *Circulation.* 2012;126:343–348; Sherwood MW, Douketis JD, Patel MR, et al. Outcomes of temporary interruption of rivaroxaban compared with warfarin in patients with nonvalvular atrial fibrillation. *Circulation.* 2014;129(18):1850–1859; Garcia D, Alexander JH, Wallentin L, et al. Management and clinical outcomes in patients treated with apixaban versus warfarin undergoing procedures. *Blood.* 2014;124(25):3692–3698.

and electrophysiology procedure. 9% of patients with temporary interruption of oral AC therapy received bridging anticoagulation therapy. Periprocedural 30-day rate of stroke or systemic embolism was 0.36%.[15]

ARISTOTLE (comparing apixaban with warfarin) reported periprocedural TE and bleeding risk for 30 days postprocedure. 33% of ARISTOTLE patients (mean CHADS$_2$ score 2.1 with temporary interruption and 2.2 without temporary interruption of AC) underwent invasive procedure or surgery. Most commonly performed procedures included dental work, colonoscopy, ophthalmologic surgery, and upper endoscopy. Anticoagulation was not interrupted in 38% of procedures and bridging anticoagulation therapy was used in 12% of procedures. Periprocedural stroke or systemic embolism risk was 0.46%[16] (Table 8.1).

For the purpose of defining risk for periprocedural TE, the American College of Chest Physicians (ACCP) using CHADS$_2$, and the American College of Cardiology (ACC) using CHA$_2$DS$_2$-VASc, have categorized patients with nonvalvular atrial fibrillation (NVAF) into low TE risk (<5%/year), moderate TE risk (5%–10%/year), and high TE risk (>10%/year). The ACCP defined low TE risk for patients with CHADS$_2$ score ≤2, moderate TE risk CHADS$_2$ score 3–4, and high TE risk CHADS$_2$ score ≥5. Any patient with CHADS$_2$ score <5 and recent (≤3 months) transient ischemic attack (TIA)/stroke or prior TE during temporary interruption of vitamin K

antagonist (VKA) were also considered high TE risk. The ACC defined low TE risk for patients with CHADS$_2$-VASc ≤ 4 and no prior history of TIA or stroke, moderate TE risk with CHADS$_2$-VASc score 5–6 and no recent (≤3 months) ischemic stroke, TIA or systemic embolism, and high TE risk with CHA$_2$DS$_2$-VASc score ≥ 7 or recent (≤3 months) TE. Although both ACCP and ACC TE risk stratifying categorizations seem reasonable and practical, neither have been prospectively evaluated in the periprocedural setting[1,17] (Table 8.2).

Periprocedural Bleeding Risk

Estimating periprocedural bleeding risk can be quite challenging. Factors that should be taken into account include (1) patient-related factors that may increase bleeding risk, (2) the inherent bleeding risk of the procedure, and (3) the clinical consequences of bleeding should it occur.[17]

Major bleeding has been variably defined but has commonly included bleeding that (1) is fatal, (2) results in a significant fall in hemoglobin (≥2–3 g/dL), (3) requires transfusion of ≥2 units of packed red blood cells, (4) requires intravenous vasoactive drugs, (5) is intracranial or intraocular (with compromised vision), and (6) requires surgical intervention to control.[18]

Patient-related factors that may increase periprocedural bleeding may potentially be assessed using the HAS-BLED score with a score ≥ 3 highly predictive of

TABLE 8.2
Perioperative Thromboembolic Risk

Thromboembolic Risk	ACCP	ACC
High (>10%/year)	• $CHADS_2 \geq 5$ • Recent (≤3 months) TIA or ischemic stroke • Rheumatic valvular heart disease • Prior TE during TI of VKA	• $CHADS_2$-VASc ≥ 7 • Recent (≤3 months) ischemic stroke, TIA, or SE • Rheumatic valvular heart disease
Moderate (5%–10%/year)	• $CHADS_2$ 3–4	• $CHADS_2$-VASc 5–6 • No recent (≤3 months) ischemic stroke, TIA, or SE
Low (<5%/year)	• $CHADS_2 \leq 2$ • No prior TIA or ischemic stroke	• $CHADS_2$-VASc ≤ 4 • No prior ischemic stroke, TIA, or SE

ACCP, American College of Chest Physicians; *ACC*, American College of Cardiology; *SE*, systemic embolism; *TE*, thromboembolism; *TI*, temporary interruption; *TIA*, transient ischemic attack; *VKA*, vitamin K antagonist.
Adapted from Douketis J, Spyropoulos AC, Spencer FA, et al. Perioperative management of antithrombotic therapy: antithrombotic therapy and prevention of thrombosis, 9th ed: American College of Chest Physicians Evidence-based Clinical Practice Guidelines. *Chest.* 2012;141(2 suppl):e326S–e350S; Doherty JU, Gluckman TJ, Hucker WJ, et al. 2017 ACC Expert consensus decision pathway for periprocedural management of anticoagulation in patients with nonvalvular atrial fibrillation. A report of the American college of cardiology clinical expert consensus document task force. *J Am Coll Cardiol.* 2017;69(7):871–898.

TABLE 8.3
HAS-BLED Bleeding Risk Score

Letter	Clinical Characteristic	Points
H	**H**ypertension (SBP > 160 mm Hg)	1
A	**A**bnormal renal function (chronic dialysis, renal transplant, Cr > 2.26 mg/dL)	1
	Abnormal liver function (chronic hepatic disease or bilirubin > 2× upper limit of normal + AST/ALT/alk phos >3× upper limit of normal)	1
S	**S**troke	1
B	**B**leeding history or predisposition (anemia)	1
L	**L**abile INRs (therapeutic time in range < 60%)	1
E	**E**lderly (>65 years old)	1
D	**D**rugs • Antiplatelet/NSAIA • Excessive alcohol use (≥8 drinks/week)	1 1

ALT, alanine aminotransferase; *AST*, aspartate transaminase; *alk phos*, alkaline phosphatase; *Cr*, creatinine; *INR*, international normalized ratio; *NSAIA*, nonsteroidal antiinflammatory agent; *SBP*, systolic blood pressure.
Adapted from Pisters R, Lane DA, Nieuwlaat R, de Vos CB, Crijns HJGM, Lip GYH, et al. A novel user-friendly score to assess 1-year risk of major bleeding in patients with atrial fibrillation. *Chest.* 2010;138(5):1093–1100.

bleeding events[17,19,20] (Table 8.3). Additional patient-related factors that should be taken into account include prior recent (≤3 months) bleeding event, history of periprocedural bleeding from similar procedure or while receiving parenteral bridging anticoagulation, deficiency in platelet number or function, concomitant antiplatelet drug use, and supratherapeutic INR for the VKA-treated patient.[17,19]

The inherent bleeding risk of procedures has most commonly been defined as either low risk (<2% risk of major bleeding within 2 days) or high risk (>2% risk of major bleeding within 2 days). Although some general consensus of opinion exists regarding low and high bleeding risk procedures, some differences of opinion exist, and for some procedures, estimated bleeding risk has not been well defined. General consensus of frequently performed high bleeding risk procedures include coronary artery bypass grafting, abdominal aortic aneurysm repair, transurethral resection of the

prostate, kidney biopsy, major orthopedic surgery, major cancer surgery, major abdominal surgery, and intracranial or spinal procedures[16,21-23] (Table 8.4). Additional factors that may affect procedural bleeding risk include operator experience, medical center procedural volume, and available ancillary supportive services.

TABLE 8.4
Bleeding Risk of Elective Procedures

	PERIPROCEDURAL BLEEDING RISK	
	Low	**High**
Cardiopulmonary	• Bronchoscopy ± biopsy • Noncoronary angiography • Electrophysiologic study • SVT/atrial fib ablation • Pacemaker/ICD implantation	• CABG • Heart valve replacement • AAA repair
General surgery	• Cholecystectomy • Abdominal hernia repair • Carpal tunnel repair • Hemorrhoidal surgery • Axillary node dissection • GI endoscopy ± biopsy	• Major cancer surgery • Major abdominal surgery • PEG replacement • Polypectomy, variceal treatment, biliary sphincterotomy, pneumatic dilatation • Endoscopic fine-needle aspiration • Liver biopsy
Urologic/gynecologic	• Hydrocele repair • Bladder/prostate biopsy • D and C • Abdominal hysterectomy	• TURP • Kidney biopsy
Orthopedic	• Arthroscopy	• Hip replacement • Knee replacement • Hand/foot/shoulder surgery
Neurosurgical		• Laminectomy • Intracranial surgery • Neuraxial anesthesia • Lumbar puncture
Others	• Tooth extraction • Cataract/noncataract surgery • Cutaneous/thyroid/breast/lymph node biopsies • Minor dermatologic procedures	

AAA, abdominal aortic aneurysm; *CABG*, coronary artery bypass grafting; *D and C*, dilatation and curettage; *GI*, gastrointestinal; *ICD*, implantable cardioverter-defibrillator; *PEG*, percutaneous endoscopic gastrostomy; *SVT*, supraventricular tachycardia; *TURP*, transurethral resection of prostate.

Adapted from Douketis J, Spyropoulos AC, Spencer FA, et al. Perioperative management of antithrombotic therapy: antithrombotic therapy and prevention of thrombosis, 9th ed: American College of Chest Physicians Evidence-based Clinical Practice Guidelines. *Chest.* 2012;141(2 suppl):e326S–e350S; Spyropoulos AC, Douketis JD. How I treat anticoagulated patients undergoing an elective procedure or surgery. *Blood.* 2012;120(15):2954–2962; Liew A, Douketis J. Perioperative management of patients who are receiving a novel oral anticoagulant. *Intern Emerg Med.* 2013;8:477–484; Heidbuchel H, Verhamme P, Alings M, et al. European heart rhythm association practical guide on the use of new oral anticoagulants in patients with non-vascular atrial fibrillation. Antithrombotic Therapy and Prevention of Thrombosis, 9th ed: American College of Chest Physicians Evidence-Based Clinical Practice Guidelines. *Europace.* 2013;15:625–651.

IDENTIFICATION OF SURGICAL PROCEDURES AT LOW RISK FOR BLEEDING

Some invasive procedures and operations are at low enough bleeding risk that they may be performed safely without interruption of VKAs. In the BRUISE CONTROL (Bridge or Continue Coumadin for Device Surgery Randomized) trial, patients with an annual TE risk of 5% or more undergoing permanent pacemaker or defibrillator surgery were randomized to uninterrupted warfarin or warfarin interruption with heparin bridging. 89% of patients had atrial fibrillation or flutter with a mean CHADS$_2$ score of 3.4. Those patients randomized to uninterrupted warfarin were to have an INR ≤3.0 (or <3.5 with mechanical valve) at the time of surgery. Those randomized to heparin bridging discontinued warfarin and began either LMWH (stopped >24 h before surgery) or UFH (stopped 4 h before surgery). Either LMWH or UFH was started 24 h after surgery and continued until the INR became therapeutic. Those patients randomized to warfarin interruption and heparin bridging had a significantly increased incidence of device-pocket hematoma. There was no significant difference in TEs[24] (Fig. 8.3). The safety and cost-effectiveness of continued warfarin administration at the time of permanent pacemaker or defibrillator surgery has been shown in other studies.[25,26]

The safety of performing simple dental extraction and cataract surgery without interruption of warfarin has been shown.[27,28] Other procedures that can potentially be safely performed without warfarin interruption, or those in which interruption of warfarin should be considered, are listed in Table 8.4.

DOACs have a shorter half-life and more rapid onset of action than VKAs. Many expected that parenteral bridging anticoagulation would not be necessary in patients requiring temporary periprocedural interruption of a DOAC. The Dresden NOAC registry assessed DOAC and heparin bridging use in patients who underwent an invasive procedure or surgery (of which 10% were major high bleeding risk procedures). 81% of patients were receiving a DOAC for stroke prevention in NVAF. The use of heparin bridging led to a significantly higher risk of major bleeding (especially in patients who underwent a major high bleeding risk procedure) without significant reduction in cardiovascular events.[29] More information on the appropriate use of parenteral anticoagulation with DOACs is needed, especially in light of the black box warning of increased stroke risk with discontinuation of DOACs.

Despite these findings and recommendations, a significant number of clinicians still interrupt anticoagulation or interrupt anticoagulation and administer parenteral bridging anticoagulation in surgical procedures at low risk for perioperative bleeding[12] (Fig. 8.4).

ANTICOAGULATION INTERRUPTION BEFORE SURGERY

Vitamin K Antagonists

When a decision to interrupt oral anticoagulation has been made, adequate time must be allowed preprocedurally to achieve normalization or near-normalization of coagulation. Warfarin, the most commonly prescribed VKA, inhibits the synthesis of clotting factors II, VII, IX, and X and proteins C and S. Warfarin's

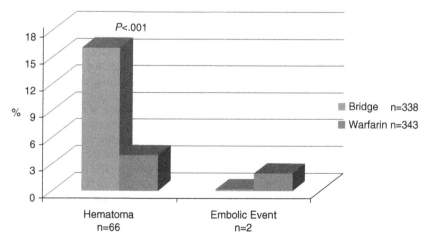

FIG. 8.3 BRUISE CONTROL results. (Adapted from Birnie DH, Healey JS, Wells GA, et al. Pacemaker or defibrillator surgery without interruption of anticoagulation. *N Engl J Med.* 2013;368:2084–2093.)

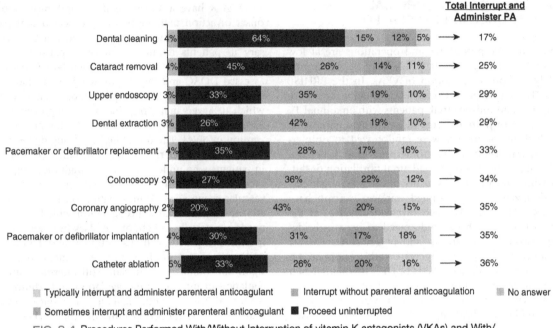

Total Interrupt and
Administer PA

Dental cleaning	4%	64%	15%	12%	5%	→	17%
Cataract removal	4%	45%	26%	14%	11%	→	25%
Upper endoscopy	3%	33%	35%	19%	10%	→	29%
Dental extraction	3%	26%	42%	19%	10%	→	29%
Pacemaker or defibrillator replacement	4%	35%	28%	17%	16%	→	33%
Colonoscopy	3%	27%	36%	22%	12%	→	34%
Coronary angiography	2%	20%	43%	20%	15%	→	35%
Pacemaker or defibrillator implantation	4%	30%	31%	17%	18%	→	35%
Catheter ablation	5%	33%	26%	20%	16%	→	36%

▨ Typically interrupt and administer parenteral anticoagulant ▨ Interrupt without parenteral anticoagulation ▨ No answer

▨ Sometimes interrupt and administer parenteral anticoagulant ■ Proceed uninterrupted

FIG. 8.4 Procedures Performed With/Without Interruption of vitamin K antagonists (VKAs) and With/Without Parenteral anticoagulation (PA). (From Flaker G, Theriot P, Binder L, et al. A survey of the management of periprocedural anticoagulation in contemporary practice. *J Am Coll Cardiol.* 2016;68:217–226.)

elimination half-life is 36–42 h. Less frequently pre-scribed VKAs acenocoumarol and phenprocoumon have elimination half-lives of 8–11 h and 96–104 h, respectively.[30]

To achieve normalization of the INR at the time of surgery, warfarin should typically be discontinued at least 5 days preprocedurally. When feasible, obtaining an INR the day before surgery may allow for admin-istration of vitamin K, or if prudent, delay of surgery should an unacceptably elevated INR be found. Time to normalization of the INR may be prolonged in patients of advancing age, of greater sensitivity to the AC effect of warfarin (i.e., lower maintenance dose of warfarin required), with decompensated heart failure, and with active cancer.[31]

Direct Oral Anticoagulants

Currently, the direct thrombin inhibitor dabigatran, and three direct factor Xa inhibitors rivaroxaban, apixa-ban, and edoxaban are approved for stroke prevention in NVAF. Because of their shorter elimination half-lives compared with warfarin, the DOACs can typically be withheld for 48–72 h preprocedurally with normal-ization or near-normalization of coagulation. How-ever, some patient characteristics and specific invasive

procedures may necessitate more prolonged withhold-ing of a DOAC. Patient characteristics that may neces-sitate more prolonged preprocedural withholding of a DOAC include renal insufficiency, advancing age, low body weight, drug-drug interactions, and the admin-istration of other drugs that may increase bleeding (e.g., antiplatelet agent, nonsteroidal antiinflammatory agent).[17,32,33]

Neuraxial anesthesia, because of significant morbid-ity should spinal hematoma occur, has been considered an especially high bleeding risk procedure. The Ameri-can Society of Regional Anesthesia and Pain Manage-ment has recommended discontinuing dabigatran 4–5 days and the factor Xa inhibitors 3–5 days before a neuraxial procedure.[34] The French Working Group on Perioperative Hemostasis has recommended for neur-axial anesthesia/puncture and intracranial surgery that DOACs be withheld for up to 5 days preprocedurally.[35] European (European Heart Rhythm Association) and American (American College of Cardiology) guide-lines for the preprocedural withholding of DOACs have been recently published. Prescribed DOAC, renal function, and procedure bleeding risk will determine the preprocedure timing of DOAC discontinuation[17,32] (Table 8.5).

TABLE 8.5
Societal Guidelines for Preprocedural Discontinuation of Direct Oral Anticoagulants

	DABIGATRAN		RIVAROXABAN/APIXABAN/EDOXABAN	
Bleed Risk	**Low**	**High**	**Low**	**High**
CrCl ≥ 80 mL/min	≥24 h	≥48 h	≥24 h	≥48 h
CrCl 50–80 mL/min	≥36 h	≥72 h	≥24 h	≥48 h
CrCl 30–50 mL/min	≥48 h	≥96 h	≥24 h	≥48 h
CrC 15–30 mL/min	a	b	≥36 h	c
CrCl < 15 mL/min	d	e	f	g

a, EHRA: not indicated for use, ACC: ≥72 h; *b*, EHRA: not indicated for use, ACC: ≥120 h; *c*, EHRA: ≥48 h; ACC: consider anti-Xa level and/or ≥72 h; *d*, EHRA: not indicated for use, ACC: consider dTT and/or ≥96 h; *e*, EHRA: not indicated for use, ACC: consider dTT; *f*, EHRA: not indicated for use, ACC: consider anti-Xa level and/or ≥48 h; *g*, EHRA: not indicated for use, ACC: consider anti-Xa level and/or ≥72 h.
ACC, American College of Cardiology; *CrCl*, creatinine clearance; *dTT*, dilute thrombin time; *EHRA*, European Heart Rhythm Association.
Adapted from Heidbuchel H, Verhamme P, Alings M, et al. Updated European Heart Rhythm Association practical guide on the use of non-vitamin K antagonist anticoagulants in patients with non-valvular atrial fibrillation. *Europace*. 2015;17:1467–1507; Doherty JU, Gluckman TJ, Hucker WJ, et al. 2017 ACC Expert consensus decision pathway for periprocedural management of anticoagulation in patients with nonvalvular atrial fibrillation. A report of the American College of Cardiology clinical expert consensus document task force. *J Am Coll Cardiol*. 2017;69(7):871–898.

Need for parenteral bridging anticoagulation

Once the decision has been made to withhold anticoagulation preprocedurally, the next decision to be made is determining whether parenteral bridging anticoagulation periprocedurally is required. However, the safety and efficacy of bridging anticoagulation has been called into question, by both retrospective reviews and prospective clinical trials.

Siegel et al. performed a systematic review and meta-analysis of studies to determine the safety and efficacy of periprocedural bridging anticoagulation in patients who required the temporary interruption of VKA therapy before elective surgery. The predominant indication for anticoagulation was atrial fibrillation (44%) but also included patients with mechanical heart valves (24%), previous venous thromboembolism (22%), and other indications (10%). Patients who received heparin bridging had a significantly increased risk of periprocedural overall and major bleeding but similar TE risk compared with patients who did not receive heparin bridging.[36]

Ayoub et al. performed a similar meta-analysis of exclusively atrial fibrillation patients of intermediate thromboembolic risk (mean CHADS$_2$ score 2.49 for no heparin bridging and 2.34 for heparin bridging groups) who required temporary interruption of warfarin before an elective invasive procedure or surgery. Patients who received heparin bridging had a significantly increased overall and major bleeding risk without significant reduction in mortality, stroke, or thromboembolic risk compared with patients who did not receive bridging anticoagulation[37] (Fig. 8.5).

In the randomized, double-blind BRIDGE (Bridging Anticoagulation in Patients Who Require Temporary Interruption of Warfarin Therapy for an Elective Procedure or Surgery) trial, patients receiving warfarin for atrial fibrillation who were at moderate risk for TE (mean CHADS$_2$ score 2.3) and who had preprocedural interruption of warfarin were randomized to either parenteral bridging anticoagulation with dalteparin or placebo. A low rate of TE, not significantly different between placebo and dalteparin, was noted. A significantly higher rate of major bleeding occurred for those patients bridged with dalteparin[6] (Fig. 8.6). Patients undergoing major surgical procedures associated with significant periprocedural bleeding risk (intracardiac, neurosurgical, and carotid) were excluded and those at high risk for TE (CHADS$_2$ score ≥ 5) were underrepresented. The BRIDGE trial suggests that patients with atrial fibrillation at low to moderate TE risk during temporary interruption of warfarin before surgery, who are undergoing a low to moderate bleeding risk surgery, are under most circumstances unlikely to benefit from parenteral bridging anticoagulation.

Direct Oral Anticoagulants

Since the DOACs have short half-lives (7–14 h with preserved renal function), in the majority of circumstances, no parenteral bridging anticoagulation will be required. Situations that might warrant parenteral bridging anticoagulation include the need for additional procedures, more prolonged DOAC-free interval (e.g., neuraxial anesthesia), and patient inability to take

All-cause mortality

Study or Subgroup	No Bridge Events	Total	Bridge Events	Total	Weight	Odds Ratio M-H, Random, 95% CI	Odds Ratio M-H, Random, 95% CI
Benjamin 2015	3	1766	1	514	24.1%	0.87 [0.09, 8.41]	
Billett 2010	384	4532	1	265	25.7%	24.44 [3.42, 174.63]	
BRIDGE 2015	5	918	4	895	29.1%	1.22 [0.33, 4.56]	
Tomic 2012	0	1093	14	1944	21.1%	0.06 [0.00, 1.02]	
Wysokinski 2008	0	182	0	204		Not estimable	
Total (95% CI)		**8491**		**3822**	**100.0%**	**1.29 [0.15, 11.52]**	
Total events	392		20				

Heterogeneity: Tau^2 = 3.83; Chi^2 = 14.24, df = 3 (P = .003); I^2 = 79%
Test for overall effect: Z = 0.23 (P = .82)

0.01 0.1 1 10 100
Favours [No Bridge] Favours [Bridge]

Major bleeding

Study or Subgroup	No Bridge Events	Total	Bridge Events	Total	Weight	Odds Ratio M-H, Random, 95% CI	Odds Ratio M-H, Random, 95% CI
Benjamin 2015	20	1766	18	514	24.6%	0.32 [0.17, 0.60]	
Billett 2010	74	4532	4	265	15.6%	1.08 [0.39, 2.99]	
BRIDGE 2015	12	918	29	895	23.5%	0.40 [0.20, 0.78]	
Douketis 2015	16	1033	26	391	24.9%	0.22 [0.12, 0.42]	
Wysokinski 2008	4	182	6	204	11.4%	0.74 [0.21, 2.67]	
Total (95% CI)		**8431**		**2269**	**100.0%**	**0.41 [0.24, 0.68]**	
Total events	126		83				

Heterogeneity: Tau^2 = 0.17; Chi^2 = 8.29, df = 4 (P = .08); I^2 = 52%
Test for overall effect: Z = 3.44 (P = .0006)

0.01 0.1 1 10 100
Favours [No Bridge] Favours [Bridge]

FIG. 8.5 Heparin bridging in atrial fibrillation patients. *CI*, confidence interval. (From Ayoub, Nairooz R, Almomani A, Marji M, Paydak H, Maskoun W. Perioperative heparin bridging in atrial fibrillation patients requiring temporary interruption of anticoagulation: evidence from meta-analysis. *J Stroke Cerebrovasc Dis.* 2016;20(9):2215–2221.)

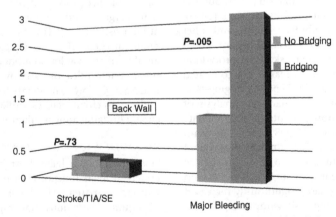

FIG. 8.6 The BRIDGE trial. *SE*, systemic embolism; *TIA*, transient ischemic attack. (Adapted from Douketis JD, Spyropoulos AC, Kaatz S, et al. Perioperative bridging anticoagulation in patients with atrial fibrillation. *N Engl J Med.* 2015:373:823–833.)

oral medications postoperatively.[17] For those patients unable to take medications by mouth, rivaroxaban and apixaban can be crushed and administered via nasogastric tube.[38,39]

Warfarin

Warfarin, because of its far longer half-life (36–42 h) compared with the DOACs, will require longer time to washout preprocedurally and to become therapeutic when reinitiated postprocedurally. Therefore, there may be a need for parenteral bridging anticoagulation in those patients with higher TE risk and lower periprocedural bleeding risk (Tables 8.2 and 8.4).

For those patients at low periprocedural TE risk ($CHADS_2 \leq 2$, CHA_2DS_2-VASc ≤ 4, and no prior TIA, stroke, or systemic embolism), under most circumstances, parenteral bridging anticoagulation will not be required.[1,17]

For those patients at moderate periprocedural TE risk ($CHADS_2$ 3–4, CHA_2DS_2-VASc 5–6, or prior TIA, stroke, or systemic embolism ≥ 3 months), the need for parenteral bridging anticoagulation is unclear.[1,17] The 2017 ACC Expert Consensus, using periprocedural bleeding risk, has advised against bridging anticoagulation for patients at moderate TE risk but higher periprocedural bleeding risk. For those patients without significant bleeding risk but prior TIA, stroke, or systemic embolism, bridging anticoagulation may be considered. For those patients without a history of TIA, stroke, or systemic embolism, bridging anticoagulation was not recommended.[17]

For those patients at high TE risk ($CHADS_2 \geq 5$, CHA_2DS_2-VASc ≥ 7, or recent ≤ 3 months TIA, stroke, or systemic embolism), bridging anticoagulation may be warranted.[1,17] Ideally, for patients who have had recent (≤ 3 months) TE event and are undergoing an elective procedure, postponement of the elective procedure for 3 months following the TE event should be considered[1,17] (Fig. 8.7).

Bridging anticoagulation recommendations

When a decision has been made to initiate perioperative bridging anticoagulation, additional decisions to be made include (1) which bridging agent to use (and at what dose) and (2) when to initiate and discontinue preoperative and/or postoperative bridging.

To date, no specific parenteral agent, dosing regimen, or perioperative timing of initiation or discontinuation has been proven superior. Most commonly, either LMWH or UFH are used. LMWH is easier to administer and requires no laboratory monitoring. Intravenous UFH is less expensive to administer,

requires no dosing adjustment for significant renal insufficiency, and can be more readily reversed. Intravenous UFH is preferred when the creatinine clearance is <30 mL/min.[1,17]

Most commonly therapeutic (full-dose) parenteral regimens are administered. Typical regimens are for the LMWHs enoxaparin 1 mg/kg subcutaneous every 12 h and dalteparin 100 units/kg subcutaneous every 12 h (both dose adjusted for significant renal insufficiency) and for intravenous UFH achieving an activated partial thromboplastin time (aPTT) of 1.5–2.0 times the control aPTT. Although therapeutic parenteral regimens are most commonly administered, alternative bridging regimens have been proposed, including the following:

- Low (prophylactic) dose
  - most commonly used for postoperative venous thromboembolism prevention
  - enoxaparin 40 mg subcutaneous daily
    dalteparin 5000 units subcutaneous daily
    UFH 5000–7000 units subcutaneous twice daily
- Intermediate dose
  - enoxaparin 40 mg subcutaneous twice daily
    dalteparin 5000 units subcutaneous twice daily[1]

Parenteral bridging anticoagulation can be initiated 24 h or more following the discontinuation of Coumadin, generally when the INR initially falls below the therapeutic indication range (typically INR < 2 for patients with NVAF).[1]

Both ACCP and ACC have recommended discontinuing therapeutic dose UFH 4–6 h before surgery and therapeutic dose LMWH 24 h before surgery (and possibly more than 24 h with significant renal insufficiency). When clinically warranted, the residual AC effect of UFH can be assessed by aPTT and of LMWH by antifactor Xa level.[1,17]

Because of current evidence suggesting an increased risk of periprocedural bleeding with bridging anticoagulation, and no significant improvement in TE risk, the conservative use of bridging anticoagulation seems warranted for most patient circumstances.

Reinitiation of bridging anticoagulation postprocedure

Several factors will affect postprocedural bleeding risk including (1) timing of reinitiation of bridging anticoagulation, (2) AC type and regimen, (3) procedure performed (and intraprocedural findings), and (4) procedural complications.[1]

When to initiate postprocedural anticoagulation must take into account postprocedural hemostasis, certain patient clinical characteristics (e.g., recent bleed history, abnormal platelet function, antiplatelet drug use),

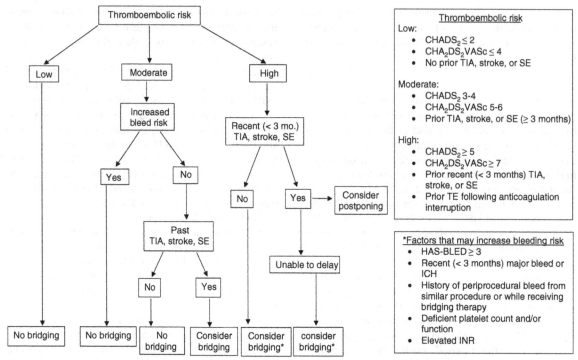

FIG. 8.7 Periprocedure Bridging Following Warfarin Discontinuation. *ICH*, intracranial hemorrhage; *INR*, international normalized ratio; *SE*, systemic embolism; *TE*, thromboembolism; *TIA*, transient ischemic attack. (Adapted from Douketis J, Spyropoulos AC, Spencer FA, et al. Perioperative management of antithrombotic therapy: antithrombotic therapy and prevention of thrombosis, 9th ed: American College of Chest Physicians Evidence-based Clinical Practice Guidelines. *Chest.* 2012;141(2 suppl.):e326S–e350S; Doherty JU, Gluckman TJ, Hucker WJ, et al. 2017 ACC Expert consensus decision pathway for periprocedural management of anticoagulation in patients with nonvalvular atrial fibrillation. A report of the American College of Cardiology clinical expert consensus document task force. *J Am Coll Cardiol.* 2017;69(7):871–898.)

and the clinical consequences should significant postprocedural bleeding occur.[1,17]

ACCP and ACC have similar recommendations for resuming postprocedural bridging anticoagulation for patients whom the benefit of decreased TE risk with bridging anticoagulation outweighs the risk of postprocedural bleeding. Once adequate postprocedure hemostasis has been achieved, and factors that could increase postprocedure bleeding risk have been mitigated, one may reasonably consider resuming therapeutic dose LMWH or UFH 24 h after non–high bleeding risk procedure and 48–72 h after high bleeding risk procedure[1,17] (Table 8.6).

Reinitiation of Direct Oral Anticoagulant postprocedure

Because therapeutic anticoagulation will be achieved within 4 h of receiving the first full dose of a DOAC,

principles guiding reinitiation of a DOAC postprocedure are similar to those for reinitiation of bridging anticoagulation with LMWH and UFH. Once adequate hemostasis has been achieved, and factors that could increase postprocedure bleeding risk have been addressed, it is reasonable to resume a DOAC 24 h after a non–high bleeding risk procedure and 48–72 h after a high bleeding risk procedure.[17] Because of rapid onset of anticoagulation following the first full dose of a DOAC, bridging anticoagulation is generally not required. The administration of reduced-dose DOAC postprocedure has not been well studied (Table 8.6).

Reinitiation of warfarin postprocedure

The ACCP and ACC have similar recommendations for the reinitiation of warfarin following an invasive procedure or surgery. Once adequate hemostasis has been achieved, warfarin can be reinitiated 12–24 h

TABLE 8.6
Reinitiation of Anticoagulation Postprocedure

Anticoagulant	Procedure Bleeding Risk	Initiation Interval Postprocedure
LMWH		
• Enoxaparin 1 mg/kg SC q 12 h[a]	Low	≥24 h[b]
• Dalteparin 100 units/kg SC q 12 h[a]	High	≥48–72 h[b]
UFH	Low	≥24 h[b]
• aPTT 1.5–2.0× control aPTT	High	≥48–72 h[b]
DOAC	Low	≥24 h[b]
	High	≥48–72 h[b]
Warfarin	Low	12–24 h[b,c]
• Usual preprocedure therapeutic dose	High	12–24 h[b,c]

aPTT, activated partial thromboplastin time; *CrCl*, creatinine clearance; *DOAC*, direct oral anticoagulant; *LMWH*, low molecular weight heparin; *SC*, subcutaneous; *TE*, thromboembolic; *UFH*, unfractionated heparin.
[a]Adjust dose for significant renal insufficiency (consider UFH for CrCl < 30 mL/min).
[b]When postprocedure hemostasis is achieved and factors that could increase postprocedure bleeding risk are corrected.
[c]Consider bridging anticoagulation for postprocedure high TE risk and low bleeding risk until therapeutic INR is achieved.
Adapted from Douketis J, Spyropoulos AC, Spencer FA, et al. Perioperative management of antithrombotic therapy: antithrombotic therapy and prevention of thrombosis, 9th ed: American College of Chest Physicians Evidence-based Clinical Practice Guidelines. *Chest.* 2012;141(2 suppl.):e326S–e350S; Doherty JU, Gluckman TJ, Hucker WJ, et al. 2017 ACC Expert consensus decision pathway for periprocedural management of anticoagulation in patients with nonvalvular atrial fibrillation. A report of the American College of Cardiology clinical expert consensus document task force. *J Am Coll Cardiol.* 2017;69(7):871–898.

postprocedure, typically at the patient's usual preprocedure therapeutic dose. Achieving an INR ≥2 will generally take between 5 and 7 days. Bridging anticoagulation for patients at significant postprocedure TE risk and low bleeding risk can be considered until a therapeutic INR has been achieved[1,17] (Table 8.6).

SUMMARY

Physicians frequently perform invasive procedures or surgery for patients with atrial fibrillation who are receiving oral anticoagulation to minimize their stroke risk. Before performing surgery, a decision must be made whether to discontinue anticoagulation before surgery, and if so, whether to then initiate parenteral bridging anticoagulation. These fundamental decisions must balance periprocedural bleeding risk with thromboembolic risk during the temporary interruption of anticoagulation. These decisions are most challenging when patients at high thromboembolic risk off anticoagulation are to undergo a high bleeding risk invasive procedure or surgery.

Thromboembolic risk during temporary interruption of anticoagulation can be estimated using the $CHADS_2$ and CHA_2DS_2-VASc scores and patient medical history. High $CHADS_2$ and CHA_2DS_2-VASc score,

recent thromboembolic TIA/stroke, rheumatic heart valve disease, and a history of TE during prior periprocedural interruption of anticoagulation suggest increased thromboembolic risk.

Periprocedural bleeding risk must take into account patient-related factors that may increase bleeding risk, the inherent bleeding risk of the procedure, and the clinical consequences of bleeding should it occur. The HAS-BLED score may assist in defining patient-related risk factors that can potentially increase periprocedural bleeding. Many procedures are of low bleeding risk and can potentially be performed when patients are fully anticoagulated.

Parenteral bridging anticoagulation, for most patient circumstances, should generally be avoided. Patients at high thromboembolic risk during temporary interruption of anticoagulation and low procedural bleeding risk, patients requiring additional procedures or prolonged anticoagulation free interval, and patients unable to take oral anticoagulation postoperatively may benefit from parenteral bridging anticoagulation.

The increasingly prescribed DOACs, because of their shorter half-lives and more rapid onset of action compared with warfarin, frequently make decision-making for patients undergoing invasive procedure or surgery who are receiving oral anticoagulation less difficult.

REFERENCES

1. Douketis J, Spyropoulos AC, Spencer FA, et al. Perioperative management of antithrombotic therapy: antithrombotic therapy and prevention of thrombosis, 9th ed: American College of chest Physicians evidence-based clinical practice guidelines. *Chest.* 2012;141(2 suppl): e326S–e350S.
2. Steinberg BA, Peterson ED, Kim S, et al. Outcomes registry for better informed treatment of atrial fibrillation (ORBIT-AF) investigators and patients. *Circulation.* 2015; 131:488–494.
3. Garcia DA, Regan S, Henault LE, et al. Risk of thromboembolism with short-term interruption of warfarin therapy. *Arch Int Med.* 2008;168(1):63–69.
4. Rechenmacher SJ, Fang JC. Bridging anticoagulation primum non nocere. *J Am Coll Cardiol.* 2015;66:1392–1403.
5. Baron TH, Kamath PS, McBane RD. Management of antithrombotic therapy in patients undergoing invasive procedures. *N Engl J Med.* 2013;368(22):2113–2124.
6. Douketis JD, Spyropoulos AC, Kaatz S, et al. Perioperative bridging anticoagulation in patients with atrial fibrillation. *N Engl J Med.* 2015;373:823–833.
7. Cannegieter SC, Rosendaal FR, Briet E. Thromboembolic and bleeding complications in patients with mechanical heart valve prostheses. *Circulation.* 1994;89:635–641.
8. Cannegieter SC, Rosendaal FR, Wintzen AR, et al. Optimal oral anticoagulant therapy in patients with mechanical heart valves. *N Engl J Med.* 1995;333:11–17.
9. Kearon C, Hirsh J. Management of anticoagulation before and after elective surgery. *N Engl J Med.* 1997;336: 1506–1511.
10. Salem DN, Daudelin DH, Levine H, et al. Antithrombotic therapy in valvular heart disease. *Chest.* 2001;119: 207S–218S.
11. Gage BF, Waterman AD, Shannon W, et al. Validation of clinical classification schemes for predicting stroke: results from the national registry of atrial fibrillation. *J Am Med Assoc.* 2001;285(22):2864–2870.
12. Flaker G, Theriot P, Binder L, et al. A survey of the management of periprocedural anticoagulation in contemporary practice. *J Am Coll Cardiol.* 2016;68:217–226.
13. January CT, Wann LS, Alpert JS, et al. 2014 AHA/ACC/HRS guideline for the management of patients with atrial fibrillation: executive summary. *J Am Coll Cardiol.* 2014;64:2246–2280.
14. Healey JS, Eikelboom J, Douketis J, et al. Periprocedural bleeding and thromboembolic events with dabigatran compared with warfarin. *Circulation.* 2012;126:343–348.
15. Sherwood MW, Douketis JD, Patel MR, et al. Outcomes of temporary interruption of rivaroxaban compared with warfarin in patients with nonvalvular atrial fibrillation. *Circulation.* 2014;129(18):1850–1859.
16. Garcia D, Alexander JH, Wallentin L, et al. Management and clinical outcomes in patients treated with apixaban vs. warfarin undergoing procedures. *Blood.* 2014;124(25):3692–3698.
17. Doherty JU, Gluckman TJ, Hucker WJ, et al. 2017 ACC Expert concensus decision pathway for periprocedural management of anticoagulation in patients with nonvalvular atrial fibrillation. A report of the American College of Cardiology clinical expert consensus document task force. *J Am Coll Cardiol.* 2017;69(7):871–898.
18. Mehran R, Rao SV, Bhatt DL, et al. Standardized bleeding definitions for cardiovascular clinical trials. *Circulation.* 2011;123:2736–2747.
19. Omran H, Bauersachs R, Rübenacker S, Goss F, Hammerstingl C. The HAS-BLED score predicts bleedings during bridging of chronic oral anticoagulation. *Thromb Haemost.* 2012;108:65–73.
20. Pisters R, Lane DA, Nieuwlaat R, de Vos CB, Crijns HJGM, Lip GYH. A novel user-friendly score to assess 1-year risk of major bleeding in patients with atrial fibrillation. *Chest.* 2010;138(5):1093–1100.
21. Spyropoulos AC, Douketis JD. How I treat anticoagulated patients undergoing an elective procedure or surgery. *Blood.* 2012;120(15):2954–2962.
22. Liew A, Douketis J. Perioperative management of patients who are receiving a novel oral anticoagulant. *Intern Emerg Med.* 2013;8:477–484.
23. Heidbuchel H, Verhamme P, Alings M, et al. European heart rhythm association practical guide on the use of new oral anticoagulants in patients with non-valvular atrial fibrillation. Antithrombotic therapy and prevention of thrombosis, 9th ed: American College of Chest physicians evidence-based clinical practice guidelines. *Europace.* 2013;15:625–651.
24. Birnie DH, Healey JS, Wells GA, et al. Pacemaker or defibrillator surgery without interruption of anticoagulation. *N Engl J Med.* 2013;368:2084–2093.
25. Coyle D, Coyle K, Essebag V, et al. Cost effectiveness of continued-warfarin versus heparin-bridging therapy during pacemaker and defibrillator surgery. *J Am Coll Cardiol.* 2015;65:957.
26. Cheng A, Nazarian S, Brinker JA, et al. Continuation of warfarin during pacemaker or implantable cardioverter-defibrillator implantation: a randomized clinical trial. *Heart Rhythm.* 2011;8:536–540.
27. Bajkin BV, Popovic SL, Selakovic SD. Randomized, prospective trial comparing bridging therapy using low-molecular-weight heparin with maintenance of oral anticoagulation during extraction of teeth. *J Oral Maxillfac Surg.* 2009;67:990–995.
28. Katz J, Feldman MA, Bass EB, et al. Study of medical testing for cataract surgery team. Risks and benefits of anticoagulant and antiplatelet medication use before cataract surgery. *Ophthalmology.* 2003;110:1784–1788.
29. Beyer-Westendorf J, Gelbricht V, Forster K, et al. Periinterventional management of novel oral anticoagulants in daily care: results from the prospective Dresden NOAC registry. *Eur Heart J.* 2014;35:188–196.
30. Ufer M. Comparative pharmacokinetics of vitamin K antagonists: warfarin, phenprocoumon and acenocoumarol. *Clin Pharmacokinet.* 2005;44(12):1227–1246.

31. Hylek EM, Regan S, Go AS, Hughes RA, Singer DE, Skates SJ. Clinical predictors of prolonged delay in return of the international normalized ratio to within the therapeutic range after excessive anticoagulation with warfarin. *Ann Intern Med.* 2001;135:393–400.

32. Heidbuchel H, Verhamme P, Alings M, et al. Updated European Heart Rhythm Association practical guide on the use of non-vitamin K antagonist anticoagulants in patients with non-valvular atrial fibrillation. *Europace.* 2015;17:1467–1507.

33. Dubois V, Dincq AS, Douxfils J, et al. Perioperative management of patients on direct oral anticoagulants. *Thromb J.* 2017;15:14.

34. Narouze S, Benzon HT, Provenzano DA, et al. Interventional spine and pain procedures in patients on antiplatelet and anticoagulant medications: guidelines from the American society of regional anesthesia and pain medicine, the European society of regional anaesthesia and pain therapy, the American academy of pain medicine, the international neuromodulation society, and the World Institute of Pain. *Reg Anesth Pain Med.* 2015;40:182–212.

35. Albaladejo, Bonhomme F, Blais N, et al. Management of direct oral anticoagulants in patients undergoing elective surgeries and invasive procedures: updated guidelines from the French Working Group on Perioperative Hemostasis (GIHP) – September 2015. *Anaesth Crit Care Pain Med.* 2017;36:73–76.

36. Siegal D, Yudin J, Kaatz S, et al. Periprocedural heparin bridging in patients receiving vitamin K antagonists: systematic review and meta-analysis of bleeding and thromboembolic rates. *Circulation.* 2012;126:1630–1639.

37. Ayoub K, Nairooz R, Almomani A, Marji M, Paydak H, Maskoun W. Perioperative heparin bridging in atrial fibrillation patients requiring temporary interruption of anticoagulation: evidence from meta-analysis. *J Stroke Cerebrovasc Dis.* 2016;20(9):2215–2221.

38. Bristol-Myers Squibb Company, Pfizer Inc. *Apixaban Prescribing Information.* 2012. Available at: http://www.accessdata.fda.gov/drugsatfda_doc/label/2012/2012155s000lbl.pdf.

39. Bayer Healthcare, Janssen Pharmaceuticals, Inc. *Rivaroxaban Prescribing Information.* 2013. Available at: http://www.accessdata.fda.gov/drugsatfda_docs/label/2013/022106s004lbl.pdf.

CHAPTER 9

Special Situations: Anticoagulation for Cardioversion

CHAD WARD, MD • MICHAEL C. GIUDICI, MD, FACC, FACP, FHRS

ANTICOAGULATION BEFORE CARDIOVERSION

Current recommendations state that all patients with atrial fibrillation lasting longer than 48 h or of unknown duration should be anticoagulated before cardioversion. According to the 2014 AHA/ACC/HRS guidelines for the management of patients with atrial fibrillation,[1] it is a class I indication for patients with atrial fibrillation longer than 48 h or unknown duration to be anticoagulated for at least 3 weeks before cardioversion.[2] This is regardless of the CHA_2DS_2-VASc score and irrespective of chemical or electrical cardioversion. Studies have found rates of thromboembolism to be anywhere from 1% to 5% in the first month following cardioversion.[3–5] In a nonrandomized retrospective series of 572 electrical cardioversions, anticoagulation reduced the frequency of thromboembolic complications from 4% to 0.67% of cardioversion attempts.[2]

The rationale for anticoagulation before cardioversion is a result of the increased risk of atrial thrombi in atrial fibrillation. One study reported that 13% of atrial fibrillation patients of short duration have atrial thrombi identified via transesophageal echocardiogram (TEE).[6] A wealth of data suggest that the left atrial appendage is the primary site of thrombus formation.[7–9] Unfortunately, if therapeutic anticoagulation is not achieved, embolization of thrombi can occur with any duration of atrial fibrillation (paroxysmal, persistent, or permanent).[10]

Factors that increase prevalence of atrial thrombi include mitral stenosis, left ventricular systolic dysfunction, enlargement of the left atrium or left atrial appendage, and spontaneous echo contrast.[11] The resolution of thrombi with a course of anticoagulation decreases the risk of embolization and stroke events.[12] Collins et al. followed up patients with nonrheumatic atrial fibrillation treated with 4 weeks of precardioversion anticoagulation with warfarin (Fig. 9.1). Serial TEE was done and it was demonstrated that 90% had resolution of atrial thrombi after 4 weeks of anticoagulation. Furthermore, no new thrombi were identified.[13]

No patients had thromboembolic events between studies. It was therefore concluded that the mechanism of benefit with a course of anticoagulation before cardioversion is thrombus resolution and prevention rather than thrombus stabilization.

It has been shown that the risk for embolic complications is highest shortly after cardioversion (Fig. 9.2). Most events occur within 10 days of cardioversion, and most occur in patients who have not been properly anticoagulated in the pericardioversion period.[14] Diabetes and hypertension are independent risk factors for embolization early after cardioversion. The risk for thromboembolism decreased significantly in patients with anticoagulation for 4 weeks before cardioversion.

Instances where it is acceptable to perform cardioversion without a course of anticoagulation beforehand are rare. When hemodynamic instability is present, emergent cardioversion should be performed regardless of prior anticoagulation status. In this instance, anticoagulation should be initiated as soon as possible and continued for 4 weeks after cardioversion.[1] The other instance where anticoagulation may not be necessary before cardioversion is when atrial fibrillation duration is definitely less than 24 h and the patient otherwise has low thromboembolic risk.

However, recent studies have reexamined the safety of cardioversion of atrial fibrillation lasting less than 48 h. The Finnish CardioVersion study focused on cardioversion of acute atrial fibrillation to determine the incidence and risks of thromboembolic complications. The study looked at over 5000 cardioversions in patients with atrial fibrillation lasting less than 48 h. The study concluded that in general the risk of thromboembolic events after cardioversion of acute atrial fibrillation is quite low. However, patients with conventional risk factors for thromboembolism need periprocedural anticoagulation.[15]

There are slight differences in the guidelines made by different professional organizations. The 2014 AHA/ACC/HRS guidelines state that high-risk features such

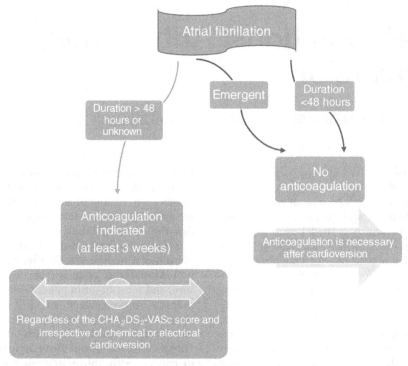

FIG. 9.1 Anticoagulation before cardioversion.

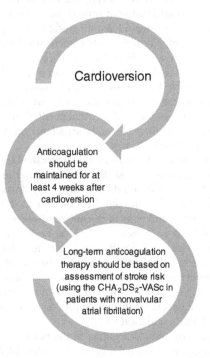

FIG. 9.2 Anticoagulation following cardioversion.

as mitral stenosis and prior thromboembolism necessitate consideration of long-term anticoagulation. The decision to initiate anticoagulation at the time of cardioversion should be based on the CHA_2DS_2-VASc risk score.[1] The European Society of Cardiology recommendations state that a heparin infusion should be started before cardioversion followed by infusion of subcutaneous low molecular weight heparin (LMWH). Oral anticoagulation should be started after cardioversion and continued lifelong in patients at risk for stroke based on $CHADS_2$ or CHA_2DS_2-VASc scores (Fig. 9.1).[16]

The Role of Transesophageal Echocardiogram

Guidelines also indicate a class IIa recommendation to perform TEE before cardioversion and proceed to cardioversion if no left atrial thrombus is identified.[1] Instances where one might consider this approach include patients who are symptomatic from atrial fibrillation and would not tolerate the obligate 3–4 weeks of anticoagulation. One may also choose this method if there is concern for bleeding complications from a precardioversion course of anticoagulation. Additionally, it is well known that deferment of conversion promotes adverse electrical atrial remodeling.[17] This delay potentially makes restoration of sinus rhythm more difficult and is another reason to consider TEE and prompt cardioversion.[18] The X-VeRT trial, which compared rivaroxaban and vitamin K antagonists for cardioversion, placed patients into two groups—early (1–5 days after randomization) or delayed (3–8 weeks after randomization). Success of cardioversion in the early group was similar to the success of cardioversion in the delayed cardioversion group. However, it is important to note the design of the study: the decision to pursue early versus late cardioversion was made by the local investigator. Furthermore, review of the baseline characteristics did not show a difference in duration of atrial fibrillation among the two groups.

In the ACUTE trial (Assessment of Cardioversion Using Transesophageal Echocardiography), a multicenter, randomized, prospective clinical trial enrolled 1222 patients to determine if there was any difference in treatment guided by TEE compared with the conventional treatment of 3 weeks of therapeutic anticoagulation. The data showed no significant difference between the two treatment groups in the rate of embolic events.[19] The TEE strategy decreased the mean time to cardioversion from 31 to 3 days. It is of interest that the TEE group had a significantly higher rate of sinus rhythm at 6 months. Given this evidence, it is reasonable to conclude that TEE-guided anticoagulation management is an effective alternative to conventional therapy.

Anticoagulation should be achieved before TEE, maintained up to the time of cardioversion, and for 4 weeks thereafter. Anticoagulation between TEE and cardioversion is necessary because of the risk of new thrombi formation after TEE. In patients who are not anticoagulated, the risk for embolism remains despite no evidence of atrial thrombus by TEE.[20]

A very important question arises in regard to management of patients with evidence of thromboembolic source or spontaneous echo contrast. The AHA/ACC/HRS guidelines suggest that if a thrombus is seen on TEE, the cardioversion must be postponed and 3–4 weeks of anticoagulation is required. At that point, a repeat TEE is an option: if thrombus remains, then alternative strategies should be considered such as rate control and anticoagulation.[1] This recommendation is a result of a study that followed up 174 patients with left atrial thrombi via TEE. 80% of these thrombi resolved after a median of 47 days of anticoagulation. The study concluded that a short course of anticoagulation achieves a high rate of thrombi resolution but does not prevent the need for follow-up TEE. Furthermore,

they noted that an additional course of anticoagulation had only limited benefits.[21] There are limited data in the literature studying spontaneous echo contrast in relation to cardioversion. However, one study found that the incidence of cerebral embolism and/or death is 22% when spontaneous echo contrast is seen in atrial fibrillation patients.[22] Thus it could be inferred that one should treat the risks associated with spontaneous echo contrast similar to visualized thrombi and avoid cardioversion when present.

Direct Oral Anticoagulation

There has been increasing popularity in recent years of direct oral anticoagulants (DOACs).[23] Recent studies, including a large observational cohort study with over 60,000 patients, demonstrated safety and effectiveness in comparison with warfarin (Table 9.1).[24] There was no significant difference in ischemic stroke in comparison with warfarin. Furthermore, apixaban and dabigatran had significantly fewer rates of death and major bleeding compared with warfarin.

It is a class IIa recommendation to use direct oral anticoagulation with dabigatran, rivaroxaban, or apixaban for 3 weeks before anticoagulation.[25–27] Data from the Randomized Evaluation of Long-Term Anticoagulation Therapy (RE-LY) trial compared dabigatran with warfarin in more than 18,000 patients. The study provided evidence for superiority of dabigatran over warfarin in prevention of chronic thromboembolism and stroke. In addition, major bleeding within 30 days of cardioversion on dabigatran was comparable with warfarin.[25] Many groups insist on performing TEE in patients on DOACs before cardioversion. This RE-LY study also showed that a TEE performed on a patient cardioverted on dabigatran did not lower the risk compared with cardioversion in patients who did not undergo TEE.

The X-VeRT trial was the first prospective randomized trial to compare rivaroxaban and vitamin K antagonists in atrial fibrillation patients undergoing elective cardioversion. The study found comparable rates of safety (major bleeding) and efficacy (stroke, transient ischemic attack, peripheral embolism, myocardial infarction, and cardiovascular death). Perhaps just as important was the finding that a significantly shorter time to cardioversion was achieved with rivaroxaban in comparison with vitamin K antagonists.[28]

Guidelines recommend that patients at high risk for thromboembolism (mechanical valves, CHA_2DS_2-VASc score ≥ 2) should receive IV heparin or LMWH, or a DOAC in the pericardioversion period followed by long-term anticoagulation. If warfarin is chosen,

TABLE 9.1
Studies Demonstrating Safety and Effectiveness of Direct Oral Anticoagulation in Atrial Fibrillation

Study Name	Direct Oral Anticoagulant	Sample Size (Patients)	Conclusion of Study
Dabigatran Versus Warfarin in Patients With Atrial Fibrillation: An Analysis of Patients Undergoing Cardioversion (from RE-LY trial)	Dabigatran	1270	Stroke and major bleeding within 30 days of cardioversion on dabigatran were low and comparable with those on warfarin with or without TEE guidance
Rivaroxaban Versus Vitamin K Antagonists for Cardioversion in Atrial Fibrillation (X-VeRT)	Rivaroxaban	1504	Comparable rates of major bleeding and stroke, TIA, peripheral embolism, MI, and cardiovascular death compared with VKA. Shorter time to cardioversion was achieved with rivaroxaban
Outcomes After Cardioversion and Atrial Fibrillation Ablation in Patients Treated with Rivaroxaban and Warfarin in the ROCKET AF Trial	Rivaroxaban	321	No difference in long-term stroke rates or survival following cardioversion in patients treated with rivaroxaban compared with warfarin
Efficacy and Safety of Apixaban in Patients After Cardioversion for Atrial Fibrillation: Insights from the ARISTOTLE Trial	Apixaban	540	Similar rates of cardiovascular events after cardioversion of atrial fibrillation between warfarin and apixaban

MI, myocardial infarction; *TEE*, transesophageal echocardiography; *TIA*, transient ischemic attack; *VKA*, vitamin K antagonists.

heparin or LMWH should be continued until the international normalized ratio (INR) is therapeutic. However, in the case of DOACs, unfractionated heparin or LMWH is not typically used. The AHA/ACC/HRS guidelines note that anticoagulation with DOACs is achieved promptly in contrast to warfarin. Furthermore, given the rapid onset of action, bridging with parenteral anticoagulation therapy is not needed during initiation.[1] An example of this practice is seen in the X-VeRT trial where in patients randomized to the rivaroxaban group any previous anticoagulation was stopped and rivaroxaban was started at least 4 h before cardioversion.[28]

In a subgroup analysis of those undergoing cardioversion in the ROCKET AF trial (Rivaroxaban Once-daily, oral, direct Factor Xa inhibition Compared with vitamin K antagonism for prevention of stroke and Embolism Trial in Atrial Fibrillation), there was no difference in patients treated with rivaroxaban or warfarin in long-term stroke rates or survival following cardioversion.[26] The ARISTOTLE trial (Apixaban for Reduction in Stroke and Other Thromboembolic Events in Atrial Fibrillation) demonstrated similar rates of cardiovascular events after cardioversion of atrial fibrillation between warfarin and apixaban.[27] Therefore, there are data to support the choice of each of the commonly used DOACs—dabigatran, rivaroxaban, or apixaban—as an alternative to warfarin for anticoagulation before or after cardioversion. The benefit of these

anticoagulants is that they do not require serial laboratory test monitoring. In addition, diet modification and appropriate dosing (which can sometimes take weeks to determine with warfarin) is not a factor. As long as patients are reliable and have not missed any doses of their DOAC, there is no need to delay cardioversion, which is occasionally the case because of a subtherapeutic INR in patients on warfarin.

ANTICOAGULATION AFTER CARDIOVERSION

The 2014 AHA/ACC/HRS guidelines[1] for the management of patients with atrial fibrillation state that long-term anticoagulation therapy should be based on assessment of stroke risk (using the CHA_2DS_2-VASc in patients with nonvalvular atrial fibrillation). The duration of atrial fibrillation does not affect the decision-making process. The rationale for postcardioversion anticoagulation is a result of atrial stunning, frequent recurrence of atrial fibrillation, and a hypercoagulable state that occurs after cardioversion.

This phenomenon of atrial stunning occurs as a result of transient atrial contractile dysfunction that develops after cardioversion and may last up to 4 weeks, until the complete recovery of atrial mechanical function.[29] Manning et al. utilized pulsed Doppler echocardiography after cardioversion to demonstrate that it took 3 weeks for atrial function to return to that of a control group. Data show that the duration of atrial fibrillation positively correlates with the duration of the left atrial contractile dysfunction.[30]

For atrial fibrillation of less than 2 weeks, function returns in 24 h. Atrial fibrillation of 2–6 weeks duration necessitated 1 week for return of normal atrial function. Longer durations of atrial fibrillation take up to 1 month for atrial recovery. Left atrial contractility can be reduced by up to 75% with decreased left appendage flow velocities.

The mechanism (Fig. 9.2) behind atrial stunning after cardioversion is thought to be a tachycardia-induced atrial cardiomyopathy, caused by impaired cellular handling of calcium.[31–33] It then makes sense then that reduced left atrial appendage function occurs regardless of the method of cardioversion, whether it be spontaneous, electrical, or chemical. One study has shown electrical cardioversion to have greater stunning than spontaneous or pharmacologic cardioversion. Interestingly, there was no association between the amount of energy used and the degree of stunning.[34] Unsuccessful cardioversion does not cause the same atrial dysfunction as seen in a successful cardioversion.[35]

Further evidence to support anticoagulation after return to sinus rhythm comes from the high reported rates of atrial fibrillation after cardioversion. Long-term follow-up of patients with implantable monitoring devices found that 88% of patients had recurrence of atrial fibrillation on stored electrocardiograms despite optimal antiarrhythmic therapy.[36] In over half of these patients, atrial fibrillation episodes lasted longer than 48 h, putting patients at great risk for forming thrombi as described above.

As we discussed, it is not just atrial stunning that puts one at increased risk for embolic events after atrial fibrillation and cardioversion: there is also a hypercoagulable state resulting from cardioversion.[37] Oltrona et al. described increased plasma levels of thrombin-antithrombin complex, a marker of thrombin generation after pharmacologic cardioversion to sinus rhythm. Another study measured plasma levels of fibrin D-dimer (a marker of thrombus formation) and plasma fibrinogen (associated with stroke and thromboembolism). The authors concluded that atrial fibrillation itself is the cause for the hypercoagulable state and that cardioversion did not significantly affect the markers of coagulation. In this study, the group on warfarin before cardioversion had lower markers of coagulation, indicating that it is protective against thromboembolism during cardioversion.[38]

SUMMARY

Atrial fibrillation lasting longer than 48 h or of unknown duration should be anticoagulated for at least 3 weeks before cardioversion regardless of the CHA_2DS_2-VASc score and irrespective of chemical or electrical cardioversion. The rationale for anticoagulation before cardioversion is due to the increased risk of atrial thrombi in atrial fibrillation. Factors that increase prevalence of atrial thrombi include mitral stenosis, left ventricular systolic dysfunction, and enlargement of the left atrium or left atrial appendage. Embolic complications are highest shortly after cardioversion. Two situations where anticoagulation is not necessary before cardioversion are emergent cardioversion for hemodynamic instability and when atrial fibrillation duration is definitely less than 48 h and the patient otherwise has low thromboembolic risk. In this instance anticoagulation should be initiated as soon as possible and continued for 4 weeks after cardioversion.

Guidelines allow for TEE followed by cardioversion if no left atrial thrombus is identified. This option is ideal for patients symptomatic from atrial fibrillation who would not tolerate the 3-week course of anticoagulation or if there is concern for bleeding complications from anticoagulation.

There has been increasing popularity in recent years of novel oral anticoagulants; large trials have provided data in support of the safety and effectiveness in comparison with warfarin. It is a class IIa recommendation to use direct oral anticoagulation with dabigatran, rivaroxaban, or apixaban for 3 weeks before anticoagulation. Serial laboratory testing, dose adjustments, and diet modification are not necessary, which are significant advantages of novel oral anticoagulants over warfarin.

Anticoagulation should be maintained for at least 4 weeks after cardioversion. Long-term anticoagulation therapy after cardioversion should be based on assessment of stroke risk. The rationale for postcardioversion anticoagulation is the presence of atrial stunning, frequent recurrence of atrial fibrillation, and a hypercoagulable state that occurs after cardioversion.

REFERENCES

1. January CT, Wann LS, Alpert JS, et al. 2014 AHA/ACC/HRS guideline for the management of patients with atrial fibrillation: executive summary: a report of the American College of Cardiology/American Heart Association Task Force on practice guidelines and the Heart Rhythm Society. *Circulation*. 2014;130(23):2071–2104.

2. Gallagher MM, Hennessy BJ, Edvardsson N, et al. Embolic complications of direct current cardioversion of atrial arrhythmias: association with low intensity of antico-agulation at the time of cardioversion. *J Am Coll Cardiol.* 2002;40(5):926–933.

3. Hall JI, Wood DR. Factors affecting cardioversion of atrial arrhythmias with special reference to quinidine. *Br Heart J.* 1968;30(1):84–90.

4. Korsgren M, Leskinen E, Peterhoff V, Bradley E, Varnauskas E. Conversion of atrial arrhythmias with DC shock: primary results and a follow-up investigation. *Acta Med Scand Suppl.* 1965;(suppl 431):1–40.

5. Oram S, Davies JP. Further experience of electrical conversion of atrial fibrillation to sinus rhythm: analysis of 100 patients. *Lancet.* 1964;1(7346):1294–1298.

6. Weigner MJ, Thomas LR, Patel U, et al. Early cardioversion of atrial fibrillation facilitated by transesophageal echocardiography: short-term safety and impact on maintenance of sinus rhythm at 1 year. *Am J Med.* 2001;110(9):694–702.

7. Blackshear JL, Odell JA. Appendage obliteration to reduce stroke in cardiac surgical patients with atrial fibrillation. *Ann Thorac Surg.* 1996;61(2):755–759.

8. Manning WJ, Silverman DI, Keighley CS, Oettgen P, Douglas PS. Transesophageal echocardiographically facilitated early cardioversion from atrial fibrillation using short-term anticoagulation: final results of a prospective 4.5-year study. *J Am Coll Cardiol.* 1995;25(6):1354–1361.

9. Tsai LM, Chen JH, Lin LJ, Yang YJ. Role of transesophageal echocardiography in detecting left atrial thrombus and spontaneous echo contrast in patients with mitral valve disease or non-rheumatic atrial fibrillation. *J Formos Med Assoc.* 1990;89(4):270–274.

10. Giudici MC, Abu-El-Haija B. Atrial fibrillation in common problems in cardiology. In: Chatterjee K, Vandenberg BF, eds; 2016:xiii. 319 pp.

11. Klein AL, Grimm RA, Murray RD, et al. Use of transesophageal echocardiography to guide cardioversion in patients with atrial fibrillation. *N Engl J Med.* 2001;344(19):1411–1420.

12. Pritchett EL. Management of atrial fibrillation. *N Engl J Med.* 1992;326(19):1264–1271.

13. Collins LJ, Silverman DI, Douglas PS, Manning WJ. Cardioversion of nonrheumatic atrial fibrillation. Reduced thromboembolic complications with 4 weeks of precardioversion anticoagulation are related to atrial thrombus resolution. *Circulation.* 1995;92(2):160–163.

14. Gentile F, Elhendy A, Khandheria BK, et al. Safety of electrical cardioversion in patients with atrial fibrillation. *Mayo Clin Proc.* 2002;77(9):897–904.

15. Airaksinen KE, Grönberg T, Nuotio I, et al. Thromboembolic complications after cardioversion of acute atrial fibrillation: the FinCV (Finnish CardioVersion) study. *J Am Coll Cardiol.* 2013;62(13):1187–1192.

16. European Heart Rhythm Association, European Association for Cardio-Thoracic Surgery, Camm AJ, et al. Guidelines for the management of atrial fibrillation: the Task Force for the Management of Atrial Fibrillation of the European Society of Cardiology (ESC). *Eur Heart J.* 2010;31(19):2369–2429.

17. Toso E, Blandino A, Sardi D, et al. Electrical cardioversion of persistent atrial fibrillation: acute and long-term results stratified according to arrhythmia duration. *Pacing Clin Electrophysiol.* 2012;35(9):1126–1134.

18. Abu-El-Haija B, Giudici MC. Predictors of long-term maintenance of normal sinus rhythm after successful electrical cardioversion. *Clin Cardiol.* 2014;37(6):381–385.

19. Klein AL, Grimm RA, Jasper SE, et al. Efficacy of transesophageal echocardiography-guided cardioversion of patients with atrial fibrillation at 6 months: a randomized controlled trial. *Am Heart J.* 2006;151(2):380–389.

20. Black IW, Fatkin D, Sagar KB, et al. Exclusion of atrial thrombus by transesophageal echocardiography does not preclude embolism after cardioversion of atrial fibrillation. A multicenter study. *Circulation.* 1994;89(6):2509–2513.

21. Jaber WA, Prior DL, Thamilarasan M, et al. Efficacy of anticoagulation in resolving left atrial and left atrial appendage thrombi: a transesophageal echocardiographic study. *Am Heart J.* 2000;140(1):150–156.

22. Bernhardt P, Schmidt H, Hammerstingl C, Lüderitz B, Omran H. Patients with atrial fibrillation and dense spontaneous echo contrast at high risk a prospective and serial follow-up over 12 months with transesophageal echocardiography and cerebral magnetic resonance imaging. *J Am Coll Cardiol.* 2005;45(11):1807–1812.

23. Barnes GD, Ageno W, Ansell J, et al. Recommendation on the nomenclature for oral anticoagulants: communication from the SSC of the ISTH. *J Thromb Haemost.* 2015;13(6):1154–1156.

24. Larsen TB, Larsen TB, Skjøth F, Nielsen PB, Kjældgaard JN, Lip GY. Comparative effectiveness and safety of non-vitamin K antagonist oral anticoagulants and warfarin in patients with atrial fibrillation: propensity weighted nationwide cohort study. *BMJ.* 2016;353:i3189.

25. Nagarakanti R, Ezekowitz MD, Oldgren J, et al. Dabigatran versus warfarin in patients with atrial fibrillation: an analysis of patients undergoing cardioversion. *Circulation.* 2011;123(2):131–136.

26. Piccini JP, Stevens SR, Lokhnygina Y, et al. Outcomes after cardioversion and atrial fibrillation ablation in patients treated with rivaroxaban and warfarin in the ROCKET AF trial. *J Am Coll Cardiol.* 2013;61(19):1998–2006.

27. Flaker G, Lopes RD, Al-Khatib SM, et al. Efficacy and safety of apixaban in patients after cardioversion for atrial fibrillation: insights from the ARISTOTLE trial (apixaban for reduction in stroke and other thromboembolic events in atrial fibrillation). *J Am Coll Cardiol.* 2014;63(11):1082–1087.

28. Cappato R, Ezekowitz MD, Klein AL, et al. Rivaroxaban vs. vitamin K antagonists for cardioversion in atrial fibrillation. *Eur Heart J.* 2014;35(47):3346–3355.

29. Manning WJ, Leeman DE, Gotch PJ, Come PC. Pulsed Doppler evaluation of atrial mechanical function after electrical cardioversion of atrial fibrillation. *J Am Coll Cardiol.* 1989;13(3):617–623.

30. Manning WJ, Silverman DI, Katz SE, et al. Impaired left atrial mechanical function after cardioversion: relation to the duration of atrial fibrillation. *J Am Coll Cardiol.* 1994;23(7):1535–1540.

31. Sun H, Gaspo R, Leblanc N, Nattel S. Cellular mechanisms of atrial contractile dysfunction caused by sustained atrial tachycardia. *Circulation.* 1998;98(7):719–727.

32. Schotten U, Ausma J, Stellbrink C, et al. Cellular mechanisms of depressed atrial contractility in patients with chronic atrial fibrillation. *Circulation.* 2001;103(5):691–698.

33. Sanders P, Morton JB, Morgan JG, et al. Reversal of atrial mechanical stunning after cardioversion of atrial arrhythmias: implications for the mechanisms of tachycardia-mediated atrial cardiomyopathy. *Circulation.* 2002;106 (14):1806–1813.

34. Harjai K, Mobarek S, Abi-Samra F, et al. Mechanical dysfunction of the left atrium and the left atrial appendage following cardioversion of atrial fibrillation and its relation to total electrical energy used for cardioversion. *Am J Cardiol.* 1998;81(9):1125–1129.

35. Falcone RA, Morady F, Armstrong WF. Transesophageal echocardiographic evaluation of left atrial appendage function and spontaneous contrast formation after chemical or electrical cardioversion of atrial fibrillation. *Am J Cardiol.* 1996;78(4):435–439.

36. Israel CW, Grönefeld G, Ehrlich JR, Li YG, Hohnloser SH. Long-term risk of recurrent atrial fibrillation as documented by an implantable monitoring device: implications for optimal patient care. *J Am Coll Cardiol.* 2004;43(1):47–52.

37. Oltrona L, Broccolino M, Merlini PA, Spinola A, Pezzano A, Mannucci PM. Activation of the hemostatic mechanism after pharmacological cardioversion of acute nonvalvular atrial fibrillation. *Circulation.* 1997;95(8):2003–2006.

38. Lip GY, Rumley A, Dunn FG, Lowe GD. Plasma fibrinogen and fibrin D-dimer in patients with atrial fibrillation: effects of cardioversion to sinus rhythm. *Int J Cardiol.* 1995;51(3):245–251.

CHAPTER 10

Anticoagulation for Ablation Procedures

MICHAEL C. GIUDICI, MD, FACC, FACP, FHRS • BRIA GIACOMINO, DO

For many years warfarin was the only oral anticoagulant (AC) used for chronic therapy in patients with atrial fibrillation (AF) and risk factors for ischemic stroke. Patients scheduled for ablation procedures would taper warfarin to present for their ablation procedure with a normal or near-normal international normalized ratio (INR), and a transesophageal echocardiogram (TEE) would be performed before the procedure to rule out left atrial thrombus. Heparin was then administered during the ablation procedure and warfarin was resumed postprocedure. Bridging with low molecular weight heparin (LMWH) injections was sometimes used until a therapeutic INR was achieved.

Just as the practice has evolved in device patients to continue therapeutic anticoagulation during device implantation,[1] data on the safety and efficacy of continuing therapeutic anticoagulation through AF ablation procedures have accumulated.[2-6] The introduction of the "novel" ACs, dabigatran, rivaroxaban, and apixaban (direct oral anticoagulants [DOACs]), has allowed for more anticoagulation options, as these have varying half-lives and response in renal insufficiency. At the same time, so many choices make it more cumbersome to study each scenario and determine the optimal strategy. Considerations for anticoagulation before, during, and after AF ablation are as follows: (1) Which agent should I use before the procedure? Do I continue a DOAC or switch to warfarin for the procedure as it is more easily reversed if a complication occurs? (2) Do I stop the AC before the procedure and, if so, how many days? (3) If I continue the AC through the procedure, I can possibly avoid the preprocedure TEE which could decrease costs and patient discomfort.[7] What is the risk/benefit ratio? (4) During the procedure, should I give heparin before or after the transseptal puncture and what dose? (5) Should I give heparin as a bolus and infusion, or repeat boluses? (6) How high should my activated clotting time (ACT) be maintained during the procedure? (7) Should I administer protamine at the end of the procedure to assist with groin hemostasis? (8) After the procedure, when should I resume warfarin or a DOAC? (9) If the

procedure is successful, how long does this patient need to be on AC? Do the various risk scores apply to someone who no longer has AF? This last question is currently under study and we will not know the answer for a few years. (10) Do the answers to these questions change if the patient has persistent AF versus paroxysmal AF? One of my old colleagues used to frequently say "if it was easy, everyone would be doing it!"

1. **Which agent should I use before the procedure?** The study of Lakkireddy et al.[3] suggested that dabigatran had a higher complication rate than warfarin, but that was with the agent administered until the morning of the procedure and resumed 3 h after sheaths were pulled. A more recent study at Johns Hopkins[8] found no increased risk with the DOACs and, in fact, had fewer minor hemorrhages and total adverse events compared with the warfarin group.

2. **Do I stop the AC before the procedure and, if so, how many days?** It is currently suggested that DOACs be held 1–2 days before the ablation procedure and be resumed the morning after the procedure.[9] With this in mind, we usually continue warfarin through the procedure and have patients stop DOACs one full day before the procedure. For paroxysmal AF patients or for patients who are not on chronic AC, we usually start warfarin 2 weeks before the procedure so that they have a therapeutic INR on the day of the ablation procedure. With this strategy of anticoagulation and the use of intracardiac echocardiography (ICE) to monitor for thrombus and guide transseptal punctures, we do not routinely perform preablation TEEs.

3. **During the procedure, should I give heparin before or after the transseptal puncture and what dose?** We administer 10,000 U of heparin as soon as the sheaths are in place and before the transseptal puncture. Thrombus has tended to form on the J-wire of the transseptal sheath, and this avoids carrying thrombus over to the left side of the heart. Because ICE is guiding the transseptal puncture, the risk of perforation is very low.[10]

4. **Should I give heparin as a bolus and infusion, or repeat boluses?** That is operator-dependent. The guidelines suggest a bolus of 100 U/kg followed by a heparin infusion of 10 U/kg/h with ACT checked every 10–15 min until an ACT of 300–350 s is reached and every 30 min thereafter.[11] A recent survey of 78 centers from 20 European countries showed significant variation in anticoagulation practices.[12] Of note in that survey was that the highest-volume centers did not do any pre- or postprocedure bridging and usually continued oral anticoagulation through the procedure.

5. **How high should my ACT be maintained during the procedure?** This number has crept up over the years. In addition to more experience with AF ablation, some of the increase has been driven by technologies. Depending of what catheter system is used, the recommendations vary considerably. If radiofrequency (RF) ablation is being performed using an open-irrigated tip catheter, an ACT range of 200–250 s has been shown to be adequate.[13] In fact, the rate of complications rose from 1.62% in patients with ACT < 250 s to 5.55% in those with ACT > 350 s. Using the phased array multielectrode PVAC (Ablation Frontiers), the recommended ACT to begin ablation is >300 s.[14] The recommendations for the Arctic Front cryoballoon (Medtronic) is >350 s.[15]

6. **Should I administer protamine at the end of the procedure to assist with groin hemostasis?** Although there is no strong consensus as to whether to let the ACT drift down to <200 s and pull sheaths or administer protamine, it appears to be safe to give protamine and this may decrease vascular complications.[16] Over the years our laboratory has performed AF ablation with and without protamine administration. We currently dose protamine by dividing the last ACT by 10—an ACT of 300 would result in a dose of 30 mg of protamine. Protamine should be avoided or given with great caution to patients on NPH insulin or those with a fish allergy, as they may be sensitized to protamine and have an allergic reaction.

7. **After the procedure, when should I resume warfarin or a DOAC?** Guidelines suggest that AC be resumed 4–6 h postprocedure.[11] If the patient is on warfarin through the procedure there is no issue. If warfarin was discontinued and is being resumed with an LMWH bridge, recommendations are to use a lower dose of LMWH to avoid bleeding complications (0.5 mg/kg twice daily). Patients who are receiving DOACs usually resume their usual dosing scheme the morning after the procedure, but at many centers the twice-daily DOACs, dabigatran and apixaban, are often resumed 3–4 h postprocedure. There are studies that support the safety of either method.[17,18]

8. **If the procedure is successful, how long does this patient need to be on AC?** Do the various risk scores apply to someone who no longer has AF?[19] As mentioned above, we do not know the answer to this question. Studies such as ASSERT[20] and Crystal-AF[21] have altered our long-standing "stop watch" approach to AF, where the clock starts at the onset of an episode of AF and risk increases over time. We are now forced to consider AF as a marker for some process—inflammatory, fibrotic, or otherwise—that makes the atrium a more likely nidus for thrombus formation.

   The current guideline recommendation is for all patients to be on anticoagulation 2 months postablation,[10] at which time decisions are made based on the individual patient's clinical course and his/her stroke risk score (CHA_2DS_2-VASc or ATRIA).

9. **Do the answers to these questions change if the patient has persistent AF versus paroxysmal AF?** Another unknown! Our work over the last 2–3 years suggests that there are more similarities than differences in atria of paroxysmal and persistent AF populations. We have been performing cryoballoon ablation in all AF patients followed by very detailed mapping of the left atrium using a high-density mapping catheter (HD, St. Jude Medical). Our work has shown that left atrial scar burden is >75% in 90% of patients with persistent AF but is also seen in 62% of patients with paroxysmal AF. We manage long-term anticoagulation based on each patient's clinical course, lifestyle, and stroke risk.

   In summary, there is much to consider in the planning of anticoagulation before ablation, during the procedure, and postprocedure. It has been shown that continuing warfarin through the procedure is not only safe but also preferred to avoid heparin bridging. The DOACs are also efficacious but require higher heparin dosing during the ablation procedure. The target ACT range during the procedure depends on the ablation technology used, and it seems the larger the object placed in the left atrium, the higher the recommended ACT.

   Studies that will attempt to answer the larger question of who truly needs chronic anticoagulation are currently in progress.

REFERENCES

1. Giudici MC, Barold SS, Paul DL, Bontu P. Pacemaker/ICD implantation without reversal of warfarin therapy. *Pacing Clin Electrophysiol.* 2004;27:368–370.
2. Wazni OM, Beheiry S, Fahmy T, et al. Atrial fibrillation ablation in patients with therapeutic international normalized ratio: comparison of strategies of anticoagulation in the periprocedural period. *Circulation.* 2007;116:2531–2534.
3. Lakkireddy D, Reddy YM, Di Biase L, et al. Feasibility and safety of dabigatran versus warfarin for periprocedural anticoagulation in patients undergoing radiofrequency ablation for atrial fibrillation: results from a multicenter prospective registry. *J Am Coll Cardiol.* 2012;59:1168–1174.
4. Maddox W, Kay GN, Yamada T, et al. Dabigatran versus warfarin therapy for uninterrupted oral anticoagulation therapy during atrial fibrillation ablation. *J Cardiovasc Electrophysiol.* 2013;24:861–865.
5. Ren JF, Marchlinski FE, Callans DJ, et al. Increased intensity of anticoagulation may reduce risk of thrombus during atrial fibrillation ablation procedures in patients with spontaneous echo contrast. *J Cardiovasc Electrophysiol.* 2005;16:474–477.
6. Vazquez SR, Johnson SA, Rondina MT. Peri-procedural anticoagulation in patients undergoing ablation for atrial fibrillation. *Thromb Res.* 2010;126:e69–e77.
7. Di Biase L, Briceno DF, Trivedi C, et al. Is transesophageal echocardiogram mandatory in patients undergoing ablation of atrial fibrillation with uninterrupted novel oral anticoagulants? Results from a prospective multicenter registry. *Heart Rhythm.* 2016;13:1197–1202.
8. Armbruster HL, Lindsley JP, Moranville MP, et al. Safety of novel oral anticoagulants compared with uninterrupted warfarin for catheter ablation of atrial fibrillation. *Ann Pharmacother.* 2015;49:278–284.
9. Knight BP. Anticoagulation for atrial fibrillation ablation – what is the optimal strategy? *J Am Coll Cardiol.* 2012;59:1175–1177.
10. Dauod EG, Kalbfletch SJ, Hummel JD. Intracardiac echocardiography to guide transseptal left heart catheterization for radiofrequency catheter ablation. *J Cardiovasc Electrophysiol.* 1999;10:358–363.
11. Calkins H, Brugada J, Packer DL, et al. HRS/EHRA/ECAS Expert consensus statement on catheter and surgical ablation of atrial fibrillation: recommendations for personnel, policy, procedures, and follow-up. *Europace.* 2007;9:335–379.
12. Chen J, Todd DM, Hocini M, et al. Current periprocedural management of ablation for atrial fibrillation in Europe: results of the European Heart Rhythm Association survey. *Europace.* 2014;16:378–381.
13. Winkle RA, Mead RH, Engel G, et al. Atrial fibrillation ablation using open-irrigated tip radiofrequency: experience with intraprocedural activated clotting times < 210 seconds. *Heart Rhythm.* 2014;11:963–968.
14. Anselmino M, Gaita F. Unresolved issues in transcatheter atrial fibrillation ablation – silent cerebrovascular ischemias. *J Cardiovasc Electrophysiol.* 2013;24:129–131.
15. Su W, Kowal R, Kowalski M, et al. Best practice guide for cryoablation in atrial fibrillation: the compilation experience of more than 3000 procedures. *Heart Rhythm.* 2015;12:1658–1666.
16. Conte G, de Asmundis C, Baltogiannis G, et al. Periprocedural outcomes of prophylactic protamine administration for reversal of heparin after cryoballoon ablation of atrial fibrillation. *J Interv Card Electrophysiol.* 2014;41:129–134.
17. Stepanyan G, Badhwar N, Lee RJ, et al. Safety of new oral anticoagulants for patients undergoing atrial fibrillation ablation. *J Interv Card Electrophysiol.* 2014;40:33–38.
18. Maan A, Heist EK, Ruskin JN, Mansour M. Practical issues in the management of novel oral anticoagulants – cardioversion and ablation. *J Thorac Dis.* 2015;7:115–131.
19. Chao T, Lin Y, Chang S, et al. Can oral anticoagulants be stopped safely after successful atrial fibrillation ablation? *J Thorac Dis.* 2015;7:172–177.
20. Healey JS, Connolly SJ, Gold MR, et al. Subclinical atrial fibrillation and the risk of stroke. *N Engl J Med.* 2012;366:120–129.
21. Sanna T, Diener H, Passman RS, et al. Cryptogenic stroke and underlying atrial fibrillation. *N Engl J Med.* 2014;370:2478–2486.

CHAPTER 11

Surgical and Implanted Devices for the Left Atrial Appendage

SANDEEP GAUTAM, MD, MPH • JOSHUA PAYNE, MD, MPH

There are several reasons why nonpharmacologic treatments of atrial fibrillation (AF), specifically elimination or obstruction of the left atrial appendage (LAA), are gaining popularity. It is well known that AF is associated with thromboembolic cerebrovascular events, increasing the risk of thromboembolism and stroke by three- to fivefold.[1,2] In addition, although the precise mechanism for stroke in AF remains elusive, there were two separate lines of evidence that suggest that stroke in AF is related to clot formation in the LAA. The first of these include clinical trial data, which demonstrate the success of stroke prevention in AF with anticoagulation, first with vitamin K antagonists[3–6] and then with direct-acting oral anticoagulants (OACs).[7–10] The second line of evidence involves transesophageal echocardiogram (TEE) data showing that the LAA is the source for most left atrial thrombus. Given these data, it is logical to think that elimination of the LAA could eliminate or greatly reduce the risk of stroke in patients with AF.

In addition, although OACs are the mainstay of prevention and treatment of thromboembolic events in AF, several studies have also shown that oral anticoagulation is underutilized, particularly in patients at higher risk of stroke based on $CHADS_2$ and $CHAD_2VASc$ scores with common explanations being prior bleeding, patient refusal, high bleeding risk, and frequent falls or frailty.[3,11] In short, for a number of reasons, many patients do not receive the benefit of anticoagulation. Consequently, this has led to the pursuit of nonpharmacologic methods to reduce risk of stroke associated with nonvalvular AF that would theoretically limit the bleeding risk accompanying systemic anticoagulation.

PHYSIOLOGY OF COAGULATION IN ATRIAL FIBRILLATION

Kamel and colleagues recently performed an elegant analysis of thromboembolic stroke in AF using Hill's criteria of causation, concluding that the association between AF and stroke fulfills the criteria of strength of association, consistency, and plausibility, but not other criteria such as specificity, temporality, biologic gradient, and accordance with experimental results. They have proposed an updated model for the mechanisms of stroke in AF (Fig. 11.1), with greater emphasis on systemic factors and atrial substrate,[2] suggesting a multipronged approach to reduce thromboembolic risk of AF. Lip and colleagues have similarly suggested that abnormal changes in flow, vessel wall, and blood constituents combine to create a prothrombotic state in AF,[4] especially in the region of the LAA (Fig. 11.2).

These data suggest that thromboembolism in AF cannot be prevented by a single strategy or approach. Exclusion of the LAA is a structural approach to reduce, if not eliminate, stroke risk in AF.

IMPORTANCE OF LEFT ATRIAL APPENDAGE IN ATRIAL FIBRILLATION–ASSOCIATED THROMBOEMBOLISM

The LAA is a fingerlike blind structure on the lateral aspect of the left atrium, between the left upper pulmonary vein and the left ventricle. The LAA is the remnant of the original embryonic left atrium that develops during the third week of gestation, with the main smooth-walled LA cavity developing later from the outgrowth of the pulmonary veins. The LAA is a long, tubular, hooked trabeculated structure with pectinate muscles, lined by endothelium. The cavities between the pectinate muscles appear as "lobes" and "twigs".[5] LAA remodeling is often seen in chronic AF, with dilation and stretching along with endocardial fibroelastosis.[5,6] The narrow neck and relatively large body of the LAA, along with the trabeculated structure, promote local blood stasis, especially during AF. Despite the possibility of nonarrhythmic thromboembolic causative factors in AF, at least 90% of thrombi in AF originate in the LAA.[7–9]

In a study of 932 patients with drug refractory AF undergoing catheter-based ablation, Di Biase et al. utilized cardiac CT or MRI to describe four different LAA morphologies, namely chicken wing (48%), cactus

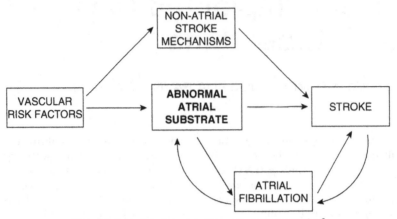

FIG. 11.1 Updated model of thromboembolic stroke.[2]

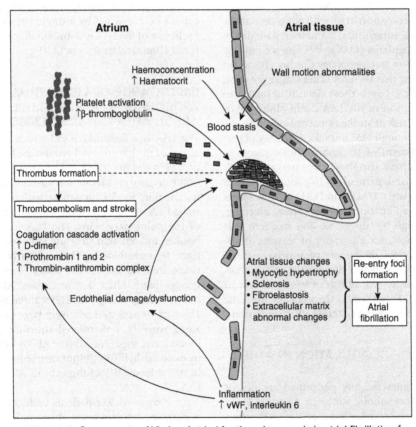

FIG. 11.2 Components of Virchow's triad for thrombogenesis in atrial fibrillation.[4]

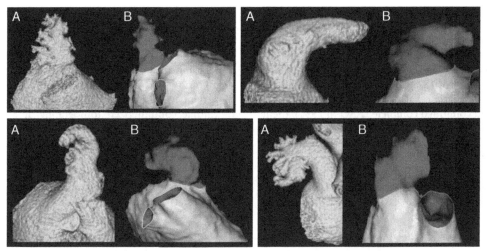

FIG. 11.3 Cardiac CT **(A)** and MRI **(B)** LAA morphology subtypes: cactus (top left), chicken wing (top right), windsock (lower left), cauliflower (lower right).[10]

(30%), windsock (19%), and cauliflower (3%). The chicken wing morphology had the lowest prevalence of stroke/transient ischemic attack (TIA) (Fig. 11.3). Using this as the reference group in a multivariate model of stroke/TIA, cactus was 4.08 times, windsock was 4.5 times, and cauliflower morphology was 8 times more likely to have had a stroke/TIA.[10] Conversely, Kosiuk et al. reported that the chicken wing morphology was associated with the highest periprocedural thromboembolic risk in 2570 consecutive patients undergoing catheter-based AF ablation,[12] while Nedios et al. did not find any such difference between LAA morphologies for periprocedural thromboembolic events in 2069 patients in the Leipzig Heart Center AF Ablation Registry.[13]

In summary, specific LAA morphologies may play a role in the development of local thrombus formation, but the data are mixed and more information is needed. However, the classification of the LAA morphologies is potentially useful during LAA occluder device placement.

SURGICAL TECHNIQUES FOR LEFT ATRIAL APPENDAGE EXCLUSION

Excision of the atrial appendage (left/both) has been an integral part of the Maze procedure for surgical treatment of AF, through its multiple modifications. In a review of 565 studies of surgical ablation for AF, Je et al. reported that the LAA is excised/ligated in 100% of open Cox-Maze procedures, as compared with ~77% of patients undergoing an epicardial "Mini-Maze," and

in only ~30% patients undergoing a hybrid surgical/catheter-based ablation procedure, suggesting that exclusion of LAA during surgical AF ablation is partially determined by operator preference and presumed additional surgical risk.[14] The Left Atrial Appendage Occlude Study (LAAOS) demonstrated the safety of perioperative LAA suture/stapling during coronary artery bypass grafting.[15]

Cox et al. reported only a single late stroke in 265 patients followed up for up to 11.5 years and attributed this low event rate to a combination of extremely low recurrence of AF as well as removal of LAA.[16] In a similar long-term follow-up of 177 out of 198 patients undergoing Maze procedure (lone or concomitant), Prasad et al. found only a single thromboembolic stroke, despite discontinuation of oral anticoagulation in >90% patients.[17] Tsai et al., in a metaanalysis of seven studies including 3653 patients undergoing LAA occlusion (LAAO), found an improvement in acute and long-term stroke and mortality in the LAAO group, without any increase in perioperative bleeding.[18] On the contrary, a recent single-center, large-scale, propensity matched analysis of prophylactic LAA exclusion in patients undergoing non-AF-related cardiac surgery did not find a significant difference in long-term stroke risk in the LAA exclusion cohort (unadjusted hazard ratio, 1.08; 95% CI, 0.74–1.60). Only 45% of patients in each group had prior AF.[19] The study was limited by lack of information on anticoagulation status during follow-up and the absence of assessment of complete LAA exclusion.

To prevent thrombus formation in the LAA, surgical removal or exclusion should theoretically not allow blood flow from the left atrium into the remnant appendage. However, the efficacy of surgical LAA exclusion is dependent on the exclusion technique. In a retrospective study of 137 patients with prior surgical LAA exclusion, Kanderian et al. performed postoperative TEE studies and confirmed complete LAAO in 73% patients with left atrial excision but in only 23% of patients with suture exclusion. Interestingly, flow was present into the LAA in all 12 patients who had undergone exclusion by stapling. Even more important, LAA thrombus was found in 41% patients with unsuccessful LAA exclusion compared with none with excision (Fig. 11.4).[20]

The AtriClip device (Atricure, West Chester, Ohio) is a self-closing, sterile, implantable stapling device placed epicardially at the base of the LAA (Fig. 11.5). The EXCLUDE trial tested the AtriClip device in 71 patients undergoing open cardiac surgery, with successful placement in 70 patients, and 98.4% complete LAAO in 61 patients who underwent left atrial imaging by TEE or cardiac computerized tomography at 3 months.[21] Based on the results of this trial, the AtriClip device was approved by FDA in 2011. Although subsequent studies also confirmed acceptable LAAO,[22] and mechanical closure of the LAA is reaching the mainstream,[23] the limiting factor for this technique remains the need for open/thoracoscopic epicardial access.

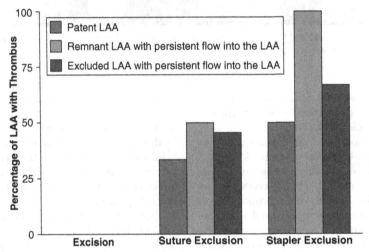

FIG. 11.4 Presence of left atrial appendage (LAA) thrombus with unsuccessful surgical LAA closure by the three techniques: excision, suture exclusion, and stapler exclusion.[20]

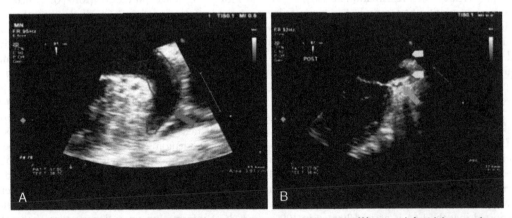

FIG. 11.5 Intraoperative transesophageal echocardiogram demonstrating **(A)** patent left atrial appendage (LAA) before AtriClip device placement (*red arrow* [light gray in print version]) and **(B)** echocardiographic evidence of LAA exclusion after clip placement (*orange arrow* [dark gray in print version]; *yellow arrowheads* [white in print version] indicate pulmonary veins).[21]

To summarize the surgical procedures for LAAO, complete LAA excision should be considered the gold standard technique. Intraoperative left atrial imaging by TEE is essential to ensure complete LAAO without patency/remnant (>1 cm stump). The AtriClip device is extremely promising with excellent medium-term (3 months) LAAO. Data regarding safety of discontinuation of anticoagulation following surgical LAA exclusion are conflicting and hampered by lack of prospective studies as well as inadequate information about completeness of LAA exclusion.

LARIAT DEVICE

The LARIAT device (SentreHEART, Redwood City, California) is a percutaneous alternative to thoracoscopic or open epicardial clipping of the LAA. This catheter-based device consists of a snare with a pretied suture that is guided epicardially over the LAA. The device consists of a 15-mm compliant occlusion balloon catheter, magnet-tipped guidewires, and a 12-F suture delivery device. The procedure involves both percutaneous epicardial and transseptal access followed by placement of the endocardial magnet-tipped guidewire in the apex of the LAA, connection of the epicardial and endocardial magnet-tipped guidewires for stabilization of the LAA, and snare capture of the LAA for LAA ligation (Fig. 11.6).

Bartus et al.[24] reported the initial clinical experience with the LARIAT device, with successful implantation in 85 of 89 patients and 95% complete LAAO by TEE at 3 months. There were three major procedural complications, two related to pericardial access (one right ventricular puncture and one vascular bleed) and one related to transseptal puncture (pericardial perforation), all treated with percutaneous drainage. A subsequent multicenter retrospective study of 154 patients undergoing LARIAT device placement was more sobering, with 94% procedural success but 9.7% major procedural complications,

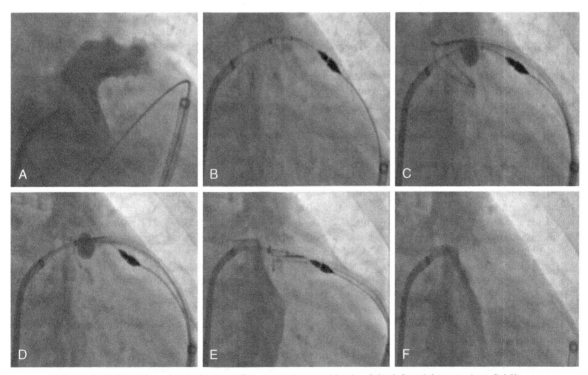

FIG. 11.6 Left atrial angiography identifies the ostium and body of the left atrial appendage (LAA) **(A)**. Attachment of the magnet-tipped endocardial and epicardial guidewires **(B)** allows for the LARIAT suture delivery device to be guided over the LAA by the magnet-tipped epicardial guidewire using an over-the-wire approach **(C)**. After verification of the correct position of the snare with the balloon catheter **(D)**, a left atrial (LA) angiogram is performed before the release of the pretied suture to exclude the existence of a remnant trabeculated LAA lobe **(E)**. A final LA angiogram is performed to verify LAA exclusion **(F)**.[24]

and 4.8% thrombi at the LAA stump and 20% residual leak in 63 patients with TEE follow-up. Two patients had an ischemic stroke.[25] The LARIAT device was originally cleared by the FDA to deliver a pre-tied stitch (suture) to aid in soft tissue closure during surgery and is being used off-label for LAAO. In July 2015, the FDA released a safety communication alerting healthcare providers and patients about reports of patient deaths and other serious adverse events during its use for LAAO.[26]

The LARIAT device is currently also being evaluated in the ongoing aMAZE randomized controlled trial for concurrent use with catheter-based pulmonary vein isolation for persistent AF, looking for any effect on recurrence of AF at 12 months.[27]

The LARIAT device seems to provide reasonable acute success for LAAO but is limited by the need for epicardial access, procedural complications, and variable long-term durable LAA exclusion.

LEFT ATRIAL APPENDAGE OCCLUSION DEVICES

The pursuit of endovascular LAAO began after a realization that the LAA was readily accessible during radio frequency ablation for AF.[28] Stroke risk reduction in nonvalvular AF by means of endocardial LAAO was first attempted in 2001 using the Percutaneous Left Atrial Appendage Transcatheter Occlusion (PLAATO) device (Appriva Medical Inc). The PLAATO device consisted of a self-expanding nickel titanium (nitinol) cage with a polytetrafluoroethylene membrane covering the atrial side of the device and struts attached to anchors for stability within the LAA. A nonrandomized study of 111 patients revealed high procedural success and technical occlusion of the LAA.[29] Another observational, multicenter prospective study of 64 patients showed a lower-than-expected annual stroke rate of 3.8% compared with the predicted stroke rate of 6.6% determined by the study populations $CHADS_2$ score of 2 or greater.[30] Despite this limited but encouraging data, the device was withdrawn from market.

Several devices have since been developed and share similar procedural and structural characteristics. The procedures generally involve introducing prosthetic material into the LAA via a transvenous catheter delivery system into the left atrium by transseptal puncture. The prosthetic material blocks blood flow into the LAA and becomes endothelialized over time providing a mechanical barrier between the LA and LAA, theoretically eliminating the risk of embolic stroke from appendage. The most well-studied device to date is the Watchman.

WATCHMAN DEVICE

The Watchman (Boston Scientific, Marlborough, Massachusetts) is composed of a self-expanding nitinol frame with a semipermeable membrane of polyethylene terephthalate lining the atrial side with 10 fixation anchors on the appendage side for device stabilization. Manufactured in five sizes ranging from 21 to 33 mm to accommodate different LAA sizes, the device is delivered via a 14F sheath via transseptal puncture into the left atrium under fluoroscopic and ultrasound guidance.[31] The Watchman was approved by the FDA in 2015 after completion of two large randomized trials showing high procedural success rate and favorable results when compared with warfarin, the PROTECT-AF trial and the PREVAIL trial.[26]

The WATCHMAN Left Atrial Appendage System for Embolic Protection in Patients with Atrial Fibrillation (PROTECT-AF) study compared the Watchman device with standard therapy with warfarin (target international normalized ratio of 2–3) in patients with a CHADS score >1. A total of 707 patients were randomized in a 2:1 fashion with 463 patients in the device arm and 244 patients in the control group. After placement, patients in the device arm were treated with aspirin 325 mg daily and warfarin for at least 45 days. At this point, a TEE was performed to evaluate the success of occlusion, device stability, residual atrial septal shunting, and device-associated thrombus. After confirming technical success, warfarin was discontinued and clopidogrel 75 mg daily was prescribed for 6 months, followed by monotherapy with aspirin to be continued indefinitely. If residual shunt was detected, warfarin was continued until resolution observed on serial TEE.

The device was successfully implanted in 91% of patients undergoing the procedure. At the 45-day follow-up period, 86% of patients met criteria to transition to dual antiplatelet therapy (DAPT) with aspirin and Plavix. This improved to 92% at 6 months. A primary efficacy composite of stroke, TIA, cardiovascular death, and systemic embolism was similar in both groups, achieving noninferiority (Fig. 11.7A); however, primary safety endpoints of major bleeding, pericardial effusion, and device embolization were more common in the intervention group (Fig. 11.7B). The most common adverse event related to device placement was serious pericardial effusion requiring drainage, occurring in 22 (4.8%) patients, with a trend toward declining adverse event rates with operator experience.[32] The Watchman device was considered to be noninferior to control (warfarin) therapy for all stroke and all-cause mortality (Fig. 11.7C and D).

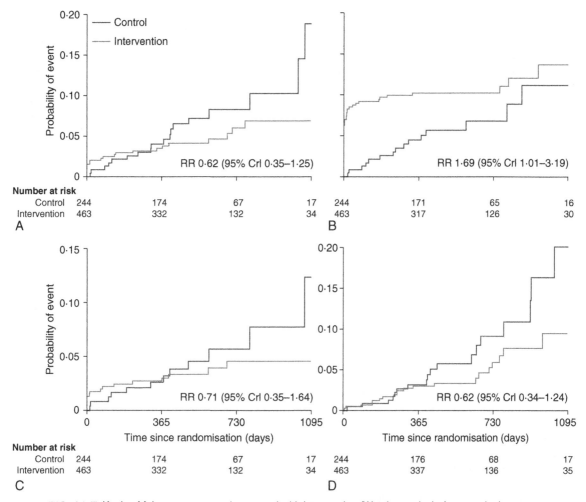

FIG. 11.7 Kaplan Meier curve comparing control with intervention (Watchman device) groups in the PROTECT-AF trial.[32] **(A)** Primary efficacy endpoint; **(B)** primary safety endpoint; **(C)** all stroke; and **(D)** all-cause mortality.

The trend of improved safety outcomes with operator experience was further observed in ongoing studies of a Continued Access Protocol (CAP) Registry that was established after the completion of the PROTECT-AF trial. At a mean of 3.8 years of follow-up, noninferiority for the primary efficacy event rate was maintained, and prespecified criteria for superiority (2.3 events/100 patient-years vs. 3.8 events/100 patient-years, rate ratio: 0.60 at a 95% credible interval, 0.41–1.05) are met. Rates of both cardiovascular and all-cause mortality were reduced in the intervention arm. Additionally, with more bleeding events occurring in the warfarin group over time, adverse event rates were similar in the two arms, damping device safety concerns.[33]

Concerns about the relatively low risk patients enrolled in the PROTECT-AF trial, and the relatively high procedural risks, led to a second large randomized trial, Prospective Randomized Evaluation of the Watchman Left Atrial Appendage Closure Device in Patients With Atrial Fibrillation Versus Long-Term Warfarin Therapy (PREVAIL). This trial randomized 407 patients in a 2:1 fashion with 269 in the interventional group and 138 in the control group. The device placement and postinterventional anticoagulation protocols were identical to PROTECT-AF. Versus PROTECT-AF, procedural success in PREVAIL improved from 90.9% to 95.1%. At 18 months of follow-up, a primary composite endpoint of stroke, systemic embolism, and cardiovascular death was similar but did not meet non-inferiority criteria. A second coprimary endpoint of stroke or systemic embolism at >7 days, however, did achieve noninferiority. Additionally, safety endpoints were significantly lower in PREVAIL compared with PROTECT-AF with fewer pericardial effusions requiring either percutaneous or surgical drainage and peri-procedural stroke. Interestingly, 39.1% of devices were placed by novice operators, and there was no signifi-cant difference in procedural success or complication rates between experienced and novice operators within this study.[34] Additional long-term follow-up data were reported later, with eight additional ischemic strokes in the Watchman group, thus not meeting the noninferi-ority efficacy endpoints.[35]

After analyzing these data, the Watchman device was approved by the FDA in March 2015 for patients with nonvalvular AF who are (1) at increased risk of stroke and systemic embolism on the basis of $CHADS_2$ or CHA_2DS_2-VASc scores; (2) deemed by their physi-cians to be suitable for warfarin therapy; and (3) have an appropriate rationale to seek a nonpharmacologic alternative to warfarin.

As with PROTECT-AF, a Continued Access Registry (CAP2) was created after the PREVAIL trial, providing a longer follow-up period for these patients. In addi-tion to the ongoing CAP and CAP2 registries, a large, prospective, international registry (EWOLUTION) was created containing information from 1021 patients receiving a Watchman implant. 30-day postimplant data have been published, showing a higher procedural success rate than PROTECT-AF and PREVAIL (98.5%) with a lower adverse event rate of 2.7%.[36]

The largest set of Watchman procedural outcomes was recently published using data collected by the manufacturer post–FDA approval.[37] A total of 3822 implants were completed in a 15-month period by 382 physicians at 169 centers. The reported implanta-tion success rate was 95.6%. Procedural complication rates were low despite 50% of the procedures being completed by new providers. As with other studies, the most common complication was pericardial effusion requiring either percutaneous or surgical drainage in 1% of patients. Although the observed complication rate was quite low, there was a concern for underreport-ing of adverse effects as the data were based solely on the procedural report by the manufacturer's clinical specialists.[38]

Regarding newer/direct oral anticoagulant medi-cations (NOACs), there have been no randomized controlled trials comparing LAAO with systemic anticoagulation with NOACs. An indirect comparison in the form of a metaanalysis comparing aggregate outcomes of several large randomized trials, including PROTECT-AF and PREVAIL, found that both NOACs and Watchman were superior to warfarin in hemor-rhagic stroke prevention. There was no difference in outcomes between NOACs and Watchman, but there was a trend toward higher ischemic stroke rates with Watchman (odds ratio [OR] 2.60 [0.60–13.96]) and trends toward higher hemorrhagic stroke with NOACs (OR = 0.44 [0.09–2.14]).[39]

PATIENT SELECTION AND APPROVAL

In 2015, after publication of the PROTECT-AF long-term follow-up and PREVAIL outcomes, the Food and Drug Administration approved the Watchman device for patients with nonvalvular AF who are at a high risk of stroke deemed by a $CHADS_2$ or $CHADS_2VASc$ score, are suitable for long-term anticoagulation, but have a rationale for seeking a nonpharmacologic alternative.[40] One year later, the Centers for Medicare and Medicaid Services rendered a similar approval with some modifi-cations. Patients are eligible if they have a $CHADS_2 \geq 2$ or $CHADS_2VASc$ of ≥3, are suitable for short-term anti-coagulation with warfarin, but are determined to be ineligible for long-term anticoagulation by an indepen-dent, noninterventional physician. Additionally, it was stipulated that the procedure must be performed in a center with a structural heart disease and/or electro-physiology program and by an interventional cardiolo-gist, electrophysiologist, or cardiovascular surgeon with manufacturer training and experience with transseptal puncture. Patients are also to be enrolled in a national registry.[41]

These approvals are in line with the European Soci-ety of Cardiology guidelines that provide a IIB (level of evidence B) indication for percutaneous LLA closure in patients with nonvalvular AF who are at high risk of stroke with contraindications to long-term antico-agulation.[42] Fig. 11.8 outlines a proposed algorithm for stroke reduction strategy in patients with nonvalvular AF. The American cardiology societies have yet to incor-porate the use of LAAO devices within their guidelines but are expected in coming updates.

AMPLATZER DEVICE

The Amplatzer Cardiac Plug (ACP) (St. Jude Medical, Minneapolis, MN, USA) (Fig. 11.9C,D) was introduced in 2008 with a design based on previous models used

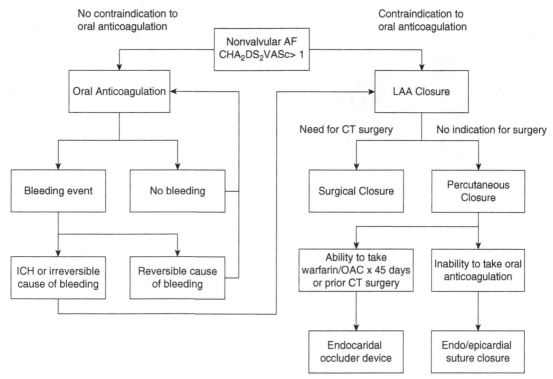

FIG. 11.8 Treatment algorithm for stroke risk reduction in patients with nonvalvular atrial fibrillation (AF).[44] *LAA*, left atrial appendage; *OAC*, oral anticoagulant; *ICH*, Intracranial hemorrhage.

for procedures such as atrial septal defect closure. The non-LAA-specific devices were initially used off-label, with notable procedural success, but with a high rate of device embolization.[43]

The ACP is a designated LAAO device made of a self-expanding, flexible nitinol mesh "lobe" with six pairs of hooks for anchoring into the LAA with a disk on the atrial side connected by a thin waist. The device is made in widths ranging from 16 to 30 mm, all with a length of 6.5 mm. The flexible lobe is designed to accommodate various LAA depths and anatomy, while the disk is designed to seal the LAA ostium traction applied by the wedged lobe, termed the "pacifier principle."[28,44-46]

In a multicenter, retrospective study of 1047 patients, there was a high procedural success rate with the ACP of 97% and with a procedural adverse event rate of 4.98%, the largest complication being pericardial tamponade (n = 13). The annual rate of stroke was 2.3%, which was a 59% reduction from predicted stroke rate determined by the study population's CHA_2DS_2-VASc score. Additionally, there was also a 61% reduction in

the annual rate of major bleeding.[45] As with other trials, postprocedural TEE was used to detect peridevice leak and confirm placement within the LAA. A second-generation ACP, the Amulet, is now available and was designed to minimize complications and simplify delivery. The device is preloaded on the delivery system unlike the first-generation ACP, saving time, reducing manipulation in vivo, and theoretically reducing risk of air embolism.

Outcome and efficacy data regarding the Amulet are limited to observational studies such as one by Kleinecke et al. that included 50 patients who received implantation over a period of 11 months.[47] Procedural success as achieved in 49 (98%) patients. There were major periprocedural adverse events in 4 (8%) patients, including one device embolization, two effusions requiring pericardiocentesis, and a retropharyngeal hematoma from TEE. At 12 months of follow-up, there were three ischemic strokes. Bleeding complications occurred in eight patients while on DAPT with aspirin and clopidogrel including gastrointestinal (GI) bleeding and subarachnoid hemorrhage. Preliminary results

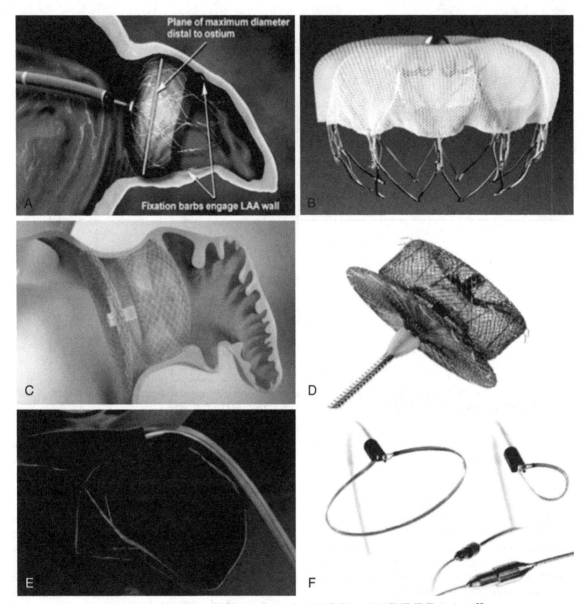

FIG. 11.9 Watchman **(A,B)**, Amplatzer Amulet **(C,D)**, and LARIAT **(E,F)** devices.[56]

from a postmarket observational study of 1073 patients from 64 international sites reported a device implantation success rate of 98.8%. Major adverse event rates within 7 days of implantation were low, with ischemic stroke occurring in 3 patients (0.3%), pericardial effusion requiring drainage in 5 (0.5%), embolization in 1 patient (0.1%), and bleeding in 10 patients (0.9%). There were three deaths, one attributed to nondevice-related complications.[48]

A prospective trial is currently enrolling that will randomize patients who are LAAO candidates to either the Amplatzer Amulet or Watchman in a 1:1 ratio, designed for noninferiority with endpoints similar to previous LAA device studies. The primary efficacy measures are ischemic stroke or systemic embolism with 18 months of implant. Primary safety measures will be all-cause death, procedure-related complications, and major bleeding within 12 months of implant. Implantation success rate will be determined at 45 days postimplant by TEE evaluation of residual flow around the devices. Patients will be followed up for 5 years postimplant (ClinicalTrials.gov identifier: NCT02879448).[49]

WAVECREST DEVICE

The WaveCrest (Coherex Medical, Salt Lake City, UT, USA) is a recently developed device with limited real-world data. Similar to other LAAO devices, it consists of a nitinol frame with a polytetrafluoroethylene cover on the left atrial side. It is secured by a foam layer with extending, flexible nitinol anchors. It has a uniquely shorter design to fix more proximally in the LAA and may be an option for patients with a smaller LAA in which other available devices are too large.[28,44] A safety and feasibility trial, WAVECREST I, was completed in 2015. Seventy-three patients with a mean CHADS$_2$ score of 2.5 and a contraindication to warfarin were implanted with a success rate of 96% (70/73), with pericardial tamponade in two patients (2.7%).[44,50]

PERIPROCEDURAL AND LONG-TERM ANTICOAGULATION

Despite the large amount of randomized clinical trial and registry data supporting the use of LAAO devices in patients who are not candidates for long-term anticoagulation, little evidence exists regarding placement in patients with an absolute contraindication to anticoagulation. All devices are generally placed under full anticoagulation with heparin with a goal activated clotting time ≥250 s. Additionally, the standard postprocedure protocol for WATCHMAN includes a 45-day period of warfarin, followed by DAPT for 6 months, and then aspirin indefinitely. Enomoto et al., in a retrospective cohort study, found equivalent bleeding events, device-related thrombosis, and thromboembolic events in patients treated with NOAC following Watchman device placement as compared with a control group receiving uninterrupted warfarin, suggesting that NOAC can be used safely in lieu of warfarin post–Watchman placement.[51]

There is some evidence suggesting that a 6-month course of DAPT following Watchman placement may be reasonable in patients with an absolute contraindication to warfarin (Fig. 11.10). In the ASA Plavix

Device/ patient	Heparin (ACT ≥ 250)	Low-molecular- weight heparin	ASA	Warfarin	Clopidogrel	Comments
Watchman/ Low bleeding risk	Prior to or immediately after transseptal punctures	Post-procedure till INR ≥ 2	Load 500 mg prior to procedure if not on ASA, continue 100–325 mg/day indefinitely	Start after procedure INR 2–3 till 45 days or continue till adequate occlusion[a] by TOE	Start when warfarin stopped continue till 6 months after the procedure	Some centres do not withhold warfarin and perform procedure on therapeutic INR (no data to support or dispute this approach)
Watchman/ High bleeding risk	Prior to or immediately after transseptal puncture	None	Load 500 mg prior to procedure if not on ASA, continue 100–325 mg/day indefinitely	None	Load 300–600 mg prior to procedure if not on clopidogrel, continue 1–6 months while ensuring adequate occlusion[a]	Clopidogrel often given for shorter time in extremely high-risk situations. Clopidogrel may replace long-term ASA if better tolerated
ACP	Prior to or immediately after transseptal puncture	None	Load 500 mg prior to procedure if not on ASA, continue 100–325 mg/day indefinitely	None	Load 300–600 mg prior to procedure if not on clopidogrel, continue 1–6 months while ensuring adequate occlusion[a]	Clopidogrel often given for shorter time in extremely high-risk situations. Clopidogrel may replace long-term ASA if better tolerated

ACT, activated clothing time; INR, international normalized ratio.
[a]Less than 5 mm leak.

FIG. 11.10 Regimens for management of oral anticoagulation around left atrial appendage (LAA) Occluder devices.[28] *ACP*, Amplatzer Cardiac Plug; *ACT*, activated clotting time; *INR*, international normalized ratio; *TOE*, Transesophageal echocardiogram.

Feasibility Study With Watchman Left Atrial Appendage Closure Technology (ASAP) study, patients with contraindication to anticoagulation underwent 6 months of DAPT postimplantation with no treatment with warfarin, followed by aspirin indefinitely. Of the 150 patients with nonvalvular AF evaluated over mean follow-up 14 months, periprocedural adverse outcomes occurred in 13 (8.7%) patients, ischemic stroke occurred in 3 patients (1.7% per year), and hemorrhagic stroke in 1 patient (0.6% per year). The ischemic stroke rate was less than expected (7.3% per year) based on the study population CHADS$_2$ scores and was lower than in the intervention arm in the PROTECT-AF trial (2.2%). With the lack of a control group, it is difficult to draw conclusions regarding noninferiority; however, these results do suggest that this strategy may be a reasonable option in these patients.[52]

There are no formalized protocols for ACP placement; however, patients are generally placed on DAPT for a period of 3–6 months, followed by indefinite treatment with aspirin, and are not treated with warfarin.[46,47] The Efficacy of Left atrIal Appendage Closure After GastroIntestinal BLEeding (ELIGIBLE) trial aimed to compare patients with AF and a history of GI bleeding to percutaneous LAA closure versus OACs. However, the trial was stopped because of insufficient recruitment.[53] An accompanying registry in patients not undergoing LAAO placement reported a high rate of GI rebleed and mortality in this population.[54]

To summarize, all LAAO devices require full intraprocedural anticoagulation during placement, therefore requiring that the patient be able to tolerate transient anticoagulation. Postplacement pharmacologic management with the ACP device consists of DAPT for a variable duration of few months and seems to be moving in the same direction with the Watchman device (presently requiring 45 days of warfarin, with possible equivalent results with NOAC).

COSTEFFECTIVENESS OF LEFT ATRIAL APPENDAGE OCCLUDER DEVICES
One major concern raised with LAAO devices in nonvalvular AF is the associated procedural cost versus standard medical treatment with oral anticoagulation over time with either warfarin or NOACs. This issue was addressed in a publication that used a 20-year prediction model of quality-adjusted life years based on data from PROTECT-AF, PREVAIL, and a meta-analysis of warfarin and NOAC studies. The model predicted that LAA closure would be cost-effective at 7 years versus warfarin and dominant at 10 years. Likewise, the model predicted that LAA closure would be dominant over NOACs at 5 years. This model has thus far mirrored the long-term follow-up data previously mentioned. There is upfront cost associated with the procedure and a low but present rate of device complications. Over time, the cost-effectiveness ratio is shifted by a lower long-term bleeding risk with LAA closure (Fig. 11.11).[55]

CONCLUSION
The LAA seems to be an important anatomic area for thrombus formation in the left atrium, and surgical and implantable devices may reduce the risk of stroke in selected patients. Given the large number of patients at higher risk for stroke who do not or cannot take oral anticoagulation, these nonpharmacologic methods to prevent stroke may provide benefit in these patients although more studies are needed. LAA morphology might be important in determining individual thromboembolic events. A variety of LAAO devices have been developed for prevention of thromboembolic events in AF. Of these, the Watchman device is currently FDA approved as an alternative to oral anticoagulation in high CHADS$_2$ or CHADS VASc score nonvalvular AF patients who are otherwise suitable for long-term anticoagulation with warfarin. Preliminary studies suggest high procedural implant success rates, improving complication rate, and long-term cost-effectiveness of these devices. Confirmation of complete exclusion of blood flow between left atrium and LAA is a critical part of percutaneous LAAO. Long-term stroke prevention with these data might be limited by the presence of nonatrial systemic factors for stroke in AF. However, ongoing studies of LAAO deployment without postoperative anticoagulation might unlock a niche in patients with absolute contraindication to anticoagulation.

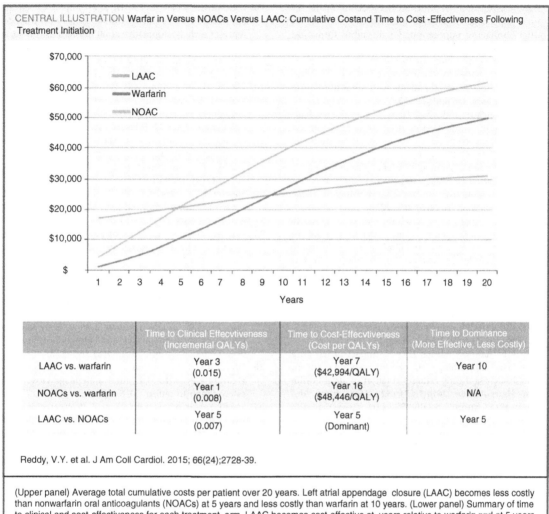

CENTRAL ILLUSTRATION Warfar in Versus NOACs Versus LAAC: Cumulative Costand Time to Cost -Effectiveness Following Treatment Initiation

	Time to Clinical Effecvtiveness (Incremental QALYs)	Time to Cost-Effecvtiveness (Cost per QALYs)	Time to Dominance (More Effective, Less Costly)
LAAC vs. warfarin	Year 3 (0.015)	Year 7 ($42,994/QALY)	Year 10
NOACs vs. warfarin	Year 1 (0.008)	Year 16 ($48,446/QALY)	N/A
LAAC vs. NOACs	Year 5 (0.007)	Year 5 (Dominant)	Year 5

Reddy, V.Y. et al. J Am Coll Cardiol. 2015; 66(24);2728-39.

(Upper panel) Average total cumulative costs per patient over 20 years. Left atrial appendage closure (LAAC) becomes less costly than nonwarfarin oral anticoagulants (NOACs) at 5 years and less costly than warfarin at 10 years. (Lower panel) Summary of time to clinical and cost-effectiveness for each treatment arm. LAAC becomes cost-effective at years relative to warfarin and at 5 years relative to NOACs achieve cost-effectiveness relative to warfarin at 16 years. ASLY = quality-adjusted life-year.

FIG. 11.11 Time to cost-effectiveness for left atrial appendage closure (LAAC) devices and oral anticoagulants.[55]

REFERENCES

1. De Caterina R, Hylek EM. Stroke prevention in atrial fibrillation: current status and near-future directions. *Am J Med.* 2011;124(9):793–799.
2. Kamel H, Okin PM, Elkind MS, Iadecola C. Atrial fibrillation and mechanisms of stroke. *Stroke.* 2016;47(3):895–900.
3. O'Brien EC, Holmes DN, Ansell JE, et al. Physician practices regarding contraindications to oral anticoagulation in atrial fibrillation: findings from the outcomes registry for better informed treatment of atrial fibrillation (OR-BIT-AF) registry. *Am Heart J.* 2014;167(4):609.e1. https://doi.org/10.1016/j.ahj.2013.12.014. http://www.ncbi.nlm.nih.gov/pubmed/24655711.
4. Watson T, Shantsila E, Lip GY. Mechanisms of thrombogenesis in atrial fibrillation: Virchow's triad revisited. *Lancet.* 2009;373(9658):155–166.
5. Stollberger C, Schneider B, Finsterer J. Elimination of the left atrial appendage to prevent stroke or embolism?: Anatomic, physiologic, and pathophysiologic considerations. *CHEST J.* 2003;124(6):2356–2362.

6. Shirani J, Alaeddini J. Structural remodeling of the left atrial appendage in patients with chronic non-valvular atrial fibrillation: implications for thrombus formation, systemic embolism, and assessment by transesophageal echocardiography. *Cardiovasc Pathol.* 2000;9(2):95–101.

7. Blackshear JL, Odell JA. Appendage obliteration to reduce stroke in cardiac surgical patients with atrial fibrillation. *Ann Thorac Surg.* 1996;61(2):755–759.

8. Cresti A, Garca-Fernndez MA, De Sensi F, et al. Prevalence of auricular thrombosis before atrial flutter cardioversion: a 17-year transoesophageal echocardiographic study. *Europace.* 2015;18(3):450–456.

9. Ussia GP, Mulè M, Cammalleri V, et al. Percutaneous closure of left atrial appendage to prevent embolic events in high-risk patients with chronic atrial fibrillation. *Cathet Cardiovasc Interv.* 2009;74(2):217–222.

10. Di Biase L, Santangeli P, Anselmino M, et al. Does the left atrial appendage morphology correlate with the risk of stroke in patients with atrial fibrillation? results from a multicenter study. *J Am Coll Cardiol.* 2012;60(6):531. http://www.ncbi.nlm.nih.gov/pubmed/22858289.

11. Hsu JC, Maddox TM, Kennedy KF, et al. Oral anticoagulant therapy prescription in patients with atrial fibrillation across the spectrum of stroke risk: insights from the NCDR PINNACLE registry. *JAMA Cardiol.* 2016;1(1):55–62. https://doi.org/10.1001/jamacardio.2015.0374.

12. Kosiuk J, Nedios S, Kornej J, et al. Impact of left atrial appendage morphology on peri-interventional thromboembolic risk during catheter ablation of atrial fibrillation. *Heart Rhythm.* 2014;11(9):1522–1527. https://doi.org/10.1016/j.hrthm.2014.05.022. http://www.ncbi.nlm.nih.gov/pubmed/24858813.

13. Nedios S, Kornej J, Koutalas E, et al. Left atrial appendage morphology and thromboembolic risk after catheter ablation for atrial fibrillation. *Heart Rhythm.* 2014;11(12):2239–2246. https://doi.org/10.1016/j.hrthm.2014.08.016. http://www.ncbi.nlm.nih.gov/pubmed/25128733.

14. Je HG, Shuman DJ, Ad N. A systematic review of minimally invasive surgical treatment for atrial fibrillation: a comparison of the cox-maze procedure, beating-heart epicardial ablation, and the hybrid procedure on safety and efficacy. *Eur J Cardiothorac Surg.* 2015;48(4):531–541.

15. Healey JS, Crystal E, Lamy A, et al. Left atrial appendage occlusion study (LAAOS): results of a randomized controlled pilot study of left atrial appendage occlusion during coronary bypass surgery in patients at risk for stroke. *Am Heart J.* 2005;150(2):288–293.

16. Cox JL, Ad N, Palazzo T. Impact of the maze procedure on the stroke rate in patients with atrial fibrillation. *J Thorac Cardiovasc Surg.* 1999;118(5):833–840.

17. Prasad SM, Maniar HS, Camillo CJ, et al. The cox maze III procedure for atrial fibrillation: long-term efficacy in patients undergoing lone versus concomitant procedures. *J Thorac Cardiovasc Surg.* 2003;126(6):1822–1827.

18. Tsai Y, Phan K, Munkholm-Larsen S, Tian DH, La Meir M, Yan TD. Surgical left atrial appendage occlusion during cardiac surgery for patients with atrial fibrillation: a meta-analysis. *Eur J Cardiothorac Surg.* 2014;47(5):847–854.

19. Melduni R, Schaff H, Lee H, et al. Impact of left atrial appendage closure during cardiac surgery on the occurrence of early postoperative atrial fibrillation, stroke, and mortality: a propensity score–matched analysis of 10 633 patients. *Circulation.* 2017;135(4):366–378. https://doi.org/10.1161/CIRCULATIONAHA.116.021952.

20. Kanderian AS, Gillinov AM, Pettersson GB, Blackstone E, Klein AL. Success of surgical left atrial appendage closure: assessment by transesophageal echocardiography. *J Am Coll Cardiol.* 2008;52(11):924–929.

21. Ailawadi G, Gerdisch MW, Harvey RL, et al. Exclusion of the left atrial appendage with a novel device: early results of a multicenter trial. *J Thorac Cardiovasc Surg.* 2011;142(5): 1009.e1.

22. Slater AD, Tatooles AJ, Coffey A, et al. Prospective clinical study of a novel left atrial appendage occlusion device. *Ann Thorac Surg.* 2012;93(6):2035–2040.

23. Cox JL. Mechanical closure of the left atrial appendage: is it time to be more aggressive? *J Thorac Cardiovasc Surg.* 2013;146(5):1027.e2.

24. Bartus K, Han FT, Bednarek J, et al. Percutaneous left atrial appendage suture ligation using the LARIAT device in patients with atrial fibrillation: initial clinical experience. *J Am Coll Cardiol.* 2013;62(2):108–118.

25. Price MJ, Gibson DN, Yakubov SJ, et al. Early safety and efficacy of percutaneous left atrial appendage suture ligation. *J Am Coll Cardiol.* 2014;64(6):565–572.

26. US Food and Drug Administration, Use of LARIAT Suture Delivery Device for left atrial appendage closure: FDA safety communication, 2015.

27. Lee RJ, Lakkireddy D, Mittal S, et al. Percutaneous alternative to the maze procedure for the treatment of persistent or long-standing persistent atrial fibrillation (aMAZE trial): rationale and design. *Am Heart J.* 2015;170(6):1184–1194. https://doi.org/10.1016/j.ahj.2015.09.019. http://www.ncbi.nlm.nih.gov/pubmed/26678640.

28. Meier B, Blaauw Y, Khattab AA, et al. EHRA/EAPCI expert consensus statement on catheter-based left atrial appendage occlusion. *Europace.* 2014;16: euu174.

29. Ostermayer SH, Reisman M, Kramer PH, et al. Percutaneous left atrial appendage transcatheter occlusion (PLAATO system) to prevent stroke in high-risk patients with non-rheumatic atrial fibrillation: results from the international multi-center feasibility trials. *J Am Coll Cardiol.* 2005;46(1):9–14.

30. Block PC, Burstein S, Casale PN, et al. Percutaneous left atrial appendage occlusion for patients in atrial fibrillation suboptimal for warfarin therapy: 5-year results of the PLAATO (percutaneous left atrial appendage transcatheter occlusion) study. *JACC Cardiovasc Interv.* 2009;2(7):594–600.

31. Saw J, Lempereur M. Percutaneous left atrial appendage closure: procedural techniques and outcomes. *JACC Cardiovasc Interv.* 2014;7(11):1205–1220.

32. Holmes DR, Reddy VY, Turi ZG, et al. Percutaneous closure of the left atrial appendage versus warfarin therapy for prevention of stroke in patients with atrial fibrillation: a randomised non-inferiority trial. *Lancet.* 2009;374(9689):534–542.

33. Reddy VY, Sievert H, Halperin J, et al. Percutaneous left atrial appendage closure vs warfarin for atrial fibrillation: a randomized clinical trial. *JAMA*. 2014;312(19):1988–1998.
34. Holmes DR, Kar S, Price MJ, et al. Prospective randomized evaluation of the watchman left atrial appendage closure device in patients with atrial fibrillation versus long-term warfarin therapy: the PREVAIL trial. *J Am Coll Cardiol*. 2014;64(1):1–12.
35. Masoudi FA, Calkins H, Kavinsky CJ, et al. 2015 ACC/HRS/SCAI left atrial appendage occlusion device societal overview. *J Am Coll Cardiol*. 2015;66(13):1497–1513. https://doi.org/10.1016/j.jacc.2015.06.028. http://www.ncbi.nlm.nih.gov/pubmed/26133570.
36. Boersma LV, Schmidt B, Betts TR, et al. Implant success and safety of left atrial appendage closure with the WATCHMAN device: peri-procedural outcomes from the EWOLUTION registry. *Eur Heart J*. 2016;37(31):2465–2474.
37. Reddy VY, Gibson DN, Kar S, et al. Post-approval US experience with left atrial appendage closure for stroke prevention in atrial fibrillation. *J Am Coll Cardiol*. 2017;69(3):253–261.
38. Saw J, Price MJ. Assessing the safety of early U.S. commercial application of left atrial appendage closure. *J Am Coll Cardiol*. 2017;69(3):262–264. https://doi.org/10.1016/j.jacc.2016.10.019. http://search.proquest.com/docview/1861146115.
39. Koifman E, Lipinski MJ, Escarcega RO, et al. Comparison of watchman device with new oral anti-coagulants in patients with atrial fibrillation: a network meta-analysis. *Int J Cardiol*. 2016;205:17–22.
40. Kavinsky CJ, Kusumoto FM, Bavry AA, et al. SCAI/ACC/HRS institutional and operator requirements for left atrial appendage occlusion. *Cathet Cardiovasc Interv*. 2016;87(3):351–362.
41. Waksman R, Pendyala LK. Overview of the food and drug administration circulatory system devices panel meetings on WATCHMAN left atrial appendage closure therapy. *Am J Cardiol*. 2015;115(3):378–384. https://doi.org/10.1016/j.amjcard.2014.11.011. http://www.ncbi.nlm.nih.gov/pubmed/25579887.
42. Kirchhof P, Benussi S, Kotecha D, et al. 2016 ESC guidelines for the management of atrial fibrillation developed in collaboration with EACTS the task force for the management of atrial fibrillation of the european society of cardiology (ESC) developed with the special contribution of the european heart rhythm association (EHRA) of the ESCEndorsed by the european stroke organisation (ESO). *Eur J Cardiothorac Surg*. 2016;50: ezw313.
43. Nietlispach F, Gloekler S, Krause R, et al. Amplatzer left atrial appendage occlusion: single center 10-year experience. *Cathet Cardiovasc Interv*. 2013;82(2):283–289.
44. Piccini JP, Sievert H, Patel MR. Left atrial appendage occlusion: rationale, evidence, devices, and patient selection. *Eur Heart J*. 2017;38(12):869–876.
45. Tzikas A, Shakir S, Gafoor S, et al. Left atrial appendage occlusion for stroke prevention in atrial fibrillation: multicentre experience with the AMPLATZER cardiac plug. *EuroIntervention*. 2015;10(10): 20140801–20140825.
46. Freixa X, Chan JLK, Tzikas A, Garceau P, Basmadjian A, Ibrahim R. The amplatzer™ cardiac plug 2 for left atrial appendage occlusion: novel features and first-in-man experience. *EuroIntervention*. 2013;8(9):1094–1098. https://doi.org/10.4244/EIJV8I9A167.
47. Kleinecke C, Park J, Gdde M, Zintl K, Schnupp S, Brachmann J. Twelve-month follow-up of left atrial appendage occlusion with amplatzer amulet. *Cardiol J*. 2017;24(2):131–138.
48. Hildick-Smith D. Results from the AMULET OBSERVATIONAL STUDY reported at TCT 2016. *Biotech Bus Week*. 2016;165.
49. St. Jude medical launches global clinical trial of amplatzer amulet in patients at an increased risk of stroke due to atrial fibrillation, M2 Pharma, September 1, 2016.
50. Reddy VY, Franzen O, Worthley S. Clinical experience with the wavecrest LA appendage occlusion device for stroke prevention in AF: acute results of the WAVECREST I trial. In: *The Heart Rhythm Society's 35th Annual Scientific Sessions.San Francisco*. 2014.
51. Enomoto Y, Gadiyaram VK, Gianni C, et al. Use of non-warfarin oral anticoagulants instead of warfarin during left atrial appendage closure with the watchman device. *Heart Rhythm*. 2017;14(1):19–24. https://doi.org/10.1016/j.hrthm.2016.10.020.
52. Reddy VY, Möbius-Winkler S, Miller MA, et al. Left atrial appendage closure with the watchman device in patients with a contraindication for oral anticoagulation: the ASAP study (ASA plavix feasibility study with watchman left atrial appendage closure technology). *J Am Coll Cardiol*. 2013;61(25):2551. http://www.ncbi.nlm.nih.gov/pubmed/23583249.
53. V.M. Yuste, ELIGIBLE (efficacy of left atrIal appendage closure after GastroIntestinal BLEeding), 2017.
54. Martin-Yuste V. Outcomes from gastrointestinal hemorrhage in oral anticoagulated patients with atrial fibrillation. Is there a target for left atrial appendage closure? *Gastroenterol Hepatol Open Access*. 2016;5(6). https://doi.org/10.15406/ghoa.2016.05.00163.
55. Reddy VY, Akehurst RL, Armstrong SO, Amorosi SL, Beard SM, Holmes DR. Time to cost-effectiveness following stroke reduction strategies in AF: warfarin versus NOACs versus LAA closure. *J Am Coll Cardiol*. 2015;66(24):2728–2739.
56. Chanda A, Reilly JP. Left atrial appendage occlusion for stroke prevention. *Prog Cardiovasc Dis*. 2017;59(6):626–635.

FURTHER READING

1. Petersen P, Godtfredsen J, Boysen G, Andersen E, Andersen B. Placebo-controlled, randomised trial of warfarin and aspirin for prevention of thromboembolic complications in chronic atrial fibrillation: the copenhagen AFASAK study. *Lancet*. 1989;333(8631):175–179.
2. Site HG. Clopidogrel plus aspirin versus oral anticoagulation for atrial fibrillation in the atrial fibrillation clopidogrel trial with irbesartan for prevention of vascular events (ACTIVE W): a randomised controlled trial. *Lancet*. 2006;367:1903–1912.

3. Stroke Prevention in Atrial Fibrillation Investigators. Warfarin versus aspirin for prevention of thromboembolism in atrial fibrillation: stroke prevention in atrial fibrillation II study. *Lancet*. 1994;343(8899):687–691.
4. Stroke Prevention in Atrial Fibrillation Investigators. Adjusted-dose warfarin versus low-intensity, fixed-dose warfarin plus aspirin for high-risk patients with atrial fibrillation: stroke prevention in atrial fibrillation III randomised clinical trial. *Lancet*. 1996;348(9028):633–638.
5. Connolly SJ, Ezekowitz MD, Yusuf S, et al. Dabigatran versus warfarin in patients with atrial fibrillation. *N Engl J Med*. 2009;2009(361):1139–1151.
6. Granger CB, Alexander JH, McMurray JJ, et al. Apixaban versus warfarin in patients with atrial fibrillation. *N Engl J Med*. 2011;365(11):981–992.
7. Patel MR, Mahaffey KW, Garg J, et al. Rivaroxaban versus warfarin in nonvalvular atrial fibrillation. *N Engl J Med*. 2011;365(10):883–891.
8. Giugliano RP, Ruff CT, Braunwald E, et al. Edoxaban versus warfarin in patients with atrial fibrillation. *N Engl J Med*. 2013;369(22):2093–2104.

CHAPTER 12

Patients Taking Oral Anticoagulants for Atrial Fibrillation With Concomitant Complex Disease States

WILLIAM J. HUCKER, MD, PHD • MITUL KANZARIA, MD •
JOHN U. DOHERTY, MD, FACC

Management of patients with nonvalvular atrial fibrillation (AF) without complex medical illnesses is relatively straightforward. Patients such as those enrolled in the landmark clinical trials have anticoagulation decisions that are often simple: evaluating the risks and benefits of anticoagulant therapy in the prevention of a thrombotic event. In clinical practice, however, patients with AF on anticoagulants frequently have other comorbid conditions. Common comorbidities such as coronary or peripheral artery disease, chronic kidney disease, an active malignancy, prior cerebrovascular accidents, obesity, or prior bleeding events all complicate the decision-making surrounding anticoagulation, and guidance on such patients is often limited. The following case scenarios and associated discussion illustrate some of the complicated decision-making that often accompanies patients with these common comorbidities when anticoagulation may be indicated.

MANAGEMENT OF ANTICOAGULANTS IN ASSOCIATION WITH ANTIPLATELET THERAPY

In patients with coronary artery disease (CAD) or peripheral arterial disease, the use of either single or dual antiplatelet therapy agents (DAPTs) increases bleeding risk and may affect the risk-benefit ratio of anticoagulation. This is an especially challenging group of patients. Ongoing or completed clinical trials will lend clarity to scenarios where direct oral anticoagulants are used with antiplatelet therapy in patients undergoing coronary stenting. Protocols that will allow maximum clinical benefit in such patients and strive to reduce risk are being devised. Challenging an old paradigm, the incremental benefit of aspirin therapy in stable patients with coronary disease is open to

question when those patients also have an indication for anticoagulation.[1]

Case

A 67-year-old man with a history of permanent AF, two transient ischemic attacks, hypertension, ischemic cardiomyopathy with placement of an ICD (implantable cardioverter-defibrillator), and CAD with a history of a coronary artery bypass grafting with previous placement of two bare metal stents (BMSs) in the saphenous vein graft to the right coronary artery a year ago who now presents with episodes of angina with walking that are relieved with nitroglycerin, and troponins are negative. The patient is currently on warfarin and clopidogrel and previously has had significant epistaxis while he was on aspirin. The patient undergoes cardiac catheterization, which shows restenosis in the previously placed stents in the saphenous vein graft (SVG) to the right coronary artery. A second-generation everolimus drug-eluting stent (DES) was placed in the SVG. The patient was discharged on aspirin, clopidogrel, and warfarin.

Case commentary: It is well known that combining antiplatelet agents with anticoagulation therapy is associated with an elevated bleeding risk. In the Randomized Evaluation of Long-Term Anticoagulation Therapy (RE-LY) trial of dabigatran or warfarin for patients with nonvalvular AF, the risk of major bleeding increased from 2.8% to 4.8% when antiplatelet agents were added to warfarin therapy. Similarly the risk of major bleeding was 2.6%/year with dabigatran 150 mg twice a day but increased to 4.4%/year with the addition of antiplatelet agents.[2] Similarly in the Apixaban for Reduction in Stroke and Other Thromboembolic Events in Atrial Fibrillation (ARISTOTLE) trial, increased bleeding was noted when aspirin was used in conjunction with either warfarin or apixaban therapy although the combination of aspirin and warfarin was associated with a higher bleeding risk than aspirin and apixaban.[3] The same concerns arise with the use of rivaroxaban or edoxaban.[4,5]

There are several different scenarios of patients with CAD requiring stenting and AF requiring anticoagulation. First, patients who have recently been treated with coronary stenting may develop new-onset AF. Second, elective stenting is undertaken in patients previously treated with anticoagulants for AF. Third, acute coronary syndromes can occur in patients with established AF taking anticoagulants. Fourth, patients may develop AF greater than 1 month after BMS or greater than 6 months after a DES, opening the door for a modification of therapy. Fifth, the patient with established AF currently taking anticoagulants can develop an acute coronary syndrome that is managed medically (Fig. 12.1).

The choice and dose of antiplatelets are important when considering prevention of recurrent events and bleeding risk. Low-dose aspirin (75–100 mg) is preferred; it provides ischemic protection with lower bleeding than higher doses. Ticagrelor and prasugrel are more potent antiplatelet agents and result in increased non-CABG-related bleeding. For this reason, many consider clopidogrel to be the preferred agent.[6] In the Trial to Assess Improvement in Therapeutic Outcomes by Optimizing Platelet Inhibition with Prasugrel-Thrombolysis in Myocardial Infarction 38 (TRITON-TIMI 38), prasugrel was associated with higher rates of TIMI major, life-threatening, and fatal bleeding with an improvement in ischemic events but no difference in mortality when compared with clopidogrel.[7] The benefits of DES versus BMS are well known, but traditionally have required longer durations of DAPT. The use of BMS may be safer than DES in patients requiring triple therapy, but certain presentations and anatomical factors (in-stent restenosis, bifurcated lesions, small vessels) may benefit with the use of a DES. Recent studies have showed that shorter duration of DAPT may be safe in patients with second-generation DES implantation. The benefits of DES need to be balanced with the increased bleeding risk of longer DAPT in patients who also need concurrent OAC.

The optimal duration of DAPT is a controversial issue, even in the absence of OAC. In the Intracoronary Stenting and Antithrombotic Regimen (ISAR-TRIPLE) trial, patients with AF who underwent placement of a DES were randomized to either 6 weeks or 6 months of triple therapy.[8] There was no significant difference in the primary composite endpoint of death, acute myocardial infarction, stent thrombosis, stroke, or TIMI major bleed. In the What is the Optimal antiplatElet

and anticoagulant therapy in patient with oral anticoagulation and coronary StenTing (WOEST) trial, an open-label, randomized trial, the comparison of triple therapy (with warfarin + clopidogrel 75 mg + low-dose aspirin) against double therapy (warfarin + clopidogrel) demonstrated lower bleeding rates, although driven mainly by lower rates of minor bleeds. Additionally, there was a lower rate of deaths in the warfarin + clopidogrel arm.[9] In the 2014 ACC/AHA guidelines, the use of clopidogrel and warfarin without aspirin was given a IIb indication.[10]

The factors to consider in determining the duration require evaluation of a patient's bleeding risk, stent thrombosis risk, and ischemic risk. Many factors need to be considered, including the patient's bleeding risk, the clinical presentation (stable angina vs. acute coronary syndromes), history of multiple myocardial infarctions, risk of stroke with AF, size of stent, location of stent, type of stent, in-stent restenosis, and more.

A recent consensus statement suggested that the following factors favor a shortening of triple therapy. They include a high bleeding risk and low atherothrombotic risk by REACH or SYNTAX scores for elective PCI and a GRACE score of ≥118 if an ACS. Conversely, factors that favor a prolongation of triple therapy are use of a first-generation DES, high atherothrombotic risk scores, stenting of the left main, proximal left anterior descending, proximal bifurcation, recurrent MI, or a low bleeding risk.[11]

The evidence from the phase 3 trials for direct-acting oral anticoagulants (DOACs) showed that apixaban, edoxaban, and low-dose dabigatran had significantly lower major bleeds when compared with warfarin. The Open-Label, Randomized, Controlled, Multicenter Study Exploring Two Treatment Strategies of Rivaroxaban and a Dose-Adjusted Oral Vitamin K Antagonist Treatment Strategy in Subjects with Atrial Fibrillation Who Undergo Percutaneous Coronary Intervention (PIONEER-AF-PCI) is the first available clinical trial comparing the use of a DOAC (rivaroxaban) with warfarin in a triple therapy regimen. In this trial, there was a decrease in a composite bleeding endpoint, including major bleeding, minor bleeding, and bleeding requiring medical attention at 12 months in the rivaroxaban group with no difference in major adverse cardiovascular events between the groups. The trial was not powered to determine differences in stroke or stent thrombosis.[12] The Randomized Evaluation of Dual Antithrombotic Therapy With Dabigatran Versus Triple Therapy With Warfarin in Patients With Nonvalvular Atrial Fibrillation Undergoing Percutaneous Coronary Intervention (RE-DUAL PCI) evaluated dabigatran in

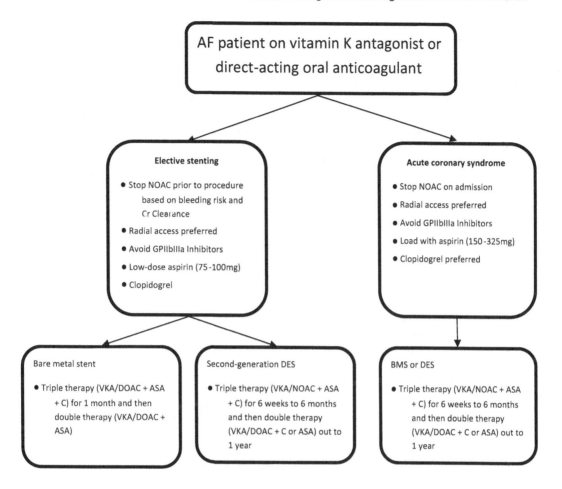

* Shorten combination therapy in patients with high bleeding risk (HAS-BLED > 3) or low atherothrombotic risk (REACH or SYNTAX score or GRACE < 118 for ACS)

* Lengthen combination therapy in patients with first-generation DES, low bleeding risk (HAS-BLED 0-2), or high atherothrombotic risk (by risk score or if stenting in left main, proximal left anterior descending, or proximal bifurcation)

* Use of proton pump inhibitors (PPI) is reasonable in patients while on triple therapy and in patients with an increased risk of gastrointestinal bleeding.

FIG. 12.1 Patients with underlying atrial fibrillation on anticoagulation requiring coronary stenting. (Adapted from Kovacs RJ, Flaker GC, Saxonhouse SJ, et al. Practical management of anticoagulation in patients with atrial fibrillation. *J Am Coll Cardiol*. 2015;65(13):1340–1360.)

both 110 mg b.i.d. and 150 mg b.i.d doses with a P2Y12 inhibitor compared with warfarin and a P2Y12 inhibitor and aspirin (for 1 month with a BMS and 3 months with a DES). The dabigatran-based regimens showed noninferiority to the warfarin-based regimen for the combined endpoint of death, thrombotic events, or unplanned revascularization. Bleeding events were less common in both dabigatran-based regimens with significant decreases in major and clinically relevant nonmajor bleeding.[13] Trials investigating the use of apixaban (AUGUSTUS) and edoxaban ENTRUST-AF-PCI are currently under way.

PATIENTS WITH A PRIOR CEREBROVASCULAR ACCIDENT OR INTRACRANIAL HEMORRHAGE

Patients with stroke ranging from ischemic stroke to intracranial hemorrhage (ICH) present an especially challenging conundrum. They may be patients who present with an acute ischemic stroke despite anticoagulant therapy, or patients who develop an ICH in the setting of prior anticoagulation. In addition, in patients who present with traumatic ICH or subdural hematoma, the question arises: for how long should anticoagulation be withheld? We describe two cases that illustrate the nuances involved with anticoagulation in these scenarios.

Case: Ischemic Stroke

A 90-year-old woman with a history of transient AF detected once in the setting of prior knee replacement surgery and a previous a history of lower gastrointestinal (GI) bleeding attributed to diverticulosis, and underlying hypertension presents to the hospital with shortness of breath and was diagnosed with pneumonia. Her home medications included aspirin, metoprolol, and a statin. Her electrocardiogram (ECG) demonstrated AF with a controlled ventricular response. On her fourth day of hospitalization, she develops slurred speech and left-sided hemiparesis. An emergent head CT reveals an acute ischemic right middle cerebral artery stroke. She receives tissue-plasminogen activator (tPA) within 2 h of the start of her symptoms and she is left with relatively mild right-sided hemiparesis.

Case commentary: This case raises several common management dilemmas regarding anticoagulation, and she may not have been anticoagulated because of two different reasons. The first is that her only prior detection of AF was in the setting of a prior surgery, which was felt to be a secondary precipitant of AF. It is common to encounter episodes of secondary AF clinically, where AF is felt to be precipitated by a postoperative state, pneumonia, alcohol abuse, or pericardial disease, to name a few causes. This condition is often considered different than AF that has no clear precipitant, although there is relatively little evidence about the long-term implications of secondary AF. In a recent analysis of patients in the Framingham Heart Study, patients with AF that occurred after a secondary precipitant had similar stroke and mortality rates to those diagnosed with AF that had no clear precipitant.[14] AF recurrence rates were lower in the secondary AF cohort; although when patients with cardiac surgery as the AF precipitant were excluded, recurrence rates were similar. This observation suggests that outside of the situation of cardiac

surgery, where there is a direct insult to the atrial myocardium, the occurrence of AF in the presence of a secondary precipitant may just be unmasking the presence of the appropriate substrate for AF, and therefore that patient's long-term risk for recurrent AF and the comorbid conditions that accompany it are elevated and similar to those with no clear reversible cause of AF. In the patient in the case above, she was admitted with pneumonia, which is a common secondary precipitant of AF, and it is not surprising that she developed recurrent AF in this situation and she unfortunately developed a stroke because of it.

The second contributing factor to her lack of anticoagulation at the time of presentation was her history of GI bleeding. The discontinuation of oral anticoagulation after a bleeding event is often associated with adverse outcomes: a direct consequence of not reinitiating anticoagulant therapy. This is especially true after a GI bleed, which is a common complication of anticoagulation. While there may be trepidation on the part of the clinician and patient to restart anticoagulation after a GI bleed, patients who had a GI bleed associated with oral anticoagulation who then resume anticoagulation have a lower risk of thromboembolism and death compared with those who did not restart. Interestingly, they had no statistically different increase in recurrent bleeding.[15] In the case above, the patient did not have GI bleeding previously in the setting of anticoagulation; however, a trial of anticoagulation in this patient despite her history of prior GI bleeding is likely safe from the hemorrhagic perspective and indicated in light of her stroke and underlying AF.

Stroke While on Anticoagulation

Had the patient mentioned above been on anticoagulation, her stroke risk would have been reduced, but not completely mitigated. Stroke or TIA while on anticoagulation for AF is relatively uncommon; however, patients with high CHA_2DS_2VASc scores have a residual stroke risk on anticoagulation, and therefore treatment strategies need to be devised to deal with these patients. One possible reason for stroke while on anticoagulation is either medication noncompliance or subtherapeutic anticoagulation while on warfarin therapy. Nevertheless true treatment failures in patients on therapeutic anticoagulation at the time of stroke do occur. Fortunately, the stroke severity is typically less if the patient was on anticoagulation at the time of the event.[16]

In the acute setting, patients taking DOACs who present with an ischemic stroke represent a challenge in treatment, namely due to the dilemma of possible thrombolytic therapy. If there is residual drug affect, thrombolytic therapy should probably not be offered, although determining whether residual drug is present is not reliably assayed with DOACs with conventional studies such as the PT/INR or PTT and may require specialized assays If the patient was on warfarin, the risk of ICH with tPA appears low if the tnternational normalized ratio (INR) is less than or equal to 1.7.[17]

The timing of anticoagulation initiation after an ischemic stroke can be challenging as well. While the risk of stroke is high in the weeks after an ischemic stroke occurs, the risk of hemorrhagic conversion is elevated as well. Risk factors for hemorrhagic conversion include large infarct size, uncontrolled hypertension, prior ICH, and hemorrhagic conversion on initial imaging. The presence of any of these factors or others may raise the likelihood of hemorrhage and will likely delay the initiation of anticoagulation. In the absence of such risk factors, initiation of anticoagulation within 14 days after a stroke is likely indicated.[18] In such patients the American Heart Association/American stroke Association guidelines recommend warfarin as a Class 1 indication with Level of Evidence A, apixaban a Class 1 recommendation Level of Evidence A, dabigatran Class 1 recommendation Level of Evidence B, or rivaroxaban a Class 2A recommendation Level of Evidence B. These guidelines came out before the FDA approval of edoxaban.[18] In patients who presented with a therapeutic INR on warfarin at the time of their stroke or TIA, consideration can be given to substituting a DOACnt. In such patients warfarin effect should be allowed to dissipate before initiating DOAC therapy.

Cryptogenic Stroke

One can easily imagine a similar case to that above where the patient was not observed to have AF, but the arrhythmia is highly suspected. Patients with stroke or TIA presumed of cardioembolic origin not previously anticoagulated often represent a challenge to clinicians because AF is not always documented at presentation. In such patients, prolonged monitoring with an implantable loop recorder may document AF.[19] There are ongoing clinical trials of rivaroxaban, dabigatran, and apixaban in patients with ischemic stroke, presumed embolic, of undetermined source in whom AF has not been documented.

Case: Intracranial Hemorrhage

A 68-year-old man with a history of persistent AF (CHA_2DS_2VASc 5: HTN, prior ischemic CVA, abdominal aortic aneurysm) who while on rivaroxaban developed word finding difficulties and decreased level of consciousness. He is brought to the emergency department where his initial blood pressure is 220/110, and an emergent head CT reveals a thalamic ICH with ventricular extension. At the time of presentation, his glomerular filtration rate is >60 mL/min.

Case commentary: ICH is the most dreaded complication of OAC therapy. Fortunately, these events are rare, however, the 30-day mortality approaching 50%.[20] In the acute setting, the presence of any anticoagulant will complicate treatment and likely worsen the bleeding. Reversal of the anticoagulant to the degree possible is indicated; the precise agents used for reversal will vary depending on the anticoagulant. The only approved agent for DOACs is the reversal agent idarucizumab for dabigatran. Other compounds are undergoing development or pending approval for the Xa inhibitors. Prothrombin-complex concentrate or fresh-frozen plasma is used for warfarin reversal.

After the acute event, there will be a need for a decision regarding whether OAC should be restarted if anticoagulation is still indicated. Given the mortality risk associated with intracranial bleeds, a cautious individualized approach to restarting anticoagulation after ICH is warranted with a careful review of factors that may increase the risk of a future hemorrhage. First, the mechanism of ICH is predictive of future events, with traumatic ICH being less likely to recur than spontaneous bleeds. Second, the location of the bleed needs to be carefully reviewed. Lobar ICHs are suggestive of amyloid angiopathy, whereas a thalamic hemorrhage is suggestive of hypertension as the cause. Amyloid angiopathy patients are at particularly high risk of hemorrhage with OAC, and therefore anticoagulation is usually avoided in these patients. Third, the presence and number of microbleeds on MRI are predictive of future hemorrhages. Finally, the presence of anticoagulation itself is a risk factor as well. In addition, assiduous control of risk factors that may have contributed to the bleed, such as hypertension, is necessary.

Limited data exist on the reinitiation of OAC after an ICH, and the reinitiation of OAC will depend on the factors discussed above. However, restarting anticoagulation after a nonlobar ICH can be considered. It is important to note that in patients with warfarin-associated ICH, resumption of anticoagulation was associated with lower risk of thrombosis and ischemic stroke, and lower risk of death without a significantly increased risk of recurrent bleeding compared with discontinuation.[21] Lobar ICH secondary to amyloid angiopathy (either spontaneous or while taking warfarin) and spontaneous subdural hematomas have a particularly high risk of rebleeding; therefore resumption of anticoagulation should likely be avoided in these situations

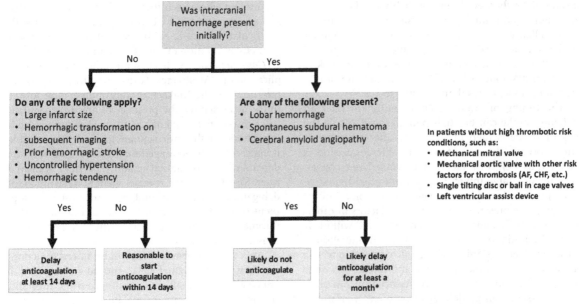

FIG. 12.2 Starting anticoagulation after stroke in the setting of atrial fibrillation.

or performed in consultation with either neurology or neurosurgical expertise. DOACs are associated with a lower risk of ICH than warfarin, but the safety of switching a patient with an ICH to a DOAC has not been evaluated. When to restart anticoagulation varies widely in observational studies (72h–30weeks), reflecting a lack of consensus. However, in patients without mechanical heart valves, guidelines recommend avoiding anticoagulation for at least 4weeks.[22] Fig. 12.2 suggests an approach to anticoagulation in the setting of ischemic stroke and ICH.

PATIENTS WITH ATRIAL FIBRILLATION AND UNDERLYING CANCER DIAGNOSIS: IMPLICATIONS FOR ANTITHROMBOTIC THERAPY

Patients with an underlying cancer diagnosis are often difficult to maintain within a therapeutic range on warfarin therapy. In addition to the AF anticoagulation indication, these patients remain at high risk of deep venous thrombosis. Nutritional status and drug-drug interactions make warfarin dosing especially challenging.

Case

A 76-year-old woman with a medical history of hypertension, heart failure, and non-insulin-dependent diabetes mellitus, with persistent AF (CHA_2DS_2-VASc score of 6) is treated with apixaban 5mg BID. She presents with a 2-week history of gross hematuria and dysuria. The patient is found to be anemic with a hemoglobin level of 9.7g/dL, down from a baseline in the 12–13g/dL range. The patient undergoes a workup by urology and is found to have a muscle-invasive urothelial carcinoma. The patient is being evaluated for radical cystectomy and chemotherapy. The patient's hemoglobin has stabilized but continues to have hematuria on a regular basis.

Case commentary: Therapeutic decisions in patients with an underlying malignancy who require anticoagulation are especially difficult. The association of a cancer diagnosis with AF is especially complex. Many of the comorbid conditions that predispose to thrombotic events in AF patients are also present in older cancer patients including heart failure, hypertension, underlying vascular disease, and diabetes. It is also well appreciated that many underlying cancers, as well as the therapies used to treat them, are associated with a prothrombotic state. Cancer patients are also more prone to bleeding. They may be thrombocytopenic from concomitant therapies or may have disease spread to areas where a bleeding event would be poorly tolerated such as the brain. We commonly use the CHA_2DS_2VASc score to denote thrombotic risk. We do not know the relative importance of these risk factors in patients with malignancy.[23] What is clear, however, is that patients with new cancer diagnoses are going to be more likely to be previously treated with DOACs for AF.[24]

Much of the experience with anticoagulants in patients with cancer comes from the treatment of venous thromboembolism (VTE) and pulmonary embolism (PE). Although DOACs have assumed a primary role in such patients without cancer, the experience in cancer patients is more limited. Low molecular weight heparin (LMWH) has emerged as the standard treatment option. There is of course little experience in the use of LMWH in preventing thromboembolic events in AF. From the experience with VTE and anticoagulation, we have learned that although therapy is effective in patients with cancer, it is associated with a higher morbidity both from recurrent VTE and anticoagulation-associated bleeding. LMWH has emerged as the standard in these patients with demonstrated superiority over warfarin because of difficulty in maintaining a therapeutic INR in cancer patients.[25,26]

Management of AF is challenging in cancer patients. There are drug-drug interactions with antiarrhythmic drugs and targeted cancer therapies. Specific cancer therapies have been associated with a higher incidence of AF including ibrutinib.[27] Clinical trials using DOACs for AF have generally excluded patients with cancer; therefore clinical experience remains limited. Some targeted therapies have also been associated with QT interval prolongation and bradycardia. On the other hand, many antiarrhythmics may interact with targeted therapies, and therefore careful attention is required to monitor for drug interactions. Traditional risk factor stratification tools such as the CHA_2DS_2VASc score have not been validated in patients with underlying cancer. Bleeding risk is certainly increased in most cancer patients who are anticoagulated; however, they may be more challenging to anticoagulate as well. For instance, a retrospective study of patients with nonvalvular AF and newly diagnosed malignancy found that only 12% of patients on vitamin K antagonists maintained a therapeutic INR.[28] This makes the idea of using DOACs in such patients attractive although there is limited clinical evidence to support their use.

As stated in a recent review of AF treatment in patients with cancer,[23] therapy needs to be individualized. Presence of intracranial tumors, underlying thrombocytopenia, and other coagulation defect that may be present in patients with hematologic malignancies may make anticoagulant therapy in balance too hazardous. Conversely, in patients with cancers associated with a very high thromboembolic risk and AF may benefit from anticoagulation even if they are assessed as low risk by tools such as CHA_2DS_2VASc.

SPECIAL PATIENT POPULATIONS AND PATIENTS WHO ARE EXCLUDED FROM CLINICAL TRIALS THAT PRESENT CHALLENGES IN ANTICOAGULATION FOR ATRIAL FIBRILLATION

Data from clinical trials guide our decision-making in everyday practice; however, the complex patients seen in clinic do not always match those included in trials. Factors such as extremes in age, renal function, hepatic function, and body mass index (BMI) are commonly underrepresented in clinical trials, and therefore the conclusions that clinicians can draw from trials for these patients are often limited. Similarly, patients on strong CYP3A4 or P-glycoprotein inhibitors or inducers are often excluded. Obviously, in many cases, several of these factors may be combined in a single patient; however, the degree of interaction between age, renal impairment, and BMI extremes when concomitantly present is even less clear. What we do know is that these effects are cumulative. When plasma concentrations of rivaroxaban were measured in patients who were very elderly (>90 years), weighed less than 40 kg, or had a CrCl of 30 or less, the levels were higher and persisted longer, especially so in patients aged >90 years who weighed <40 kg.[29-31] Accordingly, dosing recommendations for apixaban incorporate age, renal function, and body weight,[32] and rivaroxaban and edoxaban have dosing adjustments for renal function.

Case

A 68-year-old man with a history of prior substance abuse, chronic obstructive pulmonary disease, hepatitis C recently treated with ledipasvir/sofosbuvir but experienced a relapse after treatment, hypertension, diabetes mellitus, heart failure with a preserved ejection fraction, chronic kidney disease stage III, morbid obesity with a BMI of 43, and paroxysmal atrial flutter as well as AF presents to discuss anticoagulation options for his atrial arrhythmias. He has been on Coumadin in the past but had difficulty with compliance for monitoring and had wide swings in his INR with inadequate time in the therapeutic range. He was recently started on rivaroxaban.

In terms of his embolic risk, his CHADSVASC score is 4, conveying a 4.8% stroke risk per year and he warrants anticoagulation. However, the choice of agent warrants some consideration. He has a history of difficulty with Coumadin and therefore using a DOAC is reasonable. However, several factors in his medical history need to be considered when choosing an agent for this patient, namely his renal function, hepatic function, and obesity.

Renal Function

All DOACs have at least some renal clearance, and in medically complex patients, renal function can fluctuate significantly. In addition, patients with advanced renal disease (CrCl < 30 mL/min) are often excluded from clinical trials, and therefore guidance may be based on limited data. However, labeling for all DOACs will suggest dose adjustments based on renal function, and patients can be at risk for bleeding events if fluctuations in renal function occur and dose adjustments are not made. Depending on a patient's comorbidities, the renal function of a patient may be the defining comorbid condition that determines which DOAC to use. For instance, dabigatran is most dependent on renal clearance of the DOACs, whereas apixaban has recently been approved for use in hemodialysis patients. Nevertheless, the vast majority of experience for OAC in the dialysis population is with warfarin. Therefore the choice of OAC can be tailored to the renal function of the patient.

In this patient, he has a history of difficult-to-control INRs on warfarin, and therefore this is not an ideal choice even though he does have chronic kidney disease and warfarin is not affected by renal function. Dabigatran likely is not a good choice because of his renal dysfunction. Therefore a factor Xa inhibitor would likely be the best choice, and rivaroxaban, apixaban, and edoxaban all have recommended dose adjustments for his level of renal dysfunction. This will have to be monitored, and if his renal function substantially worsens, either a dose adjustment will have to be made, or he may need to be switched to another agent.

Hepatic Dysfunction

Close attention is usually paid to renal function, but liver function is often not systematically assessed. Clinicians are used to monitoring for hepatic dysfunction in a patient maintained on warfarin, but this is often less of a consideration for patients treated with a DOAC. We know, for example, that rivaroxaban is eliminated to the same extent hepatically and renally, and pharmacodynamic and pharmacokinetic properties of the drug are altered to a limited degree with mild liver impairment but to a significant degree with moderate or worse liver disease.[29] Factor Xa inhibitor use should be avoided in patients with Child-Pugh class C hepatic dysfunction,

and most agents recommend to avoid use in Child-Pugh class B hepatic impairment, or to use with caution in these patients (apixaban). In addition, factor Xa inhibitor use should be avoided in patients with any hepatic dysfunction associated with coagulopathy. For the direct thrombin inhibitor dabigatran, which is predominately cleared renally, there is no specific labeling in the United States that suggests dose adjustment or avoidance of dabigatran use in hepatic dysfunction.

In the case mentioned above, this patient has a history of hepatitis C that has been treated by ledipasvir/sofosbuvir; however, he suffered a relapse after treatment. He has no evidence of ascites; his albumin is in the normal range, and no encephalopathy. He has a mildly elevated INR; however, this may be due to the presence of rivaroxaban. Even if the elevated INR were due to hepatic dysfunction, he would be classified as Child-Pugh class A, and therefore no adjustment need to be made to rivaroxaban therapy because of hepatic dysfunction at this time.

Variations in Body Weight

Both high and low body weight individuals offer a clinical challenge, especially with the use of DOACs because without routine blood testing it is difficult to be sure for that a therapeutic state is achieved. What do we know about the obese or morbidly obese patient in terms of safety and efficacy of anticoagulant therapy? Some insights can be gained from pharmacokinetics (drug measurement) and pharmacodynamics (drug effect) in normal volunteers of various body weights. In a study of rivaroxaban, maximum concentrations of drug were similar in obese and normal weight individuals but higher in those weighing <50 kg. This resulted in a small increase in prothrombin time that was not considered clinically significant.[31] In the EINSTEIN-DVT and EINSTEIN-PE trials,[33,34] rivaroxaban was similarly effective in obese and nonobese patients. The cut-point for the diagnosis of obesity was 100 kg or greater. However, whether or not these results be extrapolated to morbidly obese patients is unclear, and the International Society for Thrombosis and Haemostasis guidelines suggest DOACs not be used in patients with a BMI > 40 or weight > 120 kg, and if they are used, peak and trough levels be measured via a drug-specific assay. If the drug levels are low, they recommend to switch to a vitamin K antagonist.[35] In the case mentioned above, this patient has an elevated BMI and therefore checking a peak and trough factor Xa level is reasonable; however based on the data from the EINSTEIN trials above, treatment with rivaroxaban is likely reasonable.

Drug Interactions

We have also relaxed our vigilance considering drug-drug interactions with the DOACs. The most concerning scenario is the combined use of drugs that are either both strong inducers and strong inhibitors of the CYP3A4 and P-glycoprotein. For rivaroxaban, strong inhibitors of both pathways mean more drug effect. Conversely, strong inducers of both lead to decreases in pharmacokinetic and pharmacodynamics effects. Strong inhibitors of one pathway or moderate inhibitors of both have lesser effects. Dabigatran is not affected by the CYP3A4 pathway, but since dabigatran is a P-gp substrate, the impact of inhibition on increasing blood levels with these drugs alone is significant. For apixaban, it should not

be given with strong CYP3A4 inhibitors but is not affected by competition for P-glycoprotein transport (Table 12.1). In the patient in the case above, he has many comorbidities and therefore a careful check of his other medications is warranted to evaluate for any possible drug interactions that may affect his rivaroxaban levels.

Anticoagulation of patients with complex disease states will continue to be a clinical challenge. Some clarity will emerge with regard to how anticoagulants should be used with antiplatelet agents in coronary interventions. Ongoing clinical trials regarding stroke will also shed light on this group of patients. The use of anticoagulation in oncology patients will continue to be challenging given the complexity of such patients and

TABLE 12.1
Drug Interactions Between DOACS and Commonly Prescribed Drugs

Medication	Mechanism	Dabigatran	Apixaban	Edoxaban	Rivaroxaban
Amiodarone	P-glycoprotein competition	↑↑	?	↑↑	− (unless CrCl < 50 mL/min)
Dronedarone	P-glycoprotein competition and CYP3A4 inhibition	↑↑↑	?	↑↑	↑
Quinidine	P-glycoprotein competition	↑↑	?	↑↑	?
Diltiazem	P-glycoprotein competition and weak CYP3A4 inhibition	−	↑↑	−	− (use with caution if CrCl < 50 mL/min)
Verapamil	P-glycoprotein competition and weak CYP3A4 inhibition.	↑↑ (reduce dose and take medications simultaneously)	?	↑↑ (reduce dose by 50%)	− (use with caution if CrCl < 50 mL/min)
Antifungals (fluconazole may have a lower impact on DOAC levels)	P-glycoprotein and BCRP competition and CYP3A4 inhibition	↑↑	↑↑	↑↑	↑↑
Cyclosporine and tacrolimus	P-glycoprotein competition	X (do Not Use)	?	↑↑	?
Rifampin Carbamazepine Phenobarbital Phenytoin St. John's wort	P-glycoprotein and BCRP and CYP3A4/CYP2 induction	↓	↓	↓ (do Not Use with Rifampin)	↓

↑, potential for increased drug effect; ↑↑, potential for greater increase in drug effect; ↑↑↑, potential for greatest increase in drug effect; ↓, potential for diminished drug effect; −, no interaction; ?, drug effect not known or not studied; x, do not use.
DOAC, direct-acting oral anticoagulant.

the wide variety of pharmacotherapy that these patients are subjected to. A good understanding of the metabolism of these agents, and their interactions with other agents, and as well as the need for individualized therapy when patients fall outside of the realm of those studied in clinical trials are paramount in safely anticoagulating our patients.

REFERENCES

1. Lambert M, Gislason GH, Lip GY, et al. Antiplatelet therapy for stable coronary artery disease in atrial fibrillation patients taking an oral anticoagulant: a nationwide cohort study. *Circulation*. 2014;129(15):1577–1585.
2. Connolly SJ, Ezekowitz YS, Yusuf S, et al. Dibigatran versus warfarin in patients with atrial fibrillation. *N Engl J Med*. 2009;361:1139–1151.
3. Granger CB, Alexander JH, Mcmurray JJ, et al. Apixaban versus warfarin in patients with atrial fibrillation. *N Engl J Med*. 2011;369:981–992.
4. Patel MR, Mahaffey KW, Garg J, et al. Rivaroxaban versus warfarin in nonvalvular atrial fibrillation. *N Engl J Med*. 2011;365:883–891.
5. Giugliano RP, Ruff CT, Braunwald E, et al. Edoxaban versus warfarin in patients with atrial fibrillation. *N Engl J Med*. 2013;369:2093–2104.
6. Li GY, Windecker S, Huber K, et al. Management of antithrombic therapy in atrial fibrillation patients presenting with acute coronary syndrome and/or undergoing percutaneous coronary or valve interventions: a joint consensus document of the European Society of Cardiology Working Group on Thrombosis, EHRA, EAPCI, and European Association of Acute Cardiac Care (ACCA) endorsed by the Heart Rhythm Society (HRS) and Asia-Pacific Heart Rhythm Society (APHRS). *Eur Heart J*. 2014;35:3155–3179.
7. Wivott SD, Braunwald E, McCabe CH, et al. Prasugrel versus clopidogrel in patients with acute coronary syndromes. *N Engl J Med*. 2007;357:2001–2015.
8. Fielder KA, Maeng M, Mehilli J, et al. Duration of triple therapy in patients requiring oral anticoagulation after drug-eluting stent implantation: the ISAR-TRIPLE trial. *J Am Coll Cardiol*. 2015;65(16):1619–1629.
9. Dewilde WJ, Oirbans T, Verheugt FW, et al. Use of clopidogrel with or without aspirin in patients taking oral anticoagulant therapy and undergoing percutaneous coronary intervention: an open-label, randomised, controlled trial. *Lancet*. 2013;381(9872):1107–1115.
10. Amsterdam EA, Wenger NK, Brindis RG, et al. 2014 AHA/ACC guideline for the management of patients with non-ST-elevation acute coronary syndromes: executive summary. *J Am Coll Cardiol*. 2014;64(24):2645–2687.
11. Heidbuchel H, Verhamme P, Alings M, et al. Updated Europeon Heart Rhythm Association Practical Guide on the use of non-vitamin K antagonist anticoagulants in patients with non-valvular atrial fibrillation. *Europace*. 2015;10:1467–1507.
12. Gibson CM, Mehran R, Bode C, et al. Prevention of bleeding in patients with atrial fibrillation undergoing PCI. *N Engl J Med*. 2016;375:2423–2434.
13. Cannon CO, Bhatt DL, Oldgren J, et al. Dual antithrombotic therapy with dabigatran after PCI in atrial fibrillation. *N Engl J Med*. 2017;377:1513–1524.
14. Lubitz SA, Yin X, Rienstra M, et al. Long-term outcomes of secondary atrial fibrillation in the community: the Framingham Heart Study. *Circulation*. 2015;131(19):1648–1655.
15. Chai-Adisaksopha C, Hillis C, Monreal M, et al. Thromboembolic events, recurrent bleeding and mortality after resuming anticoagulant following gastrointestinal bleeding. A meta-analysis. *Thromb Haemost*. 2015;114(4):819–825.
16. Xian Y, O'Brien EC, Liang L, et al. Association of preceding antithrombotic treatment with acute ischemic stroke severity and in-hospital outcomes among patients with atrial fibrillation. *JAMA*. 2017;317(10):1057–1067.
17. Xian Y, Liang L, Smith EE, et al. Risks of intracranial hemorrhage among patients with acute ischemic stroke receiving warfarin and treated with intravenous tissue plasminogen activator. *JAMA*. 2012;307:2600–2608.
18. Kernan WN, Ovbiagele B, Black HR, et al. Guidelines for the prevention of stroke in patients with stroke and transient ischemic attack: a guideline for healthcare professionals from the American Heart Association/American Stroke Association. *Stroke*. 2014;45(7):2160–2236.
19. Tommaso S, Diener HC, Passman RS, et al. Cryptogenic stroke and underlying atrial fibrillation. *N Engl J Med*. 2014;370:2478–2486.
20. Cervera A, Amaro S, Chamorro A. Oral anticoagulant-associated intracerebral hemorrhage. *J Neurol*. 2012;259(2):212–224.
21. Nielsen PB, Larsen TB, Skjøth F, et al. Restarting anticoagulant treatment after intracranial hemorrhage in patients with atrial fibrillation and the impact on recurrent stroke, mortality, and bleeding: a nationwide cohort study. *Circulation*. 2015;132(6):517–525.
22. Hemphill 3rd JC, Greenberg SM, Anderson CS, et al. Guidelines for the management of spontaneous intracerebral hemorrhage: a guideline for healthcare professionals from the American Heart Association/American Stroke Association. *Stroke*. 2015;46(7):2032–2060.
23. Farmakis D, Parissis J, Filippatos G. Insights into onco-cardiology: atrial fibrillation and cancer. *J Am Coll Cardiol*. 2014;63:945–953.
24. Short NJ, Connors JM. New oral anticoagulants and the cancer patient. *Oncologist*. 2014;19:82–93.
25. Letai A, Kuter DJ. Cancer, coagulation, and anticoagulation. *Oncologist*. 1999;4:443–449.
26. Linkins LA. Management of venous thromboembolism in patients with cancer: role of dalteparin. *Vasc Health Risk Manag*. 2008;4(2):279–287.
27. Asnani A, Manning A, Mansour M, et al. Management of atrial fibrillation in patients taking targeted cancer therapies. *Cardiooncology*. 2017;3:2.
28. Lee YJ, Park JK, Uhm JS, et al. Bleeding risk and major adverse events in patients with cancer on oral anticoagulation therapy. *Int J Cardiol*. 2016;203:372–378.

29. Mueck W, Schwers S, Stampfuss J. Rivaroxban and other novel oral anticoagulants: pharmacokinetics in healthy subjects, specific patient populations and relevance of coagulation monitoring. *Thromb J.* 2013;11:10.
30. van Es N, Coppens M, Schulman S, Middeldorp S, Büller HR. Direct oral anticoagulants compared with vitamin K antagonists for acute venous thromboembolism: evidence from phase 3 trials. *Blood.* 2014;124:1968–1975.
31. Kubitza D, Becka M, Zuehlsdorf M, Mueck W. Body weight has limited influence on the safety, tolerability, pharmacokinetics, or pharmacodynamics of rivaroxaban (BAY 59-7939) in healthy subjects. *J Clin Pharmacol.* 2007;47:218–226.
32. Agnelli G, Buller HR, Cohen A, et al. Oral apixaban for the treatment of acute venous thromboembolism. *N Engl J Med.* 2013;369:799–808.
33. Bauersachs R, Berkowitz SD, Brenner B, et al. Oral rivaroxaban for symptomatic venous thromboembolism. *N Engl J Med.* 2010;363:2499–2510.
34. Buller HR, Prins MH, Lensin AW, et al. Oral rivaroxaban for the treatment of symptomatic pulmonary embolism. *N Engl J Med.* 2012;366:1287–1297.
35. Martin K, Beyer-Westendorf J, Davidson BL, Huisman MV, Sandset PM, Moll S. Use of the direct oral anticoagulants in obese patients: guidance from the SSC of the ISTH. *J Thromb Haemost.* 2016;14(6):1308–1313.
36. Kovacs RJ, Flaker GC, Saxonhouse SJ, et al. Practical management of anticoagulation in patients with atrial fibrillation. *J Am Coll Cardiol.* 2015;65(13):1340–1360.

CHAPTER 13

Stroke and Atrial Fibrillation: The Neurologist's Perspective

LUCIANA CATANESE, MD • ROBERT G. HART, MD

INTRODUCTION

Atrial fibrillation (AF) is strongly associated with cardioembolic strokes, and this association is expected to increase severalfold in the near future. Despite better risk factor control in the developing countries, cardioembolic strokes are on the rise. This type of stroke carries the highest rates of both disability and death and constitutes a major public health concern. The first manifestation of AF can be stroke, but even when AF is detected, it is estimated that only half of patients with AF are prescribed oral anticoagulants worldwide. Maximizing screening and secondary prevention strategies for AF in the aging global population is therefore a public health priority.

EPIDEMIOLOGY

AF is a major public health burden that is expected to grow with the progressive aging of the world's population, the increasing prevalence of risk factors, and the use of advanced screening tools.[1] AF is a well-established risk factor for ischemic stroke, carrying a three- to fivefold increased risk of stroke.[2] The percentage of ischemic strokes associated with AF has been reported to range between 16% and 39%, and although the attributable risk is 17%, it is highly dependent on age ranging from 4.6% in those aged 50–59 years to >20% in those aged >80 years.[3-5] Although most AF-related strokes are cardioembolic (70%), some are noncardioembolic such as lacunar (15%) and large artery atherosclerosis (15%) caused by shared risk factors.[6] Although the overall incidence of ischemic stroke is decreasing, in high-income countries, cardioembolic strokes related to AF have tripled during the past 25 years and are expected to continue to climb at a similar rate by 2050, particularly in those aged ≥80 years.[7] In addition to causing major clinical strokes, AF has also been associated with asymptomatic brain embolism detected in bilateral transcranial Doppler ultrasound monitoring, silent cerebral infarction detected in neuroimaging, and transient ischemic attacks (TIA).[8-10] In a retrospective US nationwide inpatient sample analysis, the prevalence of AF in patients presenting with a TIA was reported to be 12%–17%, corresponding to a 38% increment since 2004.[10]

Recent attention has focused on the stroke risk associated with short duration, asymptomatic AF, termed subclinical atrial fibrillation (SCAF). SCAF lasting for more than 24 h was found to increase the risk of ischemic stroke and systemic embolism by over threefold.[11] Several different cutoffs for SCAF lasting <24 h and its association with increased stroke risk have been reported.[12] In view of the high overall prevalence of SCAF in the elderly population with cardiovascular risk factors, it remains uncertain whether SCAF lasting <24 h detected by cardiac monitoring after stroke is the cause of stroke or it is unrelated to the stroke etiology.

Risk factors associated with the development of AF overlap with those leading to an increased risk of ischemic stroke. Common risk factors include advanced age, male sex, hypertension, diabetes, smoking, heavy alcohol consumption, obesity, sleep apnea, elevated inflammatory markers, chronic kidney disease, and the presence of underlying cardiac diseases.[3,13] In regard to ethnicity, although the prevalence of AF is higher in white individuals of European descent, the risk of stroke once AF is diagnosed seems to be higher in Hispanics and blacks.[14] Particularly, patients with cardioembolic strokes tend to be, more often, female, older, and have underlying cardiac disease.[15] Validated prediction models such as $CHADS_2$ and $CHAD_2DS$-VASc have been developed to predict the risk of stroke based on some of the major cardiovascular risk factors. The risk of stroke recurrence within the first year is approximately 15%, which can be significantly (~70%) reduced with the use of oral anticoagulant therapy.[16] Unfortunately, even when the dysrhythmia is detected early, it is estimated that fewer than 50% of patients with AF receive oral anticoagulation worldwide.[1] The elderly are particularly affected as they are frequently perceived as fragile and at increased risk of complications despite the absence of contraindications, while they carry the highest risk for thromboembolism.[1]

PATHOPHYSIOLOGY

The strong association between stroke and AF has been established by multiple rigorous studies, but such association does not imply linear causality. Several pathophysiologic mechanisms underlie this association. Early studies demonstrated that fibrillation of the atrium can lead to regional atrial or left atrial appendage (LAA) blood stasis, thrombus formation, and subsequent embolization to the brain, and this hypothesis was presumed to be the sole contributor to this association. Although recurrent bouts of AF can lead to atrial remodeling and subsequent perpetuation of the dysrhythmia, atrial cardiomyopathies including fibrosis, elevated filling pressures, and chamber dilation have been associated with an increased thromboembolic risk even in the absence of AF.[17,18] Indeed, some atrial derangements are specifically associated with cryptogenic and not with noncardioembolic events, signaling a potential thrombogenic mechanism independent from AF.[19] Abnormal prothrombotic markers (e.g., elevated C-reactive protein, D-dimer, plasma vWF, and prothrombin fragments $1+2$) have been linked to progressive atrial and LAA dysfunction as well as vascular events and stroke in patients with and without AF.[17] Indeed, circulating plasma vWF levels and D-dimer have been shown to improve risk stratification scores in individuals with AF.[20,21] In patients with cardioembolic strokes, the combination of blood stasis from dysrhythmia, a procoagulant state, and abnormal atrial substrate together completes the Virchow-Robin triad leading to thrombogenesis.[17]

On the other hand, stroke can occasionally also precipitate AF. The notion of "neurogenic AF" was originated in animal studies where inducing strokes consistently triggered both AF and flutter.[22] In humans, strokes that affect cerebral autonomic regulatory centers (more commonly the kinsular region) are associated with new-onset AF in the absence of echocardiographic changes signaling chronic AF or underlying cardiac disease.[23] Autonomic deregulation or even a complete lack of central autonomic control over intrinsic cardiac pathways can trigger arrhythmias and if perpetuated, paroxysmal AF.[24] In addition, neuronal necrotic cell death from stroke can activate the inflammatory cascade, a phenomenon that has been shown to promote atrial remodeling and subsequently play a role in the origination and perpetuation of AF.[25] Both autonomic dysfunction and inflammatory upregulation peak in the acute stroke phase before fading away within days to weeks, a period that coincides with the highest risk of stroke recurrence and the highest detection rate of poststroke AF.[24,26,27]

Thus, the pathophysiology underlying AF-associated cardioembolic strokes is complex and involves several factors, including genetic predisposition, abnormal atrial substrate, hematologic and inflammatory derangements, and poststroke autonomic and inflammatory changes in addition to the dysrhythmia itself. Further understanding of the different mechanisms that result in cardioembolic strokes is essential for more effective future stroke preventive strategies.

CLINICAL PRESENTATION

At the onset of symptoms, AF-associated cardioembolic strokes are associated with reduced levels of consciousness and major hemispheric syndromes compared with those from atherosclerotic disease.[15] The hemispheric syndromes associated with large cerebral artery occlusions are diverse but clinically recognizable (Table 13.1). In a large retrospective study, arm weakness was reported to be more likely homogeneous rather than predominantly either proximal or distal in patients with hemispheric syndromes due to a cardioembolic source.[15] Language and visual disturbances were more frequent in the cardioembolic group compared with stroke associated with cerebrovascular atherosclerosis.[28] Indeed, as the cortex tends to be commonly involved in AF-associated stroke, the presence of cortical signs such as aphasia, apraxia, and agnosia has been shown to be highly suggestive of cardiogenic strokes.[29] The onset of symptoms is typically sudden with maximal severity at onset, reaching the peak intensity of symptoms within minutes compared with a more stuttering presentation for strokes due to atherothrombosis and small vessel disease strokes.[28] Rapid improvement of symptoms occurring because of embolus migration has also been related to cardiogenic embolic stokes (termed "the spectacular shrinking effect").[30] Although clinical findings are supportive of the underlying etiology, they are insufficiently sensitive and specific; additional data from neuroimaging and vascular imaging are required for clinical management.

TIAs occur less often with AF than with cerebrovascular atherosclerosis. AF-related TIAs tend to be of longer duration (>60 min) and are more often associated with restricted diffusion on magnetic resonance imaging (MRI) compared with those that originate from artery-artery embolism.[31]

DIAGNOSIS

Cardioembolism can be initially suspected on clinical grounds based on the onset and nature of the neurologic deficit, but its source should be explored and

TABLE 13.1
Large Vessel Ischemic Stroke Syndromes Typical of Atrial Fibrillation–Associated Stroke

Syndrome	Syndrome Characteristics	Artery Involved
Right MCA	Left hemiparesis, left hemihypesthesia or anesthesia, right gaze deviation, left-sided hemispatial neglect/apraxia/agnosia, left homonymous hemianopsia. Agitated delirium can be seen	M1 segment or both M2 segments or terminal carotid occlusion if patent ACOM
Left MCA	Right hemiparesis, right hemihypesthesia or anesthesia, left gaze deviation, aphasia (generally global at onset), right homonymous hemianopsia	M1 segment or both M2 segments or terminal carotid occlusion if patent ACOM
ACA	Predominantly leg weakness/numbness, abulia, mutism, disinhibition, perseveration, ideomotor apraxia. Grasp reflex. Transcortical motor aphasia can be seen when left side involved	ACA artery
ICA	Combined MCA+ACA syndromes	ICA anywhere from bifurcation to supraclinoid segment
PCA	Contralateral homonymous hemianopsia. In larger infarcts, contralateral motor-sensory loss, gaze deviation, cranial nerve III palsy, and aphasia. Alexia without agraphia is seen if splenium in left side is involved	PCA artery
Basilar (top)	Somnolence to coma, cortical blindness, oculomotor palsy, memory loss, delirium, vivid visual hallucinations, ataxia	Top of basilar artery or "basilarized" vertebral artery
Basilar (middle)	**"Locked-in" syndrome**: horizontal gaze palsy and quadriparesis with intact sensorium	Midbasilar artery

ACA, anterior cerebral artery; *ICA*, internal carotid artery; *MCA*, middle cerebral artery; *PCA*, posterior cerebral artery.

confirmed with neuroimaging (computed tomography [CT] and/or MRI), extracranial and intracranial vascular studies, echocardiogram, and cardiac rhythm monitoring. A thorough medical history and examination, a risk factor profile, and basic blood work including cardiac enzymes complete the stroke workup.

Acute stroke imaging with noncontrast CT reveals a linear hyperdensity along the course of the proximal middle cerebral artery (MCA), also known as the "hyperdense vessel sign (HVS)," present in about 49% of cases of acute cardioembolic strokes (Fig. 13.2).[32] The presence of an HVS suggests erythrocyte-rich clot, whereas fibrin-rich clots may be isointense on brain imaging.[33] Although acute neuroimaging, particularly brain CT, may not expose the ischemic area until several hours have passed, it effectively excludes hemorrhagic stroke as the cause for the sudden-onset neurologic deficit. In addition, a validated 10-point topographic score called the Alberta Stroke Program Early CT (ASPECT) can be quickly calculated based on initial CT imaging and is useful to select candidates for revascularization therapies.[34] In this score, one point is subtracted from the initial 10 for every region of the MCA territory that shows ischemic changes (Fig. 13.3). A score of 6 or more predicts higher response to acute

recanalization therapies, better functional outcomes at 3 months, and lower rates of hemorrhagic conversion.[35] In the subacute setting, both CT and MRI assist in the determination of the location, size, and degree (if any) of hemorrhagic transformation of the infarcted territory. In the presence of AF, strokes tend to be large and cortical, and more often bilateral because of the involvement of different cerebral vascular territories (Fig. 13.1).[36–38] After recanalization of an occluded vessel, the reperfusion of an infarcted territory with a disrupted blood-brain barrier can lead to hemorrhagic transformation. This phenomenon can be seen in up to 70% of large cardioembolic strokes.[39] Prior silent cortical-based strokes can be visualized in 15%–26% of acute stroke patients with paroxysmal AF, further supporting this diagnosis.[40] Angiographic imaging performed acutely with either CT or MRI angiography often reveals a large vessel occlusion (LVO) without significant atherosclerotic changes in the intracranial vasculature (Fig. 13.4).[15]

To exclude a large artery atherosclerotic plaque, a CT or MR angiogram is performed in most stroke patients. A carotid ultrasound to assess the degree of stenosis of the cervical carotid artery may suffice in cases where intracranial artery disease is deemed

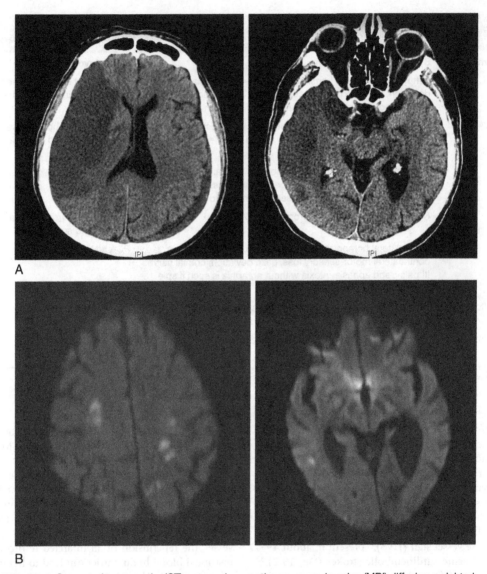

FIG. 13.1 Computed tomography (CT) scan and magnetic resonance imaging (MRI) diffusion-weighted image (DWI) sequence showing different cardioembolic stroke morphologies in patients with underlying atrial fibrillation. **(A)** CT showing a large hemispheric stroke due to occlusion of right middle cerebral artery. **(B)** Bihemispheric multiple embolic strokes on MRI DWI sequence.

unlikely. A transthoracic echocardiogram (TTE) is performed routinely in patients with risk factors for cardiogenic stroke. In contrast, a transesophageal echocardiogram (TEE) is performed in only about 20% of selected cases after an unrevealing TTE when an embolic source is highly suspected and great vessel disease has been ruled out.[29] Although TEE has a higher therapeutic yield in cryptogenic stroke patients

compared with TTE, the routine use of this modality is of uncertain cost-effectiveness. The exact duration, sequence, and type of cardiac rhythm monitoring poststroke are a matter of debate. Single EKG, 24–48-h Holter, 30-day event trigger recorder, and implantable loop recorders can detect 7.7%, 3.2%–4.5%, 16%, and 17% of AF in poststroke patients, respectively.[4,26,41] In cryptogenic stroke patients, cardiac monitoring for

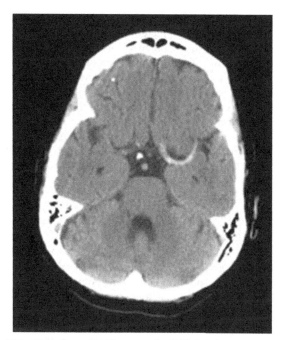

FIG. 13.2 Computed tomography (CT) showing a hyperdense vessel sign from a left middle cerebral artery embolus associated with atrial fibrillation.

30 days with an event-triggered recorder proved to be superior to standard screening strategies and of similar detection rate than long-term implantable loop recorders based on the EMBRACE and CRYSTAL-AF studies.[26,41] More recently, the FIND-AF study showed similar results with enhanced and prolonged monitoring at 6 months in all stroke patients aged 60 years or older indicating an overall high prevalence of this condition in stroke patients. According to a recent metaanalysis, subsequent combination of cardiac rhythm monitoring methods is superior to screening with a single method for the detection of new-onset AF after ischemic stroke or TIA.[4] The significance of short durations of SCAF remains uncertain, particularly when first detected several months after the index stroke.

Although the extent of the diagnostic workup is a subject of controversy, most stroke neurologists opt to perform a workup that includes a neuroimaging study, a carotid artery vascular study, TTE, and cardiac monitoring for a minimum of 30 days as suggested per guidelines.[42] Cardiogenic stroke can be confirmed in the presence of a typical clinical presentation, an embolic neuroimaging pattern, and the absence of significant atherosclerotic large vessel disease in a patient with risk factors for cardioembolism, especially AF. After a complete diagnostic workup, about

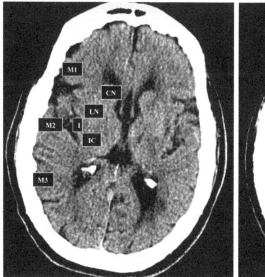
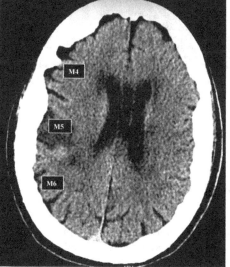

FIG. 13.3 Example of ASPECTS of 9 out of 10 with one point deducted for early ischemic changes in the M5 territory. *ASPECTS,* Alberta Stroke Program Early Computed Tomography Score; *CN,* caudate nucleus; *I,* insula; *IC,* internal capsule; *LN,* lentiform nucleus; *M1-6,* middle cerebral artery segments.

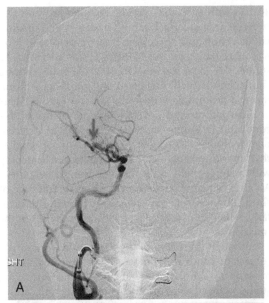

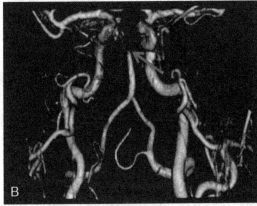

FIG. 13.4 Examples of large vessel occlusions located in the anterior and posterior circulation in patients with atrial fibrillation. **(A)** Digital subtraction angiography showing an acute right middle cerebral artery occlusion (*red arrow*). **(B)** Magnetic resonance angiogram showing a top of the basilar occlusion (*red arrow*).

25% of all ischemic strokes remain of undetermined source of which 16% have an embolic pattern on brain imaging, suggesting an occult cardiac source.[39,43] Nonlacunar cryptogenic stroke that is presumed to be embolic has been recategorized as embolic stroke of undetermined source (ESUS).[43] Although limited data are available, up to 29% of ESUS patients have been reported to have new AF on follow-up.[43] A more extensive workup can be pursued for these patients, including hypercoagulable panel, TEE, and longer-duration cardiac monitoring. The Dabigatran Etexilate

for Secondary Stroke Prevention in Patients With Embolic Stroke of Undetermined Source (RE-SPECT ESUS) and the Rivaroxaban Versus Aspirin in Secondary Prevention of Stroke and Prevention of Systemic Embolism in Patients With Recent Embolic Stroke of Undetermined Source (NAVIGATE ESUS) trials are currently enrolling patients to determine the best secondary stroke prevention strategies in this subtype of stroke. If positive results are obtained, the need for more exhaustive and costly diagnostic screening will be offset by the safety and efficacy of direct oral anticoagulants (DOACs).

ACUTE TREATMENT OF ATRIAL FIBRILLATION–ASSOCIATED STROKE

Acute stroke therapies for patients with LVOs include intravenous and intraarterial thrombolysis with recombinant tissue plasminogen (tPA) and endovascular thrombectomy with first-generation stent-retrievers with or without aspiration devices. The current therapeutic time windows are 4.5 and 6 h from symptom onset for intraintravenous and intraarterial therapies, respectively.[44,45] The selection of candidates for acute treatment is essential, and therapy depends on several factors, such as the presence of disabling stroke symptoms with a clear time of onset, age ≥ 18 years, minimal disability at baseline, small infarcts on presentation (ASPECT ≥ 6), and confirmed LVO on brain imaging.[44] A significant drawback for the administration of thrombolytic therapy is the extensive list of contraindications that attempt to exclude bleeding-susceptible patients, such as those with recent stroke before the current acute stroke and/or prior intracranial hemorrhage (ICH), which are not uncommon occurrences in AF individuals. Although antiplatelet therapy is not a contraindication for the use of thrombolytic therapy, warfarin use with an international normalized ratio (INR) > 1.7 precludes thrombolytic treatment. INR reversal in the acute ischemic stroke setting before thrombolysis is not recommended because of the potential risk of expanding thrombosis and/or increasing the risk of recurrent thromboembolism. A particularly controversial finding on baseline MRI is the presence of round, small, hypointense lesions in susceptibility weighted imaging (SWI) sequences known as cerebral microbleeds (CMBs). CMBs are common in stroke patients (~20%) and represent perivascular hemosiderin deposits secondary to leakage of hemorrhage-prone small vessels.[46] A metaanalysis of available studies has shown that the presence of pretreatment CMB is associated with an increased risk of symptomatic ICH after thrombolytic therapy for acute ischemic stroke.[46] Similar findings have been reported with the presence of moderate to severe degrees of leukoaraiosis (another marker of small vessel disease) on baseline scans.[47] To date, thrombolysis with tPA is considered to be a therapeutic option in acute stroke patients with markers of bleeding-prone small vessel disease, because the benefit is still apparent despite an increased risk of ICH.[46]

Recanalization rate of LVO with intravenous thrombolysis is about 30%–40%, whereas with a combined approach of intravenous tPA and endovascular thrombectomy, recanalization rate can reach 90%.[48] An example of complete recanalization following endovascular thrombectomy in a patient with an LVO from AF is shown in Fig. 13.5. Limited studies have explored the relationship between the presence of AF and recanalization rates. Preexisting AF was found to be an independent predictor of recanalization in acute stroke patients in two large prospective studies.[49,50] However, because of the large infarct sizes and volumes of hypoperfusion at baseline as well as more severe hemorrhagic transformation and likelihood of parenchymal hematoma after thrombolysis, the benefit in functional outcomes after treatment seems to dissipate.[51] Acute stroke therapy, particularly thrombectomy, is highly effective in patients with LVO, and despite worse imaging outcomes in AF patients, it remains the treatment of choice until more conclusive data are available.

STROKE OUTCOMES IN ATRIAL FIBRILLATION

Compared with non-AF patients, AF patients with strokes have higher rates of death at 30 days (22%) and 1 year (~40%) and disability at discharge even after acute thrombolytic therapy.[51,52] In addition to having more severe strokes at baseline, worse imaging outcomes, and higher rates of symptomatic ICH, AF patients have more medical complications (odds ratio [OR] 1.61) and higher mortality (OR 2.14) while hospitalized after stroke.[53] This effect persists beyond the immediate poststroke period with median survival rates of 1.8 years for AF patients versus 5.7 years for matched non-AF individuals (hazard ratio 2.8).[54] Furthermore, the presence of AF leads to longer hospitalizations and elevated healthcare costs after stroke compared with their counterparts without AF.[1] Women are a particularly vulnerable population because there is a higher ratio of more severe strokes compared with men, a factor that strongly correlates with long-term functional disability after stroke.[55]

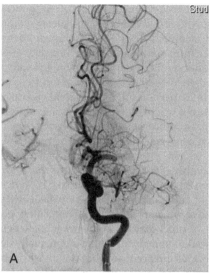

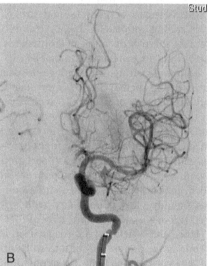

FIG. 13.5 Prethrombectomy **(A)** and postthrombectomy **(B)** digital subtraction angiography showing a case of acute left middle cerebral artery occlusion following successful thrombectomy with complete restoration of cerebral blood flow.

SECONDARY STROKE PREVENTION IN ATRIAL FIBRILLATION: ANTICOAGULATION FOR ALL? YES!

Secondary stroke prevention for most AF patients with prior strokes or TIA is fairly straightforward: anticoagulation with DOACs or vitamin K antagonists (VKA). The 10% risk of recurrent stroke/year seen in stroke patients with AF if given aspirin can be importantly reduced (relative risk reduction 60%–70%) with DOACs or VKA.[56]

As noted above, about 10% of AF patients presenting with strokes have an ipsilateral symptomatic carotid stenosis (70%–99%). Although there is no evidence from randomized trials, long-term anticoagulation after carotid endarterectomy is generally recommended. In SPAF III trial, the rate of recurrent ischemic stroke in AF patients following carotid endarterectomy was 11% per year in those randomized to aspirin versus 0% in those anticoagulated (unpublished data, R. Hart, personal communication). A similar approach is taken for AF patients presenting with lacunar strokes. The uncertain benefits of antiplatelets over anticoagulation in patients with lacunar strokes make it premature to withhold anticoagulation from AF patients with small vessel disease at present.[57] Differentiating potential sources of small subcortical infarcts is challenging and could lead to undertreatment of a potentially devastating stroke recurrence if anticoagulation is withheld. In AF patients with prior stroke or TIA who have carotid artery atherosclerosis or prior lacunar stroke, we do not favor adding antiplatelet therapy to anticoagulation because the risk of major hemorrhage is clearly increased, while the benefits are unestablished.

The timing of starting or resuming anticoagulation after stroke in AF patients relies on factors such as stroke size and the presence of poststroke hemorrhagic conversion or ICH. The recommended time ranges from 1, 3, and 6 days for TIA, mild, and moderate strokes, respectively, to a minimum period of 2 weeks for patients with severe stroke and poststroke hemorrhagic conversion or ICH.[58] Although the presence of CMBs on MRI in patients with AF-related strokes on anticoagulants (mainly VKA) is associated with a fourfold increased risk of ICH, the absolute rates of ICH remain low.[59] Hence, the benefits of anticoagulation in terms of ischemic stroke prevention seem to still surpass the risks of ICH even in this high-risk population. CMBs are only one expression of the cerebral amyloid angiopathy (CAA) spectrum, which also encompasses lobar ICH, cortical superficial siderosis, posterior predominant leukoaraiosis, and enlarged perivascular spaces. All of these imaging findings have been correlated with an increased risk of ICH, cortical superficial siderosis being the one with the highest risk. As CAA increases with age, it is not uncommon to find AF patients with coexisting conditions. As such, cardiologists should include the diagnostic possibility of CAA in the complex anticoagulation decision-making process. To date, the decision to start anticoagulation in CAA patients is made on a case-by-case basis based on nonrandomized observational studies. Several randomized studies such as NASPAF ICH are on its way. Overall, VKA

for secondary stroke prevention are to be avoided in patients with prior lobal ICH, multiple CMBs, and evidence of cortical superficial siderosis.

ATRIAL FIBRILLATION AND STROKE: MAJOR PROGRESS IN STROKE PREVENTION

Recognition of the importance and frequency of AF-associated stroke, its prevention by anticoagulation, and the development of safer, more efficacious direct-acting oral anticoagulants during the past 25 years represent major progress in stroke prevention. Previously ignored as a cause of stroke, AF-associated stroke is now the most preventable cause of disabling ischemic stroke. Although much remains to be done to capitalize on this knowledge, many of the tools are at hand, and the challenge is how best to apply them.

REFERENCES

1. Rahman F, Kwan GF, Benjamin EJ. Global epidemiology of atrial fibrillation. *Nat Rev Cardiol.* 2014;11:639–654.
2. Marini C, De Santis F, Sacco S, et al. Contribution of atrial fibrillation to incidence and outcome of ischemic stroke: results from a population-based study. *Stroke.* 2005;36:1115–1119.
3. Pistoia F, Sacco S, Tiseo C, Degan D, Ornello R, Carolei A. The epidemiology of atrial fibrillation and stroke. *Cardiol Clin.* 2016;34:255–268.
4. Sposato LA, Cipriano LE, Saposnik G, Ruiz Vargas E, Riccio PM, Hachinski V. Diagnosis of atrial fibrillation after stroke and transient ischaemic attack: a systematic review and meta-analysis. *Lancet Neurol.* 2015;14:377–387.
5. O'Donnell MJ, Xavier D, Liu L, et al. Risk factors for ischaemic and intracerebral haemorrhagic stroke in 22 countries (the INTERSTROKE study): a case-control study. *Lancet.* 2010;376:112–123.
6. Hart RG, Pearce LA, Miller VT, et al. Cardioembolic vs. noncardioembolic strokes in atrial fibrillation: frequency and effect of antithrombotic agents in the stroke prevention in atrial fibrillation studies. *Cerebrovasc Dis.* 2000;10:39–43.
7. Yiin GS, Howard DP, Paul NL, et al. Age-specific incidence, outcome, cost, and projected future burden of atrial fibrillation-related embolic vascular events: a population-based study. *Circulation.* 2014;130:1236–1244.
8. Ezekowitz MD, James KE, Nazarian SM, et al. Silent cerebral infarction in patients with nonrheumatic atrial fibrillation. The Veterans Affairs Stroke Prevention in Nonrheumatic Atrial Fibrillation Investigators. *Circulation.* 1995;92:2178–2182.
9. Cullinane M, Wainwright R, Brown A, Monaghan M, Markus HS. Asymptomatic embolization in subjects with atrial fibrillation not taking anticoagulants: a prospective study. *Stroke.* 1998;29:1810–1815.

10. Otite FO, Khandelwal P, Chaturvedi S, Romano JG, Sacco RL, Malik AM. Increasing atrial fibrillation prevalence in acute ischemic stroke and TIA. *Neurology.* 2016;87:2034–2042.
11. Van Gelder IC, Healey JS, Crijns HJ, et al. Duration of device-detected subclinical atrial fibrillation and occurrence of stroke in ASSERT. *Eur Heart J.* 2017;38(17):1339–1344.
12. Hess PL, Healey JS, Granger CB, et al. The role of cardiovascular implantable electronic devices in the detection and treatment of subclinical atrial fibrillation: a review. *JAMA Cardiol.* 2017;2:324–331.
13. Chang SN, Lai LP, Chiang FT, Lin JL, Hwang JJ, Tsai CT. The C-reactive protein gene polymorphism predicts the risk of thromboembolic stroke in atrial fibrillation: a more than 10-year prospective follow-up study. *J Thromb Haemost.* 2017;15(8):1541–1546.
14. Birman-Deych E, Radford MJ, Nilasena DS, Gage BF. Use and effectiveness of warfarin in Medicare beneficiaries with atrial fibrillation. *Stroke.* 2006;37:1070–1074.
15. Timsit SG, Sacco RL, Mohr JP, et al. Early clinical differentiation of cerebral infarction from severe atherosclerotic stenosis and cardioembolism. *Stroke.* 1992;23:486–491.
16. Freedman B, Potpara TS, Lip GY. Stroke prevention in atrial fibrillation. *Lancet.* 2016;388:806–817.
17. Watson T, Shantsila E, Lip GY. Mechanisms of thrombogenesis in atrial fibrillation: virchow's triad revisited. *Lancet.* 2009;373:155–166.
18. Heijman J, Voigt N, Nattel S, Dobrev D. Cellular and molecular electrophysiology of atrial fibrillation initiation, maintenance, and progression. *Circ Res.* 2014;114:1483–1499.
19. Kamel H, Hunter M, Moon YP, et al. Electrocardiographic left atrial abnormality and risk of stroke: Northern Manhattan study. *Stroke.* 2015;46:3208–3212.
20. Nozawa T, Inoue H, Hirai T, et al. D-dimer level influences thromboembolic events in patients with atrial fibrillation. *Int J Cardiol.* 2006;109:59–65.
21. Lip GY, Lane D, Van Walraven C, Hart RG. Additive role of plasma von Willebrand factor levels to clinical factors for risk stratification of patients with atrial fibrillation. *Stroke.* 2006;37:2294–2300.
22. Mihm MJ, Yu F, Carnes CA, et al. Impaired myofibrillar energetics and oxidative injury during human atrial fibrillation. *Circulation.* 2001;104:174–180.
23. Gonzalez Toledo ME, Klein FR, Riccio PM, et al. Atrial fibrillation detected after acute ischemic stroke: evidence supporting the neurogenic hypothesis. *J Stroke Cerebrovasc Dis.* 2013;22:e486–e491.
24. Sposato LA, Riccio PM, Hachinski V. Poststroke atrial fibrillation: cause or consequence? Critical review of current views. *Neurology.* 2014;82:1180–1186.
25. Chung MK, Martin DO, Sprecher D, et al. C-reactive protein elevation in patients with atrial arrhythmias: inflammatory mechanisms and persistence of atrial fibrillation. *Circulation.* 2001;104:2886–2891.
26. Gladstone DJ, Spring M, Dorian P, et al. Atrial fibrillation in patients with cryptogenic stroke. *N Engl J Med.* 2014;370:2467–2477.
27. Wachter R, Groschel K, Gelbrich G, et al. Holter-electrocardiogram-monitoring in patients with acute ischaemic stroke (Find-AFRANDOMISED): an open-label randomised controlled trial. *Lancet Neurol.* 2017;16:282–290.
28. Arboix A, Oliveres M, Massons J, Pujades R, Garcia-Eroles L. Early differentiation of cardioembolic from atherothrombotic cerebral infarction: a multivariate analysis. *Eur J Neurol.* 1999;6:677–683.
29. Kamel H, Healey JS. Cardioembolic stroke. *Circ Res.* 2017;120:514–526.
30. Minematsu K, Yamaguchi T, Omae T. 'Spectacular shrinking deficit': rapid recovery from a major hemispheric syndrome by migration of an embolus. *Neurology.* 1992;42:157–162.
31. Harrison MJ, Marshall J. Atrial fibrillation, TIAs and completed strokes. *Stroke.* 1984;15:441–442.
32. Forlivesi S, Bovi P, Tomelleri G, et al. Stroke etiologic subtype may influence the rate of hyperdense middle cerebral artery sign disappearance after intravenous thrombolysis. *J Thromb Thrombolysis.* 2017;43:86–90.
33. Froehler MT, Tateshima S, Duckwiler G, et al. The hyperdense vessel sign on CT predicts successful recanalization with the Merci device in acute ischemic stroke. *J Neurointerv Surg.* 2013;5:289–293.
34. Barber PA, Demchuk AM, Zhang J, Buchan AM. Validity and reliability of a quantitative computed tomography score in predicting outcome of hyperacute stroke before thrombolytic therapy. ASPECTS Study Group. Alberta Stroke Programme early CT score. *Lancet.* 2000;355:1670–1674.
35. Hill MD, Demchuk AM, Goyal M, et al. Alberta Stroke Program early computed tomography score to select patients for endovascular treatment: Interventional Management of Stroke (IMS)-III trial. *Stroke.* 2014;45:444–449.
36. Arquizan C, Lamy C, Mas JL. Simultaneous supratentorial multiple cerebral infarctions. *Rev Neurol (Paris).* 1997;153:748–753.
37. Lodder J, Bamford JM, Sandercock PA, Jones LN, Warlow CP. Are hypertension or cardiac embolism likely causes of lacunar infarction? *Stroke.* 1990;21:375–381.
38. Nah HW, Lee JW, Chung CH, et al. New brain infarcts on magnetic resonance imaging after coronary artery bypass graft surgery: lesion patterns, mechanism, and predictors. *Ann Neurol.* 2014;76:347–355.
39. Ustrell X, Pellise A. Cardiac workup of ischemic stroke. *Curr Cardiol Rev.* 2010;6:175–183.
40. Hahne K, Monnig G, Samol A. Atrial fibrillation and silent stroke: links, risks, and challenges. *Vasc Health Risk Manag.* 2016;12:65–74.
41. Sanna T, Diener HC, Passman RS, et al. Cryptogenic stroke and underlying atrial fibrillation. *N Engl J Med.* 2014;370:2478–2486.
42. January CT, Wann LS, Alpert JS, et al. 2014 AHA/ACC/HRS guideline for the management of patients with atrial fibrillation: executive summary: a report of the American College of Cardiology/American Heart Association Task Force on practice guidelines and the Heart Rhythm Society. *Circulation.* 2014;130:2071–2104.

43. Hart RG, Catanese L, Perera KS, Ntaios G, Connolly SJ. Embolic stroke of undetermined source: a systematic review and clinical update. *Stroke.* 2017;48:867–872.

44. Demaerschalk BM, Kleindorfer DO, Adeoye OM, et al. Scientific rationale for the inclusion and exclusion criteria for intravenous alteplase in acute ischemic stroke. A statement for healthcare professionals from the American Heart Association/American Stroke Association. *Stroke.* 2016;47(2):581–641.

45. Powers WJ, Derdeyn CP, Biller J, et al. 2015 American Heart Association/American Stroke Association focused update of the 2013 guidelines for the early management of patients with acute ischemic stroke regarding endovascular treatment. A guideline for healthcare professionals from the American Heart Association/American Stroke Association. *Stroke.* 2015;46:3024–3039.

46. Charidimou A, Shoamanesh A, Wilson D, et al. Cerebral microbleeds and postthrombolysis intracerebral hemorrhage risk updated meta-analysis. *Neurology.* 2015;85:927–934.

47. Pantoni L, Fierini F, Poggesi A. Thrombolysis in acute stroke patients with cerebral small vessel disease. *Cerebrovasc Dis.* 2014;37:5–13.

48. Catanese L, Tarsia J, Fisher M. Acute ischemic stroke therapy overview. *Circ Res.* 2017;120:541–558.

49. Mendonca N, Rodriguez-Luna D, Rubiera M, et al. Predictors of tissue-type plasminogen activator nonresponders according to location of vessel occlusion. *Stroke.* 2012;43:417–421.

50. Vanacker P, Lambrou D, Eskandari A, et al. Improving the prediction of spontaneous and post-thrombolytic recanalization in ischemic stroke patients. *J Stroke Cerebrovasc Dis.* 2015;24:1781–1786.

51. Saposnik G, Gladstone D, Raptis R, Zhou L, Hart RG, Investigators of the Registry of the Canadian Stroke Network and the Stroke Outcomes Research Canada Working Group. Atrial fibrillation in ischemic stroke: predicting response to thrombolysis and clinical outcomes. *Stroke.* 2013;44:99–104.

52. Seet RC, Zhang Y, Wijdicks EF, Rabinstein AA. Relationship between chronic atrial fibrillation and worse outcomes in stroke patients after intravenous thrombolysis. *Arch Neurol.* 2011;68:1454–1458.

53. Steger C, Pratter A, Martinek-Bregel M, et al. Stroke patients with atrial fibrillation have a worse prognosis than patients without: data from the Austrian Stroke Registry. *Eur Heart J.* 2004;25:1734–1740.

54. Fang MC, Go AS, Chang Y, et al. Long-term survival after ischemic stroke in patients with atrial fibrillation. *Neurology.* 2014;82:1033–1037.

55. Lang C, Seyfang L, Ferrari J, et al. Do women with atrial fibrillation experience more severe strokes? Results from the Austrian Stroke Unit Registry. *Stroke.* 2017;48:778–780.

56. Hart RG. Secondary prevention in patients with atrial fibrillation: what every neurologist should know. *Pract Neurol.* 2003:260–267.

57. Mohr JP, Thompson JL, Lazar RM, et al. A comparison of warfarin and aspirin for the prevention of recurrent ischemic stroke. *N Engl J Med.* 2001;345:1444–1451.

58. Heidbuchel H, Verhamme P, Alings M, et al. Updated European Heart Rhythm Association Practical Guide on the use of non-vitamin K antagonist anticoagulants in patients with non-valvular atrial fibrillation. *Europace.* 2015;17:1467–1507.

59. Charidimou A, Boulouis G, Shams S, Calvet D, Shoamanesh A, International M-MI. Intracerebral haemorrhage risk in microbleed-positive ischaemic stroke patients with atrial fibrillation: preliminary meta-analysis of cohorts and anticoagulation decision schema. *J Neurol Sci.* 2017;378:102–109.

CHAPTER 14

Stroke and Atrial Fibrillation in Chronic Kidney Disease and Dialysis

DAVID COLLISTER, MD • MICHAEL WALSH, MD, PHD

INTRODUCTION

Chronic kidney disease (CKD) is a common condition that is increasing in incidence and prevalence because of an aging population and an increase in diabetes, hypertension, and obesity globally. Between 8% and 16% of people globally are thought to have CKD[1] including more than 20% of people older than 60 years.[2] The importance of CKD is underscored by its strong, independent association with major cardiovascular events, which is on par with diabetes.[3]

Cardiovascular disease, including stroke, is the leading cause of death in individuals with CKD. Impaired kidney function, marked by a decline in glomerular filtration rate and/or proteinuria, is an independent risk factor for stroke.[4] Nonvalvular atrial fibrillation is an independent risk factor for ischemic stroke and is associated with CKD[5] and is likely a contributing factor to the increased risk of stroke in this population.

Estimates of the incidence of stroke in patients with CKD vary based on the degree of CKD as well as the definition of stroke (e.g., whether transient ischemic attack, ischemic stroke, and/or hemorrhagic stroke are included) and its method of ascertainment (e.g., registry or administrative database diagnostic coding, prospective clinical assessment, or imaging). However, the overall risk of stroke in patients with the most severe form of CKD, end-stage renal disease, which is treated with dialysis, is up to 10-fold greater than that in age-matched controls without kidney disease.[6–8] Despite this high burden of disease, there is controversy over the management of stroke risk in patients with advanced CKD and nonvalvular atrial fibrillation because of uncertain benefits and risks with oral anticoagulation as it is used in patients without advanced CKD. In this chapter, we will explore the risk factors for stroke in CKD and dialysis, the incidence of stroke, the outcomes of stroke, and the potential benefits and risks of preventative treatments for stroke with a focus on nonvalvular atrial fibrillation.

ISCHEMIC STROKE IN CHRONIC KIDNEY DISEASE AND DIALYSIS

Epidemiology

Ischemic strokes are common in patients with CKD and end-stage renal disease with estimated incidences that range from 10 to 50 per 1000 patient-years.[8–12] The variability in incidence rates reflects the differing patient populations of studies (CKD vs. incident and/or prevalent dialysis patients, hemodialysis vs. peritoneal dialysis patients, comorbidities) and the method of detecting ischemic strokes. For example, a retrospective cohort study of 1382 incident and prevalent hemodialysis patients from Glasgow that defined ischemic stroke by clinical diagnosis, imaging, or death certificate and included a review by two independent physicians demonstrated a stroke incidence rate of 50.1/1000 patient-years in incident dialysis patients and 41.5/1000 patient-years in prevalent dialysis patients.[9] A prospective cohort study of 1041 incident dialysis patients with adjudication of all cerebrovascular events (and use ICD-9 coding only if chart review was not possible) demonstrated a stroke incidence rate of 49/1000 patient-years with most events being ischemic strokes.[11] In contrast, in cohorts in which strokes are ascertained using administrative health data, incidences range from 10.1/1000 patient-years in Taiwan[8] and 11.2/1000 patient-years in Scotland[10] to 21.1/1000 patient-years[12] in the United States.

The accuracy of administrative data to identify strokes without confirmatory imaging and the degree to which imaging is obtained in these often chronically ill patients are two potential sources of discrepancy between prospective and administrative health data studies. However, the fact that heterogeneity exists across studies even with adjudicated events suggests factors intrinsic to the study populations also contributing to varying incidence rates. Furthermore, classifying patients with broadly varying kidney function as having CKD can lead to substantially different case-mixes. This is important since the degree of renal impairment correlates with the risk of stroke.[13]

Etiology

Patients with kidney disease have a high prevalence of traditional risk factors for ischemic stroke including older age,[8,9,14–17] an increased frequency of CKD in non-Caucasians,[15,17] a high prevalence of diabetes,[8,9,14–17] hypertension,[8,15,17] smoking, and preexisting vascular disease.[9,15] In addition to traditional risk factors, end-stage renal disease introduces disease-specific risk factors such as anemia,[17] common use of erythropoietin stimulating agents, mineral bone disorder[18] with vascular calcification, malnutrition,[17] and intradialytic hypotension but not inflammation.[19] Furthermore, CKD can cause a hypercoagulable state with increased endothelial dysfunction and thrombin activation[20] (Fig. 14.1).[21]

In addition to the high burden of vascular risk factors most patients with CKD carry, they may also have novel mechanisms of ischemic stroke. This is alluded to in some studies that demonstrate a disproportionately high rate of ischemic stroke in the vertebrobasilar territory.[22] Additionally, mechanisms of ischemic stroke that are uncommon in patients without CKD may be more common in those with CKD. These include not only small vessel disease and cardioemboli but can also include infective endocarditis,[23] thrombus from left ventricular dysfunction, vascular catheter thrombus with patent foramen ovale,[23] and rarely iatrogenic air embolism. Despite the numerous potential mechanisms for ischemic stroke, the breakdown of ischemic, hemorrhagic and carotid origins is similar in patients with and without CKD requiring dialysis as reflected by the Choices for Healthy Outcomes in Caring for End-Stage Renal Disease study[11] in which 165 of 1041 incident dialysis patients experienced a stroke over a median 2.7 years of follow-up. Of these, 76% were ischemic stroke, 12% were hemorrhagic stroke, and 12% were carotid endarterectomies. Of

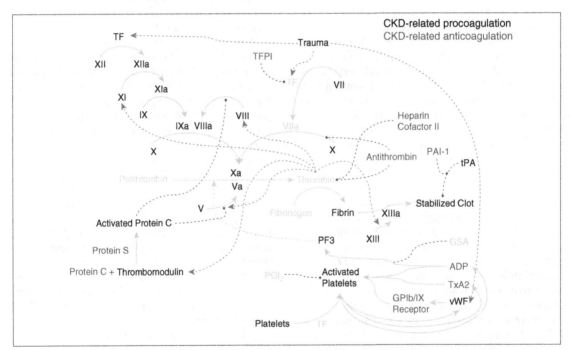

FIG. 14.1 Effects of chronic kidney disease (CKD) on coagulation factors. The classic coagulation cascade with the *dashed red lines* demonstrates a negative effect of CKD-related factors, and the *dashed slate lines* demonstrate positive effect on the indicated reaction or activation. The factors written in **red** are decreased in CKD, whereas the factors in **slate** are increased. *ADP*, adenosine diphosphate; *GPIb*, glycoprotein Ib; *GSA*, guanidinosuccinic acid; *PAI-1*, plasminogen activator inhibitor-1; *PGI₂*, prostacyclin; *TF*, tissue factor; *TFPI*, tissue factor pathway inhibitor; *tPA*, tissue plasminogen activator; *TxA2*, thromboxane A2; *vWF*, Von Willebrand factor. (From Ball T, Weelan K, McCullough PA. Chronic anticoagulation in chronic kidney disease. *J Am Coll Cardiol.* 2014;64(23):2483–2485.)

the adjudicated ischemic strokes, the stroke mechanisms were as follows: cardioembolic 28% (of which the majority were presumably nonvalvular atrial fibrillation), small vessel occlusion 20%, large artery atherosclerosis 11%, multiple causes 18%, other or undetermined 23%.

Outcomes After Stroke

Regardless of the underlying mechanism, strokes in patients with CKD are associated with an increase in morbidity[22] (cognitive dysfunction, poor functional status, impaired quality of life, peritoneal dialysis technique failure[24]) and mortality[9,12,25] in most but not in all studies[26] in CKD and dialysis. In a study of 1382 incident and prevalent hemodialysis patients from a single center in Glasgow from 2007 to 2012, 11.6% of patients experienced a stroke in follow-up with a 7-day mortality of 18.8%, 28-day mortality of 26.9%, and 1-year mortality of 56.3%, with hemorrhagic strokes having a worse prognosis worse than ischemic strokes.[9] In a study of prevalent hemodialysis patients from United States Renal Data System database that used ICD coding for stroke assessment from 2000 to 2005, a semi-Markov model with additive hazard extension showed a 30-day mortality of 17.9% for ischemic stroke and 53.4% for hemorrhagic stroke and median months of life lost of 40.7 and 34.6, respectively.[12] Poor outcomes of stroke in CKD and dialysis may be related to inferior quality of care including thrombolysis, revascularization, and stroke rehabilitation in addition to an unacceptably high cardiovascular risk that is not modifiable by standard medical therapy (e.g., statins, β-blockers, renin angiotensin blockade). For example, in the Get With The Guidelines-Stroke program which evaluated 679,827 patients admitted with ischemic strokes from 1564 US centers from 2009 to 2012, kidney failure was associated with an adjusted odds ratio of 0.72 (95% CI 0.68–0.76) of receiving 100% defect-free care defined by seven quality targets including acute care, tissue plasminogen activator, antithrombotics, deep vein thrombosis and prophylaxis, and discharge care, antithrombotics, anticoagulation, cholesterol therapy, and smoking cessation counseling, with all categories inferior for kidney failure.[27]

ATRIAL FIBRILLATION IN CHRONIC KIDNEY DISEASE AND DIALYSIS

Epidemiology

In patients with dialysis-dependent CKD, atrial fibrillation has an overall incidence rate estimated at 27/1000 patient-years but individual study estimates range from 9.7 to 59/1000 patient-years and an overall prevalence estimate of 11.6% ranging from 5.4% to 27%.[5] In patients with nondialysis-dependent CKD, nonvalvular atrial fibrillation is estimated to have an incidence of 37/1000 patient-years with relative risk increasing by 6%–16% for every decrease in estimated glomerular filtration rate of 10 mL/min and an increase of 4% for each 100 mg/g rise in urine albumin to creatinine ratio and a prevalence of 18%.[28] Nonvalvular atrial fibrillation in CKD and dialysis is driven by aging, hypertension, hypervolemia, left ventricular hypertrophy, diastolic dysfunction, and left atrial abnormalities with varying incidence and prevalence depending on diagnosis (provoked, paroxysmal, persistent, permanent) and the degree of surveillance (routine electrocardiogram monitoring, electrocardiogram monitoring guided by symptoms, Holter monitors, administrative databases). For example, in the Dialysis Outcomes and Practice Patterns Study,[29] an international sample of hemodialysis patients from 11 countries, the overall prevalence of nonvalvular atrial fibrillation predating the initiation of dialysis identified with a medical questionnaire was 12.5% and ranged from 5.6% in Japan to 24.7% in Belgium (12.5% in the United States and 19.0% in Canada) with an overall incidence of 1./100 patient-years but was defined as a hospitalization with a diagnosis of nonvalvular atrial fibrillation. Nonvalvular atrial fibrillation was associated with a variety of factors including age, ethnicity, dialysis vintage, body mass index, systolic blood pressure, dialysis duration, serum calcium, dialysate potassium, coronary artery disease, congestive heart failure, and other cardiovascular comorbidities and medications.

Based on United States Renal Data System data,[30] the incidence of nonvalvular atrial fibrillation identified by ICD-9 or Medicare claims from 1995 to 2007 in incident hemodialysis patients was 29% with an unadjusted incidence rate of 148/1000 patient-years. Similarly, using United States Renal Data System data, Winkelmayer et al.[31] showed a 7.7% prevalence of nonvalvular atrial fibrillation that was associated with age, male, comorbidity, and Caucasian ethnicity. The prevalence of nonvalvular atrial fibrillation seems to be increasing over time from 3.5% in 1989 to 10.7% in 2007 because of an increase in incident hemodialysis patients with preexisting nonvalvular atrial fibrillation, an increase in the incidence rate of nonvalvular atrial fibrillation, and improving survival in dialysis patients.[30]

A prospective cohort study from Spain that included 256 hemodialysis patients showed an incidence of nonvalvular atrial fibrillation of 12.4% with 5.9/100 patient-years associated with age, body mass index, pulse pressure, left atrium size, hemoglobin, calcium, albumin, calcification, bundle branch block, and previous transient ischemic attack/cerebrovascular accident.[32]

Only a few studies have examined echocardiographic associations including a 2003 study of 488 hemodialysis patients from five dialysis centers in Lombardy, Italy, with atrial fibrillation identified over 3 years of follow-up. Atrial fibrillation was associated with an increase in cardiovascular death (hazard ratio 2.15 95% CI: 1.27–3.64) and all-cause mortality (hazard ratio 1.65 95% CI: 1.18–2.31), and left ventricular hypertrophy was a risk factor for incident atrial fibrillation (hazard ratio 2.55 95% CI: 1.04–6.26) and left atrial dilation was a risk factor for prevalent atrial fibrillation (odds ratio 3, $P < .001$).[33]

In addition to a high burden of nonvalvular atrial fibrillation and other traditional risk factors for stroke, the hemodialysis procedure itself may precipitate stroke. In the Choices for Healthy Outcomes in Caring for End-Stage Renal Disease Study,[11] a relative large number of strokes occurred after the initiation of long-term dialysis. The risk of stroke among incident hemodialysis and peritoneal patients was evaluated over 12 months before and after dialysis initiation using United States Renal Data System databases and ICD coding excluding patients with previous stroke. There was an increased risk of stroke beginning 90 days before initiating dialysis, which peaked at 1 month afterward and gradually declined to approximately two times above baseline risk overall in follow-up.[14] The increased risk of stroke in incident hemodialysis patients is thought to be due to the hemodynamic challenge of hemodialysis, which is associated with cerebral hypoperfusion[34,35] and ischemia. Dialysis may be a cerebral "stress test" that precipitates events in individuals at risk with fixed stenoses in the cerebral circulation or induces a hypercoagulable state. In a single center study from Japan spanning 22 years, 39.5% of ischemic strokes and 34.7% of hemorrhagic strokes occurred during or 30 minutes after a dialysis session.[36] Nonvalvular atrial fibrillation has also been shown to be precipitated by hemodialysis because of volume and electrolyte shifts, vascular catheter movement, and ischemia as potential mechanisms, which may contribute the disproportional risk in incident patients, especially as a dry weight is established through ultrafiltration. Dialysate cooling has been shown to be a protective intervention against cerebral injury[37] by preventing hypotension (putatively by increasing preload) and maintaining cerebral perfusion.

Risk of Stroke Associated With Atrial Fibrillation

Importantly, nonvalvular atrial fibrillation is common in patients with CKD and is causally associated with ischemic stroke. In a systematic review of patients receiving dialysis, the overall incidence rate of strokes was 52/1000 patient-years in those with atrial fibrillation and 19/1000 patient-years in those without atrial fibrillation.[5] Nonvalvular atrial fibrillation diagnosed before patients started dialysis was associated with all-cause mortality (hazard ratio 1.16, 95% CI: 1.08–1.25, $P < .001$) and hospitalization or death because of a stroke/cerebrovascular accident (hazard ratio 1.28, 95% CI: 1.01–1.63; $P < .048$). Again, caveats regarding the methods of ascertaining the strokes and atrial fibrillation apply, as patients with atrial fibrillation may have increased vigilance for documenting strokes whereas patients with an obvious stroke may have increased surveillance for atrial fibrillation. Similarly, in patients with CKD that did not require dialysis, a systematic review and meta-analysis of 18 randomized controlled trials and observational studies including over half a million patients and greater than 40,000 cerebrovascular events demonstrated the relative risk of stroke in atrial fibrillation is 1.6-fold (95% CI: 1.4–1.9) compared with those with an estimated glomerular filtration rate less than 60 mL/min/1.73 m^2 compared with those with preserved renal function.[38]

Accurately predicting stroke and systemic embolism risk in nonvalvular atrial fibrillation is critical to framing the possible benefit of therapies and compare absolute risk reduction with potential harms, costs, and inconveniences of therapy as well as determining net clinical benefit. In the general population, risk prediction tools include the CHADS$_2$[39] and CHAD-VASc scores,[40] which have been extensively validated and, because of their simplicity and clinical utility/usability, have been universally adopted. However, these traditional risk prediction tools do not include renal dysfunction (including glomerular filtration rate and proteinuria) as an independent risk factor for stroke and systemic embolism because of the limited number of patients with CKD or dialysis in their derivation populations.

Although CKD and dialysis patients with nonvalvular atrial fibrillation are at an increased risk of stroke and systemic embolism compared with those without kidney dysfunction, including a renal variable in risk prediction tools does not seem to substantially improve their discriminatory performance.[38] This may be a reflection of the correlation between CKD and other risk factors for stroke and systemic embolism already captured by these risk prediction tools.[29] This issue is potentially important in the application of risk prediction to treatment. For example, if these risk prediction tools systematically underestimate or overestimate the incidence of stroke in patients with severe CKD, they may cause patients and health care providers to misestimate the benefits and risks of treatment. Conversely, it may point to differences in the etiology of the excess strokes in patients with CKD. These limitations are further highlighted by the uncertain efficacy of oral anticoagulation for preventing strokes in patients with atrial fibrillation and advanced CKD.

Risk of Bleeding in Chronic Kidney Disease

The limitations seen with stroke prediction are highlighted by the bleeding diatheses associated with CKD. Kidney disease is associated with defective platelet function leading to a prolonged bleeding time because of an accumulation of metabolites,[41] defective platelet adhesion[42] from altered GPIb[43,44] and GP IIb-IIIa activity[45,46] that reverses with dialysis.[47] The effects of these defects in coagulation are seen in the rates of major bleeding in patients with CKD. For example, in the Dialysis Outcomes and Practice Patterns Study, major bleeding occurred at a rate of 0.05–0.22 events per patient-year[48] in dialysis patients. Major bleeding was associated with acetylsalicylic acid and oral anticoagulation use with bleeding rates of 2.5% per person-year without therapy, 3.1% per person-year with vitamin K antagonists, 4.4% per person-year with acetylsalicylic acid, and 6.3% per person-year with combination therapy with hazard ratios of 3.50, 5.24, and 6.19, respectively.[49]

CKD and dialysis are associated with 5.24 and 1.95 times increase in gastrointestinal ulcer bleeding compared with the general population.[50] CKD was associated with an increased risk of upper gastrointestinal bleeding requiring hospitalization in the Atherosclerosis Risk in Communities Study[51] ranging from 1.51 to 7.06 times and 1.36–2.13 times the risk depending on glomerular filtration rate and albuminuria categories. Major bleeding risk is influenced by the degree of decline in glomerular filtration rate in addition to increasing albuminuria in CKD.[52] Upper gastrointestinal bleeds occur at rates of 57–328 episodes per 1000 person-years in dialysis depending on their definitions but seems to be decreasing in frequency and is not a benign event as it has an 11.8% 30-day mortality.[53]

Dialysis is also associated with an increased rate of nontraumatic subarachnoid hemorrhage (73.5 vs. 11.2 per 100,000 population in unadjusted analysis) with an increased mortality rate (38.4% vs. 21.9% $P<.001$) compared with the general population.[54]

The pathobiology linking kidney disease to bleeding is reflected in bleeding prediction tools. Kidney disease is an independent predictor of bleeding in nonvalvular atrial fibrillation patients treated with oral anticoagulation in tools such as HAS-BLED,[55] ATRIA,[56] and ORBIT-AF[57] with adjusted odd ratios of 2.86 (1.33–6.18), 2.53, 1.44 (1.21–1.72) for bleeding, respectively. Kidney disease was a variable defined in these studies as the need for dialysis, transplant or creatinine > 200 μmol/L in HAS-BLED, an estimated glomerular filtration rate < 30 mL/min/1.73 m² or dialysis in ATRIA, and estimated glomerular filtration rate < 60 mL/min/1.73 m² in ORBIT-AF. Empirically, the tendency to bleed is seen in observational studies such as the 11,173 patient study by Sood et al. that demonstrated a 14.4% cumulative risk over 3 years for a major bleeding episode that required hospitalization.[58]

THERAPIES TO PREVENT STROKES IN PATIENTS WITH CHRONIC KIDNEY DISEASE AND ATRIAL FIBRILLATION

In the general population, oral anticoagulation with a vitamin K antagonist targeting an international normalized ratio of 2–3 reduces the risk of ischemic stroke and systemic embolism by approximately 64% whereas acetylsalicylic acid reduces the risk by 22%.[59] In addition, direct oral anticoagulants (dabigatran, rivaroxaban, apixaban) are noninferior or superior compared with vitamin K antagonists with regard to ischemic stroke and systemic embolism prevention while being superior with regard to safety given less intracranial bleeding[60] with the added benefit of no need for therapeutic monitoring. In CKD and dialysis, the benefits of vitamin K antagonists are uncertain and they may have additional adverse events including vascular calcification, vitamin K antagonist–associated nephropathy, and calciphylaxis.

Studies examining the effects of oral anticoagulation in CKD and dialysis are limited to retrospective observational studies typically relying on databases of routinely collected health data or registries including pharmacies for oral anticoagulation prescriptions and hospitalization records for clinical outcomes and covariates used for model adjustment. Heterogeneity across studies can be explained by their populations (inclusion of CKD with or without glomerular filtration rate stratification; hemodialysis; peritoneal dialysis; transplant, incident, or prevalent dialysis patients; and incident or prevalent oral anticoagulation users), exposure to oral anticoagulation (not handled or handled as time varying covariate, international normalized ratio monitoring, adherence, censoring related to drug discontinuation), outcomes (transient ischemic attack, ischemic stroke, hemorrhagic stroke, any stroke, major bleeding, minor bleeding, cardiovascular mortality, all-cause mortality, a variety of composites to define net clinical benefit), and incorporation of the competing risks of mortality, transplant, and progression of CKD to end-stage renal disease. Given the inherent bias involved in offering oral anticoagulation in CKD and dialysis to healthier, adherent patients and withholding oral anticoagulation in sicker, nonadherent patients (supported by a mortality benefit of oral anticoagulation vs. no oral anticoagulation in several studies), studies have attempted to use rigorous statistical methodology to adjust for imbalances in prognostic variables between groups including propensity matching and inverse probability of treatment and censoring-weighting, but residual confounding by indication and bias (misclassification, survivorship, ascertainment, selection) remains. Several systematic reviews and meta-analyses have been performed and all demonstrate significant heterogeneity with possible benefit of oral anticoagulation for ischemic stroke/systemic embolism prevention in CKD but not in end-stage renal disease but with an increase in bleeding risk in both settings. The debate regarding oral anticoagulation for atrial fibrillation in CKD and dialysis for ischemic stroke and systemic embolism prevention is ongoing.[61,62]

Because of these limitations, the overall evidence base supporting or refuting the efficacy and safety of oral anticoagulation or antiplatelet agents in patients with advanced CKD is very limited. As such, the net clinical benefit of treatments to prevent strokes patients with CKD and atrial fibrillation is uncertain.[63]

Oral Anticoagulation in Chronic Kidney Disease or Dialysis
Studies suggesting benefit
Hart et al.[64] performed a post hoc analysis of 1936 mostly stage 3 CKD patients from the Stroke Prevention in Atrial Fibrillation III study comparing vitamin K antagonist use with an international normalized ratio of 2-3 to 1-3 mg orally daily (mean international normalized ratio 1.3) with acetylsalicylic acid 325 mg orally daily. They showed a relative risk reduction of 76% (95% C.I. 42%-90% $P = .001$) with the former

therapy with no difference in bleeding but uncertain effects estimates given early discontinuation of the study.

Olesen et al.[65] used population-based registries from Denmark including all hospital discharges with a diagnosis of nonvalvular atrial fibrillation from 1997 to 2008 and medication prescriptions up to 7 days after discharge to perform a time-dependent Cox regression analysis to determine the association between acetylsalicylic acid, vitamin K antagonist, or combination therapy with stroke (ischemic stroke or hemorrhagic stroke), systemic embolism, and bleeding adjusted for CHADS-VASc, and HAS-BLED in CKD (2.7% of cohort or 3587 patients) and end-stage renal disease (0.7% of cohort or 901 hemodialysis, peritoneal dialysis, and transplant patients). The risk of bleeding was higher with acetylsalicylic acid, vitamin K antagonist, and combination therapy compared with no therapy in both CKD and end-stage renal disease groups but only decreased stroke and systemic embolism in dialysis but not CKD.

Bonde et al.[66] performed a similar analysis that included 11,128 CKD (7.2% of cohort) and 1728 end-stage renal disease (1.1% of cohort with hemodialysis > peritoneal dialysis > transplant) patients, focusing on net clinical benefit using a variety of composites of stroke/bleeding/hospitalization/cardiovascular mortality/mortality. In high-risk CKD defined by a $CHADS_2$ score of ≥2, vitamin K antagonist use was associated with a lower risk of cardiovascular death (hazard ratio: 0.80, 95% CI: 0.74-0.88) and all-cause mortality (hazard ratio: 0.64, 95% CI: 0.60-0.69), and in low/intermediate-risk CKD defined by a $CHADS_2$ score of 0-1, vitamin K antagonist use was associated with a significantly lower risk of all-cause mortality (hazard ratio: 0.62, 95% CI: 0.49 to 0.79) and a nonsignificant trend toward lower risk of cardiovascular death. In high-risk end-stage renal disease, vitamin K antagonist use was associated with a significantly lower risk of all-cause mortality (hazard ratio: 0.85, 95% CI: 0.72 to 0.99) and nonsignificant trends toward lower risks of cardiovascular death and the composite of death/hospitalization from stroke/systemic embolism/bleeding, whereas low/intermediate-risk end-stage renal disease was nonsignificant for all outcomes.

Carrero et al.[67] used the SWEDEHEART registry, which includes 72 hospitals with admissions for cardiovascular diseases in Sweden from 2003 to 2010 with data linkage to national registries to examine the association between vitamin K antagonist use as a time-fixed variable at discharge and mortality, hospitalization for myocardial infarction, ischemic stroke, bleeding (intracranial hemorrhage, gastrointestinal, anemia, others) in those with nonvalvular atrial fibrillation determined by history or documented by electrocardiogram during admission or hospitalization across CKD stages. The study included 24,317 individuals of which 41.7%, 8.1%, and 2.0% had stages 3, 4, and 5 CKD, respectively, and 21.8% were treated with vitamin K antagonists at discharge. In each CKD category vitamin K antagonist use versus no vitamin K antagonist use was associated with a lower number of events of the composite of death, myocardial infarction, or stroke except for stage 5 CKD because of a limited power with no differences in bleeding risk.

Friberg et al.[68] used Swedish health registries to identify nonvalvular atrial fibrillation from hospitalizations and clinics between 2005 and 2010 to identify 307,351 individuals of which 13,435 had renal failure by ICD-10 codes, which included CKD, hemodialysis, peritoneal dialysis, and transplant patients. In a multivariate model adjusted for CHADS-VASc and HAS-BLED, use of a vitamin K antagonist identified by drug registry had a significantly more net clinical benefit defined by the combined endpoint of ischemic stroke or intracranial hemorrhage (hazard ratio: 0.85, 95% CI: 0.74–0.98) and ischemic stroke, intracranial hemorrhage, death (hazard ratio: 0.76, 95% CI: 0.72–0.80).

Shen et al.[69] used the United States Renal Data System database to compare outcomes by vitamin K antagonist exposure in 12,284 dialysis patients with incident nonvalvular atrial fibrillation from 2007 to 2011 defined by ICD coding. Outcomes of included death, cardiovascular death, stroke-related death, ischemic stroke, hemorrhagic stroke, gastrointestinal bleeding, and a Cox regression analysis using propensity scores and inverse probability of treatment and censoring-weighting and sensitivity analyses (intention to treat and censoring at 30 or 60 days after discontinuation of vitamin K antagonist). The results did not show any benefit or harm for any individual or composite outcome other than a decrease in all-cause mortality with vitamin K antagonist use but only 30% of vitamin K antagonist users were still on therapy at 1 year.

Studies suggesting harm

Shah et al.[70] performed a population-based retrospective cohort study that included 204,210 nondialysis-dependent and 1626 dialysis-dependent individuals aged > 65 years with hospitalizations for nonvalvular atrial fibrillation identified by ICD coding 1998–2007 in Canada and medications assessed within 30 days after discharge. Outcomes were transient ischemic attack/stroke and bleeding (intracranial hemorrhage,

gastrointestinal, eye, hematuria, unspecified), and a multivariable Cox proportional hazards model was performed with vitamin K antagonist use treated as a time-fixed variable in addition to a propensity score as a covariate. In dialysis patients, vitamin K antagonist use was not associated with a lower risk for ischemic stroke/transient ischemic attack (adjusted hazard ratio, 1.14; 95% CI: 0.78–1.67 and propensity score adjusted hazard ratio 1.17; 95% CI: 0.79–1.75) unlike nondialysis patients but was associated with a 20%–44% increased risk of bleeding (adjusted hazard ratio, 1.44; 95% CI: 1.13–1.85 and propensity score adjusted hazard ratio 1.20; 95% CI: 1.17–1.23).

Similarly, Keskar et al.[71] performed a population-based retrospective cohort study in Canada that included 6544 individuals aged > 65 years with nondialysis-dependent CKD defined as one outpatient estimated glomerular filtration rate assessment < 45 mL/min/1.73 m^2 before a hospitalization/emergency room visit with nonvalvular atrial fibrillation identified by ICD coding from 2002 to 2014 with follow-up until 2015. Medications were assessed within 30 days from hospitalization/emergency visit and censoring performed if no refill was completed after 180 + 100 days. Outcomes were hospitalization or emergency room visit for transient ischemic attack/ischemic stroke, hemorrhagic events (intracranial, gastrointestinal, nontraumatic, transfusion), and mortality with propensity score matching followed by Cox proportional hazards models stratified on 1:1 matched pairs on the basis of the logit of propensity score, CKD stage, and index date with sensitivity analyses (competing risk of death, 180 days cutoff, and oral anticoagulation as time-varying covariate in an extended Cox model). Ischemic stroke was not significantly lower among those on oral anticoagulation (hazard ratio: 1.10; 95% CI: 0.78–1.56) and was unchanged in the competing risk of death and 180 days sensitivity analyses, but in a time-varying model, the risk of ischemic stroke was higher with oral anticoagulation (hazard ratio of 1.22; 95% CI: 1.02–1.47). However, the risk for bleeding was higher in the oral anticoagulation group (hazard ratio: 1.42; 95% CI: 1.04–1.93), which persisted after accounting for the competing risk of death (hazard ratio: 1.60; 95% CI: 1.31–1.97), matching (hazard ratio: 1.66; 95% CI: 1.26–2.18), and in a time-varying analysis (hazard ratio: 2.40; 95% CI: 2.08–2.77). However, the hazard ratio for mortality was lower (hazard ratio: 0.74; 95% CI: 0.62–0.88) in those patients treated with oral anticoagulation.

This is supported by a study in which Jun et al.[72] examined emergency room or hospitalizations for major bleeding in elderly patients aged≥65 years with atrial fibrillation on vitamin K antagonists stratified by estimated glomerular filtration adjusted for CHADS-VASc, HAS-BLED, and comorbidities using multivariate Poisson regression and Alberta Kidney Disease Network databases with ICD coding. In 15,319 individuals with 1443 major bleeding events, estimated glomerular filtration rates<30 and <15 mL/min/1.73 m² were independently associated with major bleeding on warfarin but not at lesser degrees of glomerular filtration rate impairment.

A systematic review and metaanalysis of 20 observational studies comparing vitamin K antagonists with placebo for atrial fibrillation in end-stage renal disease (hemodialysis, peritoneal dialysis, estimated glomerular filtration rate<15) did not show any benefit for stroke prevention (hazard ratio 0.92 95% CI: 0.74–1.16) but did show an increase in all-cause bleeding (hazard ratio 95% CI: 1.21 1.01–1.44) and any bleeding (hazard ratio 1.21 95% CI: 0.99–1.48) but not major or gastrointestinal bleeding. This increased risk of bleeding and modified efficacy of vitamin K antagonists in CKD and end-stage renal disease may be due to altered responsiveness to vitamin K antagonists leading to lower doses, less time in therapeutic range, and a higher risk of overanticoagulation.[73,74]

Lack of consensus on use of anticoagulation for stroke prevention. Uncertainty of the benefits and risks of therapies to reduce the risk of stroke, particularly oral anticoagulants, for patients with advanced kidney disease is reflected in both the attitudes of nephrologists to anticoagulation and their documented practice patterns. Canadian nephrologists who were surveyed in

2013 six hypothetical CKD patients with varying stroke and bleeding risks showed variability in the willingness to initiate oral anticoagulation for nonvalvular atrial fibrillation ranging from 16.1% to 48.2% favoring use depending on the case.[75] Similarly, a survey of Italian nephrologists in 2010 assessing practice patterns of oral anticoagulation for atrial fibrillation in dialysis patients showed that comorbidities, previous bleeding episodes, and a history of falls drove hesitancy in the prescription of oral anticoagulation.[76] Variability in acetylsalicylic acid and oral anticoagulation use for ischemic stroke and systemic embolism prevention in nonvalvular atrial fibrillation in dialysis patients is therefore not surprising. The Dialysis Outcomes and Practice Patterns Study demonstrated acetylsalicylic acid use ranged from 17% in Japan to 46% in the United Kingdom and oral anticoagulation use ranged from 2% in Germany to 37% in Canada.[29]

This issue is also reflected in guidelines from various national and international groups. The Kidney Disease: International Guideline Organization and Canadian Cardiology Society consider the current data insufficient to recommend anticoagulation with vitamin K antagonists for stroke preventions in CKD patients with atrial fibrillation.[77,78] In contrast, the American College of Cardiology/American Heart Association/Heart Rhythm Society consider the use of a vitamin K antagonist a class IIa recommendation for patients with a creatinine clearance of less than 15 mL/min and a CHADS-VASc score of 2 or greater.[79] Meanwhile some neurologists recommend anticoagulation for those patients with moderate CKD at high risk of stroke.[80] Clearly, perspectives differ because of inconclusive evidence (Table 14.1).

TABLE 14.1
Major Studies of Warfarin for Stroke Prevention in Patients With End-Stage Renal Disease and Atrial Fibrillation

Study	Study Type	n	Receiving Warfarin (%)	Hazard Ratio for Ischemic Stroke (95% Confidence Interval)
Chan et al.[81]	Administrative data	1,671	(44.7%)	1.95 (0.99–3.84)
Lai (2010)	Retrospective observational	93	51 (54.8%)	0.26 (0.10–0.64)
Wizemann et al.[29]	Prospective observational	2,188	(16%)	<65 years 1.26 (0.45–3.68) 66–75 years 1.35 (0.69–2.63) >75 years 2.17 (1.04–4.53)
Winkelmayer et al.[31]	Administrative data	2,313	249 (10.8%)	0.92 (0.61–1.37)
Olesen et al.[65]	Administrative data	901	223 (24.7%)	0.44 (0.26–0.74)
Shah et al.[70]	Administrative data	1,626	756 (46%)	1.14 (0.78–1.67)
Shen et al.[69]	Administrative data	12,285	1838 (15%)	0.68 (0.47–0.99)

Antiplatelet agents in chronic kidney disease and dialysis. Chan et al.[81] studied 1671 incident > 90 days hemodialysis patients from Fresenius centers in the United States from 2003 to 2004 with preexisting nonvalvular atrial fibrillation identified by electronic medical records (75% accuracy compared with electrocardiogram) and assessed the association of vitamin K antagonists, clopidogrel, and acetylsalicylic acid with hospitalization/death from transient ischemic attack/stroke in follow-up. A time-varying Cox proportional hazards model that included a propensity score analysis demonstrated that vitamin K antagonist increased the risk of both ischemic stroke (hazard ratio 1.81 95% CI: 1.12 to 2.92) and hemorrhagic stroke (hazard ratio 2.22 95% CI: 1.01 to 4.91), whereas acetylsalicylic acid and clopidogrel did not significantly influence the outcomes compared to no therapy.

In the Dialysis Outcomes and Practice Patterns Study, acetylsalicylic acid use was associated with a decreased risk of stroke in all patients (relative risk 0.82, $P < .01$), but stroke mechanism subgroups including atrial fibrillation were not presented.[82]

DIRECT ORAL ANTICOAGULANTS IN CHRONIC KIDNEY DISEASE OR DIALYSIS

In a systematic review and meta-analysis of randomized controlled trials comparing direct oral anticoagulants with vitamin K antagonists in CKD (defined by a creatinine clearance of 30–50 mL/min/1.73 m^2) with outcomes including stroke, systemic embolism, and bleeding, which included ARISTOTLE,[83] RE-LY,[84] and ROCKET-AF[85] totaling 9693 patients,[86] direct oral anticoagulants were associated with a trend toward less stroke and systemic embolism (relative risk 0.64 95% CI: 0.39–1.04) with no increase in major bleeding or clinically relevant nonmajor bleeding (relative risk 0.89 95% CI: 0.68–1.16) with significant heterogeneity across agents (dabigatran, rivaroxaban, apixaban). Studies dedicated to evaluating the efficacy and safety of direct thrombin inhibitors and factor Xa inhibitors in nonvalvular atrial fibrillation are limited to CKD subgroups in randomized controlled trials with only pharmacokinetic/pharmacodynamic for rivaroxaban[87] and apixaban[88] studies in hemodialysis. However, uptake of dabigatran and rivaroxaban in end-stage renal disease is occurring as demonstrated by the Fresenius end-stage renal disease database from 2010 to 2014 of 29,977 patients with nonvalvular atrial fibrillation on hemodialysis with a 5.9% prevalence of direct oral anticoagulant including 3.1% dabigatran and 2.8% rivaroxaban with very few

events for the assessment of their efficacy but higher risks of major bleeding and minor bleeding compared with vitamin K antagonists unaffected by sensitivity analyses.[89]

LEFT ATRIAL OCCLUSION DEVICES

Left atrial occlusion devices including the WATCHMAN device have been shown to be noninferior to vitamin K antagonists for stroke and systemic embolism prevention in nonvalvular atrial fibrillation in the general population with more ischemic strokes and less hemorrhagic strokes as well as periprocedural risks that seem to be related to an operator learning curve.[90,91] Unfortunately, CKD and dialysis patients were excluded from both studies but would be ideal candidates given their inherent stroke and bleeding risks.

Patients' Values and Preferences

The poor outcomes for strokes in CKD and dialysis and the increased risks of bleeding from antiplatelet agents and oral anticoagulation and their consequences (risk of acute kidney injury, progression of CKD, blood transfusion as a sensitization event affecting transplant eligibility, morbidity, and mortality) may influence patient values and preferences in selecting appropriate therapies. Thus, the results of previous studies using probability trade-off techniques and thresholds for therapy selection[92] may not apply to CKD and dialysis, given the fundamental differences in outcomes and uncertainty regarding the efficacy of therapies for ischemic stroke and systemic embolism prevention in nonvalvular atrial fibrillation.

FUTURE DIRECTIONS

Given the clinical equipoise of oral anticoagulation in the CKD and dialysis populations for stroke and systemic embolism in nonvalvular atrial fibrillation, the call for randomized controlled trials evaluating therapies has been ongoing.[93] A study comparing vitamin K antagonists with acetylsalicylic acid for stroke prevention in nonvalvular atrial fibrillation in dialysis patients is currently planned.[94] Apixaban is also being compared with vitamin K antagonists for nonvalvular atrial fibrillation stroke prevention in dialysis in another study that is currently recruiting.[95] The WATCHMAN device is also being evaluated in CKD and dialysis in the STOP-HARM[96] study. Studies evaluating the values and preferences of CKD and dialysis patients regarding their values and preferences regarding therapies are needed.

CONCLUSIONS

Atrial fibrillation, ischemic strokes, and major bleeding are common in patients with advanced CKD. The etiology for these diseases is complex and may differ from patients without CKD, but they are important as they may inform the difference in treatments and outcomes for patients with versus without CKD. For patients with CKD, there is a current lack of high-quality evidence supporting the use of therapies known to safely and effectively prevent strokes in patients with normal renal function. This uncertainty is reflected in practice pattern variations, and high-quality evidence is urgently needed given the increasing prevalence of both CKD and atrial fibrillation globally and the devastating effects of strokes on patients with these concomitant disorders.

REFERENCES

1. Jha V, Garcia-Garcia G, Iseki K, et al. Chronic kidney disease: global dimension and perspectives. *Lancet*. 2013;382(9888):260–272.
2. Coresh J, Selvin E, Stevens LA, et al. Prevalence of chronic kidney disease in the United States. *JAMA*. 2007;298(17):2038–2047.
3. Tonelli M, Muntner P, Lloyd A, et al. Risk of coronary events in people with chronic kidney disease compared with those with diabetes: a population-level cohort study. *Lancet*. 2012;380(9844):807–814.
4. Masson P, Webster AC, Hong M, Turner R, Lindley RI, Craig JC. Chronic kidney disease and the risk of stroke: a systematic review and meta-analysis. *Nephrol Dial Transplant*. 2015;30(7):1162–1169.
5. Zimmerman D, Sood MM, Rigatto C, Holden RM, Hiremath S, Clase CM. Systematic review and meta-analysis of incidence, prevalence and outcomes of atrial fibrillation in patients on dialysis. *Nephrol Dial Transplant*. 2012;27(10):3816–3822.
6. Kuo CC, Lee CT, Ho SC, Kuo HW, Wu TN, Yang CY. Haemodialysis and the risk of stroke: a population-based cohort study in taiwan, a country of high incidence of end-stage renal disease. *Nephrology (Carlton)*. 2012;17(3):243–248.
7. Masson P, Kelly PJ, Craig JC, Lindley RI, Webster AC. Risk of stroke in patients with ESRD. *Clin J Am Soc Nephrol*. 2015;10(9):1585–1592.
8. Wang HH, Hung SY, Sung JM, Hung KY, Wang JD. Risk of stroke in long-term dialysis patients compared with the general population. *Am J Kidney Dis*. 2014;63(4):604–611.
9. Findlay MD, Thomson PC, Fulton RL, et al. Risk factors of ischemic stroke and subsequent outcome in patients receiving hemodialysis. *Stroke*. 2015;46(9):2477–2481.
10. Power A, Chan K, Singh SK, Taube D, Duncan N. Appraising stroke risk in maintenance hemodialysis patients: a large single-center cohort study. *Am J Kidney Dis*. 2012;59(2):249–257.
11. Sozio SM, Armstrong PA, Coresh J, et al. Cerebrovascular disease incidence, characteristics, and outcomes in patients initiating dialysis: the choices for healthy outcomes in caring for ESRD (CHOICE) study. *Am J Kidney Dis*. 2009;54(3):468–477.
12. Wetmore JB, Phadnis MA, Ellerbeck EF, Shireman TI, Rigler SK, Mahnken JD. Relationship between stroke and mortality in dialysis patients. *Clin J Am Soc Nephrol*. 2015;10(1):80–89.
13. Providencia R, Marijon E, Boveda S, et al. Meta-analysis of the influence of chronic kidney disease on the risk of thromboembolism among patients with nonvalvular atrial fibrillation. *Am J Cardiol*. 2014;114(4):646–653.
14. Murray AM, Seliger S, Lakshminarayan K, Herzog CA, Solid CA. Incidence of stroke before and after dialysis initiation in older patients. *J Am Soc Nephrol*. 2013;24(7):1166–1173.
15. Wetmore JB, Ellerbeck EF, Mahnken JD, et al. Stroke and the "stroke belt" in dialysis: contribution of patient characteristics to ischemic stroke rate and its geographic variation. *J Am Soc Nephrol*. 2013;24(12):2053–2061.
16. Sanchez-Perales C, Vazquez E, Garcia-Cortes MJ, et al. Ischaemic stroke in incident dialysis patients. *Nephrol Dial Transplant*. 2010;25(10):3343–3348.
17. Seliger SL, Gillen DL, Tirschwell D, Wasse H, Kestenbaum BR, Stehman-Breen CO. Risk factors for incident stroke among patients with end-stage renal disease. *J Am Soc Nephrol*. 2003;14(10):2623–2631.
18. Yamada S, Tsuruya K, Taniguchi M, et al. Association between serum phosphate levels and stroke risk in patients undergoing hemodialysis: the Q-cohort study. *Stroke*. 2016;47(9):2189–2196.
19. Sozio SM, Coresh J, Jaar BG, et al. Inflammatory markers and risk of cerebrovascular events in patients initiating dialysis. *Clin J Am Soc Nephrol*. 2011;6(6):1292–1300.
20. Nampoory MR, Das KC, Johny KV, et al. Hypercoagulability, a serious problem in patients with ESRD on maintenance hemodialysis, and its correction after kidney transplantation. *Am J Kidney Dis*. 2003;42(4):797–805.
21. Ball T, Wheelan K, McCullough PA. Chronic anticoagulation in chronic kidney disease. *J Am Coll Cardiol*. 2014;64(23):2483–2485.
22. Toyoda K, Fujii K, Fujimi S, et al. Stroke in patients on maintenance hemodialysis: a 22-year single-center study. *Am J Kidney Dis*. 2005;45(6):1058–1066.
23. Ishida K, Brown MG, Weiner M, Kobrin S, Kasner SE, Messe SR. Endocarditis is a common stroke mechanism in hemodialysis patients. *Stroke*. 2014;45(4):1164–1166.
24. Wu X, Yang X, Liu X, et al. Patient survival and technique failure in continuous ambulatory peritoneal dialysis patients with prior stroke. *Perit Dial Int*. 2016;36(3):308–314.
25. Iseki K, Fukiyama K, Okawa Dialysis Study (OKIDS) Group. Clinical demographics and long-term prognosis after stroke in patients on chronic haemodialysis. The okinawa dialysis study (OKIDS) group. *Nephrol Dial Transplant*. 2000;15(11):1808–1813.
26. Mattana J, Effiong C, Gooneratne R, Singhal PC. Outcome of stroke in patients undergoing hemodialysis. *Arch Intern Med*. 1998;158(5):537–541.

27. Ovbiagele B, Schwamm LH, Smith EE, et al. Patterns of care quality and prognosis among hospitalized ischemic stroke patients with chronic kidney disease. *J Am Heart Assoc.* 2014;3(3):e000905.
28. Abramson JL, Jurkovitz CT, Vaccarino V, Weintraub WS, McClellan W. Chronic kidney disease, anemia, and incident stroke in a middle-aged, community-based population: the ARIC study. *Kidney Int.* 2003;64(2):610–615.
29. Wizemann V, Tong L, Satayathum S, et al. Atrial fibrillation in hemodialysis patients: clinical features and associations with anticoagulant therapy. *Kidney Int.* 2010;77(12):1098–1106.
30. Goldstein BA, Arce CM, Hlatky MA, Turakhia M, Setoguchi S, Winkelmayer WC. Trends in the incidence of atrial fibrillation in older patients initiating dialysis in the United States. *Circulation.* 2012;126(19):2293–2301.
31. Winkelmayer WC, Liu J, Setoguchi S, Choudhry NK. Effectiveness and safety of warfarin initiation in older hemodialysis patients with incident atrial fibrillation. *Clin J Am Soc Nephrol.* 2011;6(11):2662–2668.
32. Vazquez E, Sanchez-Perales C, Garcia-Garcia F, et al. Atrial fibrillation in incident dialysis patients. *Kidney Int.* 2009;76(3):324–330.
33. Genovesi S, Pogliani D, Faini A, et al. Prevalence of atrial fibrillation and associated factors in a population of long-term hemodialysis patients. *Am J Kidney Dis.* 2005;46(5):897–902.
34. Hata R, Matsumoto M, Handa N, Terakawa H, Sugitani Y, Kamada T. Effects of hemodialysis on cerebral circulation evaluated by transcranial Doppler ultrasonography. *Stroke.* 1994;25(2):408–412.
35. Postiglione A, Faccenda F, Gallotta G, Rubba P, Federico S. Changes in middle cerebral artery blood velocity in uremic patients after hemodialysis. *Stroke.* 1991;22(12):1508–1511.
36. Toyoda K, Fujii K, Ando T, Kumai Y, Ibayashi S, Iida M. Incidence, etiology, and outcome of stroke in patients on continuous ambulatory peritoneal dialysis. *Cerebrovasc Dis.* 2004;17(2–3):98–105.
37. Eldehni MT, Odudu A, McIntyre CW. Randomized clinical trial of dialysate cooling and effects on brain white matter. *J Am Soc Nephrol.* 2015;26(4):957–965.
38. Zeng WT, Sun XT, Tang K, et al. Risk of thromboembolic events in atrial fibrillation with chronic kidney disease. *Stroke.* 2015;46(1):157–163.
39. Gage BF, Waterman AD, Shannon W, Boechler M, Rich MW, Radford MJ. Validation of clinical classification schemes for predicting stroke: results from the national registry of atrial fibrillation. *JAMA.* 2001;285(22):2864–2870.
40. Lip GY, Nieuwlaat R, Pisters R, Lane DA, Crijns HJ. Refining clinical risk stratification for predicting stroke and thromboembolism in atrial fibrillation using a novel risk factor-based approach: the euro heart survey on atrial fibrillation. *Chest.* 2010;137(2):263–272.
41. Jubelirer SJ. Hemostatic abnormalities in renal disease. *Am J Kidney Dis.* 1985;5(5):219–225.
42. Castillo R, Lozano T, Escolar G, Revert L, Lopez J, Ordinas A. Defective platelet adhesion on vessel subendothelium in uremic patients. *Blood.* 1986;68(2):337–342.

43. Sloand EM, Sloand JA, Prodouz K, et al. Reduction of platelet glycoprotein ib in uraemia. *Br J Haematol.* 1991;77(3):375–381.
44. Sloand JA, Sloand EM. Studies on platelet membrane glycoproteins and platelet function during hemodialysis. *J Am Soc Nephrol.* 1997;8(5):799–803.
45. Benigni A, Boccardo P, Galbusera M, et al. Reversible activation defect of the platelet glycoprotein IIb-IIIa complex in patients with uremia. *Am J Kidney Dis.* 1993;22(5):668–676.
46. Sreedhara R, Itagaki I, Hakim RM. Uremic patients have decreased shear-induced platelet aggregation mediated by decreased availability of glycoprotein IIb-IIIa receptors. *Am J Kidney Dis.* 1996;27(3):355–364.
47. Gawaz MP, Dobos G, Spath M, Schollmeyer P, Gurland HJ, Mujais SK. Impaired function of platelet membrane glycoprotein IIb-IIIa in end-stage renal disease. *J Am Soc Nephrol.* 1994;5(1):36–46.
48. Sood MM, Larkina M, Thumma JR, et al. Major bleeding events and risk stratification of antithrombotic agents in hemodialysis: results from the DOPPS. *Kidney Int.* 2013;84(3):600–608.
49. Holden RM, Harman GJ, Wang M, Holland D, Day AG. Major bleeding in hemodialysis patients. *Clin J Am Soc Nephrol.* 2008;3(1):105–110.
50. Luo JC, Leu HB, Huang KW, et al. Incidence of bleeding from gastroduodenal ulcers in patients with end-stage renal disease receiving hemodialysis. *CMAJ.* 2011;183(18):E1345–E1351.
51. Ishigami J, Grams ME, Naik RP, Coresh J, Matsushita K. Chronic kidney disease and risk for gastrointestinal bleeding in the community: the atherosclerosis risk in communities (ARIC) study. *Clin J Am Soc Nephrol.* 2016;11(10):1735–1743.
52. Molnar AO, Bota SE, Garg AX, et al. The risk of major hemorrhage with CKD. *J Am Soc Nephrol.* 2016;27(9):2825–2832.
53. Yang JY, Lee TC, Montez-Rath ME, et al. Trends in acute nonvariceal upper gastrointestinal bleeding in dialysis patients. *J Am Soc Nephrol.* 2012;23(3):495–506.
54. Sakhuja A, Schold JD, Kumar G, Katzan I, Navaneethan SD. Nontraumatic subarachnoid hemorrhage in maintenance dialysis hospitalizations: trends and outcomes. *Stroke.* 2014;45(1):71–76.
55. Pisters R, Lane DA, Nieuwlaat R, de Vos CB, Crijns HJ, Lip GY. A novel user-friendly score (HAS-BLED) to assess 1-year risk of major bleeding in patients with atrial fibrillation: the euro heart survey. *Chest.* 2010;138(5):1093–1100.
56. Fang MC, Go AS, Chang Y, et al. A new risk scheme to predict warfarin-associated hemorrhage: the ATRIA (anticoagulation and risk factors in atrial fibrillation) study. *J Am Coll Cardiol.* 2011;58(4):395–401.
57. O'Brien EC, Simon DN, Thomas LE, et al. The ORBIT bleeding score: a simple bedside score to assess bleeding risk in atrial fibrillation. *Eur Heart J.* 2015;36(46):3258–3264.
58. Sood MM, Bota SE, McArthur E, et al. The three-year incidence of major hemorrhage among older adults initiating chronic dialysis. *Can J Kidney Health Dis.* 2014;1:21. https://doi.org/10.1186/s40697-014-0021-x. eCollection 2014.

59. Hart RG, Pearce LA, Aguilar MI. Meta-analysis: antithrombotic therapy to prevent stroke in patients who have nonvalvular atrial fibrillation. *Ann Intern Med.* 2007;146(12):857–867.

60. Dentali F, Riva N, Crowther M, Turpie AG, Lip GY, Ageno W. Efficacy and safety of the novel oral anticoagulants in atrial fibrillation: a systematic review and meta-analysis of the literature. *Circulation.* 2012;126(20):2381–2391.

61. McCullough PA, Ball T, Cox KM, Assar MD. Use of oral anticoagulation in the management of atrial fibrillation in patients with ESRD: Pro. *Clin J Am Soc Nephrol.* 2016;11(11):2079–2084.

62. Keskar V, Sood MM. Use of oral anticoagulation in the management of atrial fibrillation in patients with ESRD: Con. *Clin J Am Soc Nephrol.* 2016;11(11):2085–2092.

63. Dahal K, Kunwar S, Rijal J, Schulman P, Lee J. Stroke, major bleeding, and mortality outcomes in warfarin users with atrial fibrillation and chronic kidney disease: a meta-analysis of observational studies. *Chest.* 2016; 149(4):951–959.

64. Hart RG, Pearce LA, Asinger RW, Herzog CA. Warfarin in atrial fibrillation patients with moderate chronic kidney disease. *Clin J Am Soc Nephrol.* 2011;6(11):2599–2604.

65. Olesen JB, Lip GY, Kamper AL, et al. Stroke and bleeding in atrial fibrillation with chronic kidney disease. *N Engl J Med.* 2012;367(7):625–635.

66. Bonde AN, Lip GY, Kamper AL, et al. Net clinical benefit of antithrombotic therapy in patients with atrial fibrillation and chronic kidney disease: a nationwide observational cohort study. *J Am Coll Cardiol.* 2014;64(23):2471–2482.

67. Carrero JJ, Evans M, Szummer K, et al. Warfarin, kidney dysfunction, and outcomes following acute myocardial infarction in patients with atrial fibrillation. *JAMA.* 2014;311(9):919–928.

68. Friberg L, Benson L, Lip GY. Balancing stroke and bleeding risks in patients with atrial fibrillation and renal failure: the Swedish atrial fibrillation cohort study. *Eur Heart J.* 2015;36(5):297–306.

69. Shen JI, Montez-Rath ME, Lenihan CR, Turakhia MP, Chang TI, Winkelmayer WC. Outcomes after warfarin initiation in a cohort of hemodialysis patients with newly diagnosed atrial fibrillation. *Am J Kidney Dis.* 2015;66(4):677–688.

70. Shah M, Avgil Tsadok M, Jackevicius CA, et al. Warfarin use and the risk for stroke and bleeding in patients with atrial fibrillation undergoing dialysis. *Circulation.* 2014;129(11):1196–1203.

71. Keskar V, McArthur E, Wald R, et al. The association of anticoagulation, ischemic stroke, and hemorrhage in elderly adults with chronic kidney disease and atrial fibrillation. *Kidney Int.* 2017;91(4):928–936.

72. Jun M, James MT, Ma Z, et al. Warfarin initiation, atrial fibrillation, and kidney function: comparative effectiveness and safety of warfarin in older adults with newly diagnosed atrial fibrillation. *Am J Kidney Dis.* 2016; 69(6):734–743.

73. Limdi NA, Beasley TM, Baird MF, et al. Kidney function influences warfarin responsiveness and hemorrhagic complications. *J Am Soc Nephrol.* 2009;20(4):912–921.

74. Limdi NA, Limdi MA, Cavallari L, et al. Warfarin dosing in patients with impaired kidney function. *Am J Kidney Dis.* 2010;56(5):823–831.

75. Juma S, Thomson BK, Lok CE, Clase CM, Blake PG, Moist L. Warfarin use in hemodialysis patients with atrial fibrillation: decisions based on uncertainty. *BMC Nephrol.* 2013;14:174. https://doi.org/10.1186/1471-2369-14-174.

76. Genovesi S, Rossi E, Pogliani D, et al. The nephrologist's anticoagulation treatment patterns/regimens in chronic hemodialysis patients with atrial fibrillation. *J Nephrol.* 2014;27(2):187–192.

77. Herzog CA, Asinger RW, Berger AK, et al. Cardiovascular disease in chronic kidney disease. A clinical update from kidney disease: improving global outcomes (KDIGO). *Kidney Int.* 2011;80(6):572–586.

78. Macle L, Cairns J, Leblanc K, et al. 2016 focused update of the Canadian Cardiovascular Society guidelines for the management of atrial fibrillation. *Can J Cardiol.* 2016;32(10):1170–1185.

79. January CT, Wann LS, Alpert JS, et al. 2014 AHA/ACC/HRS guideline for the management of patients with atrial fibrillation: a report of the American College of Cardiology/American Heart Association task force on practice guidelines and the Heart Rhythm Society. *J Am Coll Cardiol.* 2014;64(21):e1–e76.

80. Hart RG, Ingram AJ, Eikelboom JW. Which patients with atrial fibrillation and chronic kidney disease should receive anticoagulation-and with which anticoagulant? *Can J Cardiol.* 2017;33(2):211–213.

81. Chan KE, Lazarus JM, Thadhani R, Hakim RM. Warfarin use associates with increased risk for stroke in hemodialysis patients with atrial fibrillation. *J Am Soc Nephrol.* 2009;20(10):2223–2233.

82. Ethier J, Bragg-Gresham JL, Piera L, et al. Aspirin prescription and outcomes in hemodialysis patients: the dialysis outcomes and practice patterns study (DOPPS). *Am J Kidney Dis.* 2007;50(4):602–611.

83. Granger CB, Alexander JH, McMurray JJ, et al. Apixaban versus warfarin in patients with atrial fibrillation. *N Engl J Med.* 2011;365(11):981–992.

84. Connolly SJ, Ezekowitz MD, Yusuf S, et al. Dabigatran versus warfarin in patients with atrial fibrillation. *N Engl J Med.* 2009;361(12):1139–1151.

85. Patel MR, Mahaffey KW, Garg J, et al. Rivaroxaban versus warfarin in nonvalvular atrial fibrillation. *N Engl J Med.* 2011;365(10):883–891.

86. Harel Z, Sholzberg M, Shah PS, et al. Comparisons between novel oral anticoagulants and vitamin K antagonists in patients with CKD. *J Am Soc Nephrol.* 2014;25(3):431–442.

87. De Vriese AS, Caluwe R, Bailleul E, et al. Dose-finding study of rivaroxaban in hemodialysis patients. *Am J Kidney Dis.* 2015;66(1):91–98.

88. Mavrakanas TA, Samer CF, Nessim SJ, Frisch G, Lipman ML. Apixaban pharmacokinetics at steady state in hemodialysis patients. *J Am Soc Nephrol.* 2017;28(7):2241–2248.

89. Chan KE, Edelman ER, Wenger JB, Thadhani RI, Maddux FW. Dabigatran and rivaroxaban use in atrial fibrillation patients on hemodialysis. *Circulation.* 2015;131(11):972–979.

90. Holmes DR, Reddy VY, Turi ZG, et al. Percutaneous closure of the left atrial appendage versus warfarin therapy for prevention of stroke in patients with atrial fibrillation: a randomised non-inferiority trial. *Lancet.* 2009;374(9689):534–542.

91. Holmes Jr DR, Kar S, Price MJ, et al. Prospective randomized evaluation of the watchman left atrial appendage closure device in patients with atrial fibrillation versus long-term warfarin therapy: the PREVAIL trial. *J Am Coll Cardiol.* 2014;64(1):1–12.

92. Devereaux PJ, Anderson DR, Gardner MJ, et al. Differences between perspectives of physicians and patients on anticoagulation in patients with atrial fibrillation: observational study. *BMJ.* 2001;323(7323):1218–1222.

93. Granger CB, Chertow GM. A pint of sweat will save a gallon of blood: a call for randomized trials of anticoagulation in end-stage renal disease. *Circulation.* 2014;129(11):1190–1192.

94. *Oral Anticoagulation in Haemodialysis Patients (AVKDIAL).* 2016. clinicaltrials.gov.

95. *Trial to Evaluate Anticoagulation Therapy in Hemodialysis Patients with Atrial Fibrillation (RENAL-AF).* 2016. clinicaltrials.gov.

96. *The Strategy to Prevent Hemorrhage Associated with Anticoagulation in Renal Disease Management (STOP HARM) Trial (STOP-HARM).* 2016. clinicaltrials.gov.

Index

Note: Page numbers followed by "f" indicate figures, "t" indicate tables.